AF565104

LAPAROSCOPIC COMPLICATIONS

PREVENTION AND MANAGEMENT

LAPAROSCOPIC COMPLICATIONS

PREVENTION AND MANAGEMENT

MAX BORTEN, M.D.

ASSOCIATE PROFESSOR OF
OBSTETRICS AND GYNECOLOGY
HARVARD MEDICAL SCHOOL

ASSOCIATE OBSTETRICIAN AND GYNECOLOGIST
BETH ISRAEL HOSPITAL
BOSTON, MASSACHUSETTS

EDITED BY

EMANUEL A. FRIEDMAN, M.D., Sc.D.

PROFESSOR OF OBSTETRICS AND GYNECOLOGY
HARVARD MEDICAL SCHOOL

OBSTETRICIAN-GYNECOLOGIST-IN-CHIEF
BETH ISRAEL HOSPITAL
BOSTON, MASSACHUSETTS

B.C. DECKER INC • TORONTO • PHILADELPHIA

Publisher

B.C. Decker Inc.
3228 South Service Road
Burlington, Ontario L7N 3H8

B.C. Decker Inc.
P.O. Box 30246
Philadelphia, Pennsylvania 19103

Sales and Distribution

United States and Possessions	**The C.V. Mosby Company** 11830 Westline Industrial Drive Saint Louis, Missouri 63146
Canada	**The C.V. Mosby Company, Ltd.** 5240 Finch Avenue East, Unit No. 1 Scarborough, Ontario M1S 4P2
United Kingdom, Europe and the Middle East	**Blackwell Scientific Publications, Ltd.** Osney Mead, Oxford OX2 OEL, England
Australia	**Holt-Saunders Pty. Limited** 9 Waltham Street Artarmon, N.S.W. 2064 Australia
Japan	**Igaku-Shoin Ltd.** Tokyo International P.O. Box 5063 1-28-36 Hongo, Bunkyo-ku, Tokyo 113, Japan
Asia	**Holt-Saunders Asia Limited** 10/F, Inter-Continental Plaza Tsim Sha Tsui East Kowloon, Hong Kong

Laparoscopic Complications
Prevention and Management

ISBN 0-941158-37-3

Printed in Hong Kong

Library of Congress catalog card number: 85-073547

10 9 8 7 6 5 4 3 2 1

FOREWORD

The use of laparoscopy for gynecologic diagnosis and operative therapy has burgeoned in recent years. Laparoscopy has become ingrained as an essential component of the training and practice of the gynecologist. Improved technical resources, equipment, and skills have made it possible both to expand its applications and to permit it to be done in freestanding or outpatient ambulatory surgical units. Whereas many benefits are apparent, these trends have not always been entirely salutary. On the positive side of the ledger, earlier and more accurate diagnosis of intra-abdominal disorders has resulted; many major surgical explorations have thus been averted, and those done have often been better planned and executed because of the information obtained at laparoscopy. Improved skills and awareness should have reduced the frequency and severity of complications. However, this has not always been the case since growing confidence in and reliance on the technique lead to relaxation of safeguards and expansion of uses. Rapidly rising numbers of laparoscopic procedures may reflect that indications are being unnecessarily and inappropriately liberalized, surgical skills perhaps exceeded, and facilities undoubtedly strained. The consequences to the patient may be exposure to risks which are or ought to be avoidable.

This practical book goes far beyond any currently available to resolve the issues. Not only does it deal with instrumentation, techniques, and indications, but it addresses such critical aspects as informed consent and preoperative counseling, both essential preparations for surgery properly anticipating subsequent complications from the procedure to be undertaken. Most important, the book delves into great detail concerning what can be expected, why do complications occur, how can they be avoided, and specifically what can be done to correct them? These are matters of vital clinical value that are immediately applicable to daily practice. This volume concentrates a wealth of clinical surgical experience for rapid assimilation by the reader.

Doctor Borten has been actively involved as a busy, academically based practitioner and enthusiastic teacher of diagnostic and operative laparoscopy for many years. Physicians who have been privileged to learn from him at first hand have all developed a uniformly high level of competence and proficiency. The store of information he has heretofore been able to provide to inculcate them with delicate skill and knowledgeable attention to detail is now much more widely available through this book. Its informative text is supplemented with a large number of excellent translaparoscopic photographs and, where needed, supplementary drawings, collectively making the material presented both lucid and readily grasped. It will prove especially valuable to residents and fellows in gynecologic training programs and can be expected to aid gynecologists already in practice to sharpen their skills and thereby benefit their patients.

Emanuel A. Friedman, M.D., Sc.D.
Boston

PREFACE

It has often been said that laparoscopy is a wonderful procedure as long as everything goes right, but when complications occur it can be disastrous. I believe this to be a misconception. It appears to be based on the selective recall of only the rare major catastrophic events associated with this procedure, such as bowel perforation or aortic laceration. In perspective, however, it does not really differ from other delicate surgical techniques that require a combination of knowledge, practice, and caution for their successful completion.

As with other surgical procedures, physicians performing laparoscopy tend to master what they consider to be the best way. In due course, they become familiar with the shortcomings, risks, and complications associated with their way of carrying out the procedure. It is quite a different experience to teach laparoscopy to the uninitiated. Complications are to be expected while experience is being gathered by the novice. Teaching laparoscopy has been exciting and rewarding for me. My objective in this book is to share with the reader the experience I have been fortunate to accumulate over the years. I have approached this task with a central focus of offering practical points not only on how to avoid complications but also how to resolve them once they have arisen.

The advent of laparoscopy in gynecology can be construed as a landmark in the progressive development of the specialty. From a technique only performed by a handful of courageous gynecologists in this country, it has mushroomed into an indispensable tool in the gynecologist's armamentarium. Although it has not yet achieved its deserved recognition by the general surgeon, this should not be interpreted as a limitation of the technique itself. A chapter on nongynecologic indications for laparoscopy is included as a testimonial to its benefits. Isolated reports of the usefulness of laparoscopy in general surgery lend additional support to my belief that the day will come when general surgeons will also discover laparoscopy. It will then become, for them, as indispensable a tool as it currently is for gynecologists.

Perhaps more important than knowledge about the indications for laparoscopy are the contraindications. The old dictum *"Primum, noli nocere"* (first, do no harm) is as applicable to laparoscopy as to all other medical decisions. Personal interest or an individual operator's ability ought not to prevail when the risks of laparoscopy outweigh the benefits that can accrue to a patient. Individual chapters on diagnostic and operative indications for laparoscopy seemed appropriate, since each possesses particular risks which must be thoroughly evaluated before the procedure is recommended. The decision to employ the open versus closed laparoscopic technique has to be tailored to the primary indication for and the purpose of the laparoscopy. Both methods are described and illustrated.

The popularization of laparoscopy has unavoidably been paralleled by a proliferation of instruments, advocates of each claiming it has some particular advantage over its predecessors. A description of all available instrumentation is beyond the aim of this work. Instead, a discussion of the basic tools required to carry out laparoscopy and translaparoscopic surgery is successfully included. The need to become familiar with the peculiarities of each instrument used in performing laparoscopy cannot be sufficiently stressed. A common event is the operator's inability to complete a laparoscopy as a consequence of equipment malfunction. Similarly, lack of appropriate instrumentation may entice the laparoscopist to improvise by using other instruments available in the operating room. A compilation of suggestions that have proven useful to me on how to overcome the aforementioned inconveniences is detailed.

Different anesthetic techniques used with laparoscopy are described. This discussion ought to prove useful during the preoperative counseling of patients. It should not be interpreted as sufficient to take the place of consultation with an experienced anesthesiologist. A separate chapter detailing the most common anesthetic complications occurring in conjunction with laparoscopy is included.

Current emphasis on high turnover of cases, mostly performed as same-day outpatient surgery, results in early discharge following laparoscopy. Postoperative recovery is usually not limited to the short time patients spend in a recovery room immediately after the procedure. Baseline parameters may not be recovered until 24 to 48 hours have elapsed. The normal postoperative course is discussed in Chapter 11. Short-term postoperative side effects and the signs and symptoms of early complications are described in Chapter 24.

At the present time, laparoscopy is most commonly used for diagnostic purposes. Nevertheless, laparoscopic sterilization must be credited with the rapid popularization of laparoscopy in the United States. Over the years, it has become the method of choice for female sterilization whenever feasible. The controversy as to whether electrocoagulation methods are superior to the nonelectrical, occlusive ones or vice versa remains unresolved. Knowledge of the indications, contraindications, and complications associated with each method is essential before an intelligent selection can be made. The different methods most commonly used are described and depicted in a step-by-step fashion.

In the interest of clarity, the material dealing with complications of laparoscopy has been subdivided according to the causative instrumental factor (trocar insertion, electrical) and by the particular anatomical system injured. A description of the most likely causes of these complications, how they take place, and their early recognition and appropriate management comprise the body of Section II of this book. Attention to detail and adherence to proper technique go a long way toward preventing these unwelcome events.

While this book is concerned with laparoscopic technique and its complications, their prevention and management, I would be remiss not to mention the psychological and medicolegal aspects involved with laparoscopy. No ancillary method or technique will ever replace a thorough discussion and explanation of the procedure to be undertaken. A good doctor-patient relationship can go a long way toward reducing the ever increasing number of malpractice litigations.

Translaparoscopic photography, which is dealt with in detail, may appear as investigational and luxurious at first glance. This is definitely not so. Documentation of findings at laparoscopy ought not to be limited to the subjective description of the operator. A practical and inexpensive method for obtaining endoscopic pictures is described. All laparoscopic photographs in this book were obtained by me. While my previous experience as an amateur photographer proved helpful, similar results are not beyond the reach of the individual laparoscopist. Drawings detailing complications which could not be photographically documented complement the text description.

Gynecologists in training will undoubtedly find the content of this book helpful. It can be expected to fulfill a similar role for general surgeons in due course. My sense of satisfaction will be complete if those already performing laparoscopy find the material of value.

Max Borten, M.D.

ACKNOWLEDGEMENTS

I would like to express my appreciation to the residents, staff physicians, and operating room nurses and personnel of the Beth Israel Hospital, Boston. Their enthusiastic and patient cooperation helped me gather the pictorial information in this book.

A special note of thanks is in order to Emanuel A. Friedman to whom I am greatly indebted. Academician, teacher, and mentor of generations of physicians, his encouragement and contagious enthusiasm are responsible for the successful completion of this work. His contribution was not limited to reviewing the original manuscript; his keen insights and unparalleled ability to communicate scientific knowledge have heavily influenced the final presentation of this material. His talent has definitely enriched this book.

For her patience and efforts in typing the many drafts before the final manuscript came to fruition, Joan F. McLean deserves my appreciation.

Cynthia McCann, artist and friend, is responsible for the illustrations. Her attention to detail and cooperative spirit are greatly appreciated.

My ability to obtain the endoscopic photographs was facilitated by the cooperation of Joseph J. Houser of the Olympus Company who made sure that equipment in working condition was always available to me.

I am grateful to Dennis Boyes and Brian C. Decker who made publication of this book a surprisingly pleasant experience for me.

Finally, I wish to acknowledge the understanding and unremitting moral support of my parents, Rosa and Eisik.

Max Borten, M.D.

CONTENTS

1 INSTRUMENTATION

The popularization of laparoscopy for diagnostic and operative procedures is due mainly to technological advances that have been made over the last few decades. Much like a craftsman in any endeavor, the surgeon must know the tools he or she utilizes. The knowledge of the laparoscope and its accessories should not be a mere superficial familiarity. In-depth understanding of the advantages, limitations, and common pitfalls of each device may prove to be the key to successful completion of the procedure. The most frequent problems encountered with each device and apparatus will be discussed in detail later (see Chapter 12). This chapter will be limited to a description of standard instrumentation and alternatives.

UTERINE MANIPULATION

Thorough visualization of the posterior cul-de-sac and adnexal structures is a sine qua non of diagnostic pelvic laparoscopy. Failure to visualize and inspect every pelvic structure capable of being seen by means of an endoscopic procedure makes diagnostic laparoscopy inconclusive and operative laparoscopy hazardous. The uterine corpus is the central organ in the female pelvis and the extent of the translaparoscopic visual field is directly related to how well the uterus can be moved. The ability to manipulate the uterus in different directions (e.g., cephalo-caudally, laterally) allows the gynecologist to inspect each particular area without limitations. The ideal instrument should be capable of elevating, rotating, and projecting the uterus laterally so as to place it and the adnexal structures under tension. This should be accomplished in a gentle and atraumatic manner. An accurate estimation of uterine size and position is important for selecting the right instrument. An incorrectly fitted device will not provide adequate uterine mobility and may be the source of serious complications.

The uterus will pivot at the level of its lateral cervical ligamentous attachments. The key factors that limit uterine mobility are the degree of laxity of the ligaments holding the uterus in position and the angle of flexion of the uterine corpus with respect to its cervix. At times, simple traction applied to the cervix provides sufficient uterine displacement to allow adequate pelvic visualization.

At present, the most common instrument used to manipulate the uterus is a self-retaining cannula (used principally for testing tubal patency) interlocked to a single toothed tenaculum attached to the cervix (Figures 1.1 and 1.2). The proximal tip or olive of the cannula entering the endocervical-endometrial cavity is interchangeable with tips of different size designed to fit the cervical shape of both nulliparas and multiparas snugly. This instrument is impractical for use in a patient with a severely retroflexed uterus or with a large endometrial cavity. Its use in less than ideal circumstances can give rise to complications (see Chapter 13).

A variety of instruments were designed to overcome the problem of the ill-fitting olive tip.[1,6,9,11] Unfortunately, all of them have inherent design faults, so that each has some advantages and disadvantages when compared to the others. For example, the rigidity of the Cohen patency cannula, the versatility of the

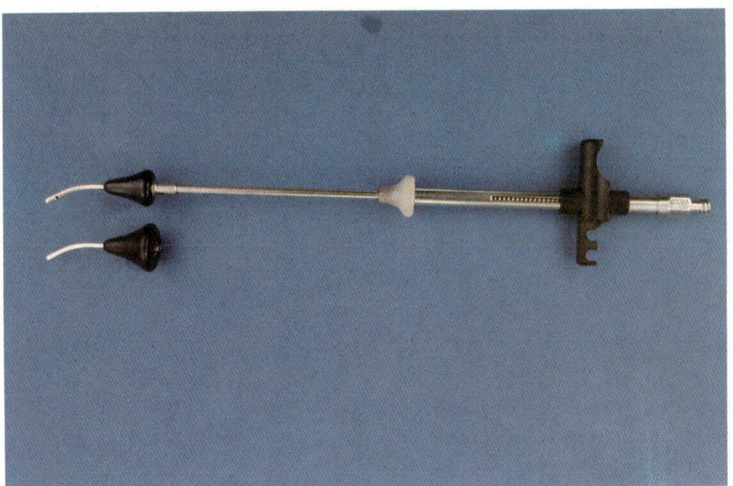

Figure 1.1 Cohen's self-retaining patent cannula is used principally for testing tubal patency. The nulliparous tip is mounted on the cannula; the larger multiparous tip used for the larger cervix is shown alongside.

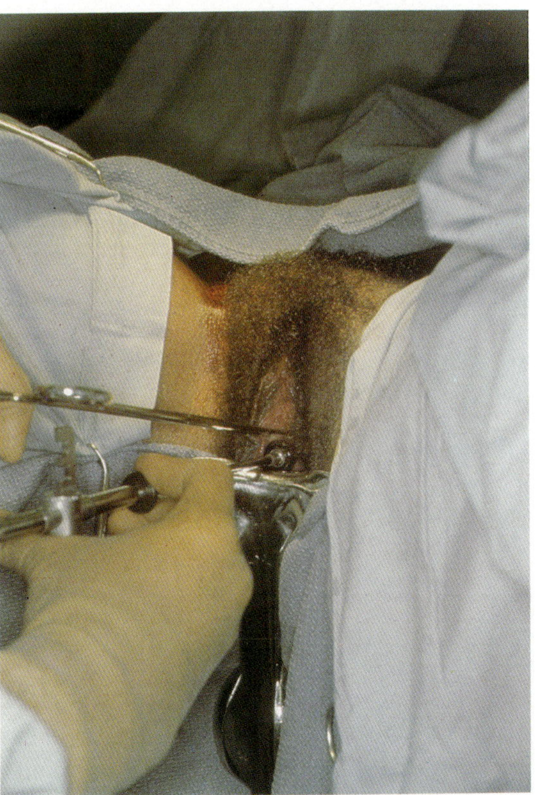

Figure 1.2 Olive tip at proximal end of the cannula is inserted into the endocervical canal and the cannula attached to the single toothed tenaculum applied to the anterior cervical lip.

Valtchev uterine mobilizer, or the flexibility of the ballooned uterine elevator cannula may prove to be particularly advantageous in selected instances, although in others they may severely limit the surgeon's ability to move the uterus. A laparoscopist should be familiar with most of the instruments available and choose the most appropriate one on an individual basis for each particular patient. Whichever instrument is utilized, it must be patent and have the capability to allow one to inject or aspirate fluid through it to carry out a tubal lavage concomitantly, when indicated.

A common feature of all these instruments is that they invade the uterine cavity. In some diagnostic laparoscopies this is inadvisable; at other times, it is absolutely contraindicated. An example of a contraindication is a diagnostic laparoscopy to rule out an ectopic pregnancy in a woman who wishes to continue the gestation if it is found to be intrauterine in location. In these instances, the uterus can be mobilized by attaching a tenaculum to the anterior or posterior cervical lip. An alternative is the use of sponge forceps or vaginal packing in order to elevate the uterus out of the pelvis. Not previously described, but rather obvious and at times very useful, is the manual mobilization of the uterus by a surgical assistant who inserts his or her fingers into the vagina preoperatively (Figure 1.3).

PNEUMOPERITONEUM

The separation of the anterior abdominal wall from the intraperitoneal organs by creating a gas compartment (pneumoperitoneum) is fundamental for

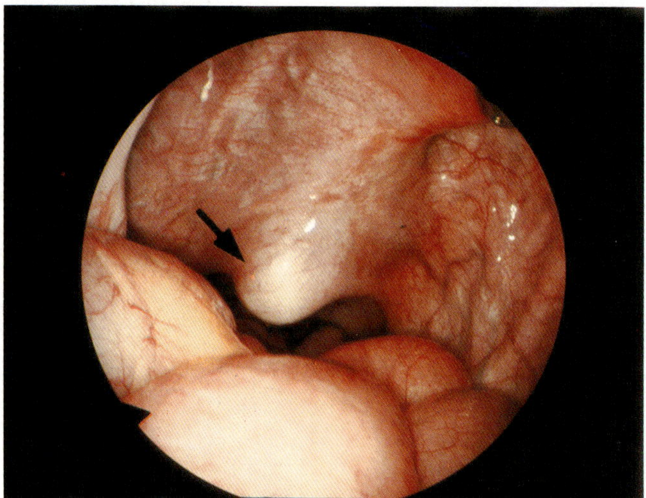

Figure 1.3 Digital mobilization of the uterus during laparoscopy. Arrow points to protrusion into the pouch of Douglas produced by the cervix being pushed towards the posterior vaginal fornix. This motion pivots the uterus out of the pelvis and permits visualization of the posterior cul-de-sac.

successful visualization of the pelvic organs and performance of translaparoscopic surgery. A variety of different distention gases (carbon dioxide, nitrous oxide, room air) and routes of insufflation (transabdominal, transfundal, via the posterior fornix) have been advocated; each has its own special advantageous feature.[7,8]

It is believed by some laparoscopists that morbidity related to producing a pneumoperitoneum can be avoided by direct insertion of the laparoscopic trocar before the gas insufflation.[2] This eliminates any complications arising from using a Verres needle, although there may be a trade-off in higher frequencies of complications from the trocar (see Chapter 16).

Whichever method is chosen, the instruments required to achieve a suitable pneumoperitoneum should be well known to the laparoscopist. In regard to the insufflation gas for peritoneal distention, the instrument's advantages and shortcomings should play an important role in its selection.

Verres Needle

The Verres cannula is a double-barrelled, spring-action stylet, automatic needle (Figures 1.4*a* and 1.4*b*). The sharply bevelled outer sleeve facilitates perforation of the fascial planes and the blunt-ended, inner hollow needle is more suited to traversing the peritoneal layer. At the same time, the blunt end serves to push aside any freely mobile intra-abdominal structure it comes into contact with, such as bowel, omentum, or ovaries. The needle is held by its spring chamber (collar) to allow free movement of the inner needle as it penetrates the different tissue planes. Two upward thrusts can generally be seen, the first as the rectus fascia is passed through and the second as the peritoneal layer is penetrated.

The Verres needle comes in diverse diameters and lengths. The usual external diameter of the most commonly used needle is 2.1 mm; needles with 1.7 mm and 2.5 mm outer dimensions are also available, but serve little practical purpose. Knowledge of the type of needle used is essential to enable one to interpret accurately the intra-abdominal pressure measured during insufflation of the distending gas. A needle with a smaller internal diameter increases the resistance and thereby registers an increase in the intra-abdominal pressure reading. By contrast, a larger bore needle has just the opposite effect. A newly developed dual-port Verres needle (Figure 1.4*c*) enables the operator to measure the intraperitoneal pressure even though the insufflation of the distending gas is discontinued.

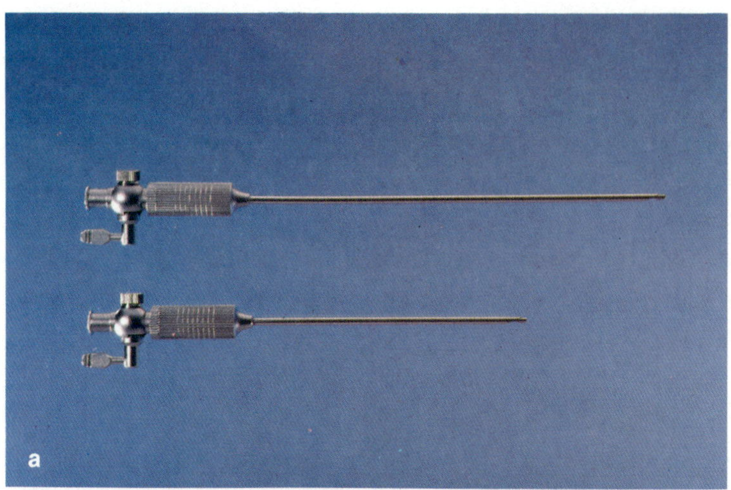

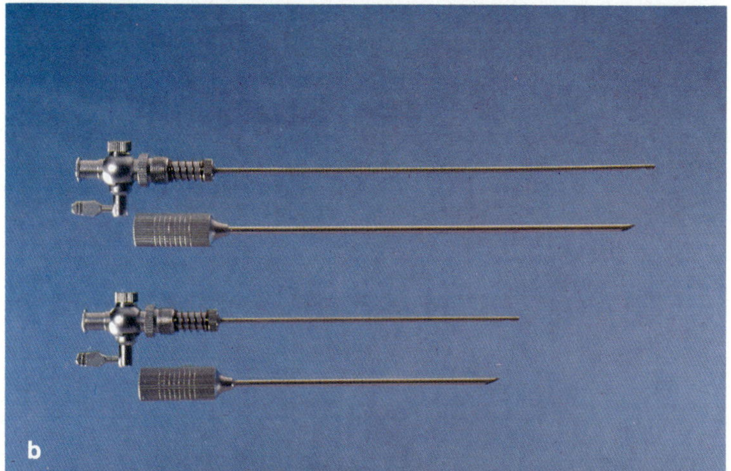

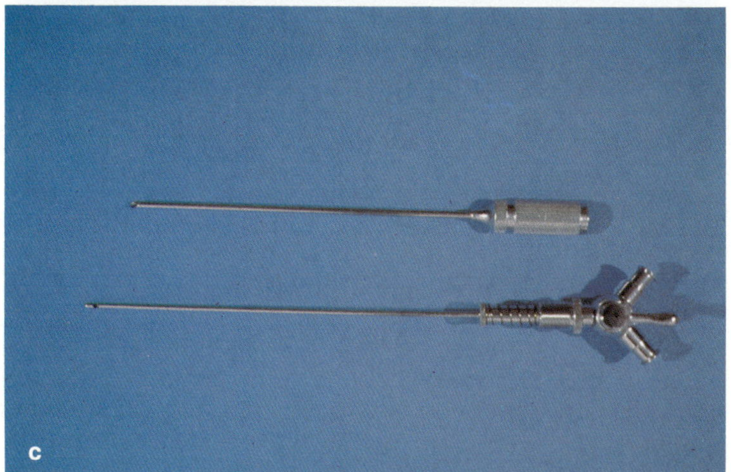

Figure 1.4 *a*. Verres needles, illustrating standard 80 mm length and longer 120 mm needle. The latter was once thought to be required in the obese patient, but is now seldom used. *b*. Verres needles disassembled, showing blunt spring-action stylet and sharply-bevelled outer sleeve. *c*. Dual-port Verres needle. The two parts enable the operator to measure the intraperitoneal pressure even though insufflation of the distending gas is discontinued.

As far as the length of the instrument is concerned, longer needles were developed for use in very obese patients. When the usual infraumbilical site of insertion is used, the standard Verres needle of 80 mm length is sufficient to traverse all the abdominal layers in nearly all cases because the wall seldom exceeds 1 to 2 cm depth in the region usually selected for puncture (see Chapter 2). As will be discussed later (see Chapter 15), failure to enter the peritoneal cavity is rarely the result of a Verres needle that is too short. Instead, it is much more likely to be caused by the improper direction used for its insertion.

Insufflation Equipment

Pneumoperitoneum was originally obtained by insufflating room air by hand into the peritoneal cavity. At present, this step of the procedure has been automated. The insufflation of the distending gas, the rate of flow, the amount delivered, and the measurement of the intra-abdominal pressure are mechanically performed by an instrument. A visual display of these functions provides the surgeon all of the aforementioned information. Whichever insufflating apparatus is used, it should conform to current safety and application standards. It must limit the insufflation of gas to 1 liter per minute on low flow and not more than 3 liters per minute on high flow. It must also include a shut-off valve which permits the interruption of gas flow into the patient's abdomen when the gas tank is being refilled. Figure 1.5 depicts a standard insufflator. The minimum information and function that a surgeon needs during the procedure are as follows: gas flow, intraperitoneal pressure, volume of gas insufflated, shut-off valves, and manual-automatic insufflation.

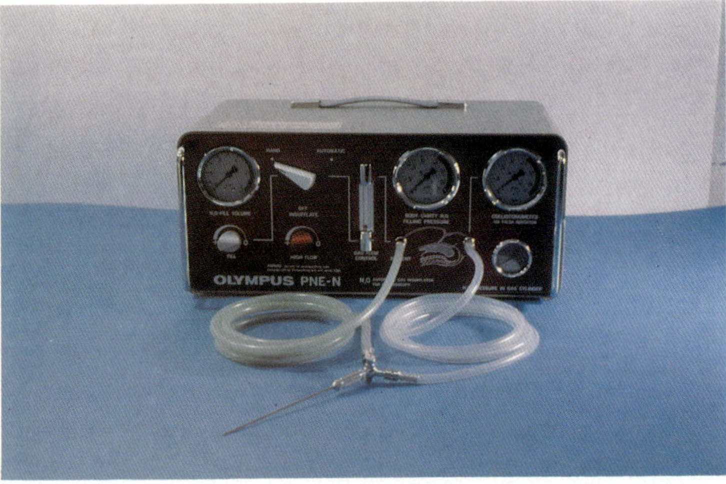

Figure 1.5 Insufflating apparatus. Visual display of the flow of gas, amount of gas delivered, intraperitoneal pressure and amount of gas reserve is seen at a glance. There are separate controls for manual or automatic insufflation, refill of the small gas tank and variable flow on the front panel.

Gas Flow. The regular flow of gas from the apparatus to the patient should be set at 1 liter per minute. A flow control guide (usually a floating plastic ball) provides a constant indication of flow activity. In machines equipped with a choice of fast or slow insufflation, the fast rate should never exceed 3 liters per minute. Manual operation should be required at all times until an adequate pneumoperitoneum is achieved. An indicator of the total volume of gas pumped by the apparatus provides the surgeon with an approximation of the gas insufflated into the patient's abdominal cavity (this is discussed later). An on-off insufflation switch is essential to allow the operator to interrupt and restart the gas insufflation instantly. A separate switch should control the passage of gas from the reserve tank into the 10 liter gas cylinder within the apparatus. Some type of indicator (dial) should record the amount of gas or pressure available in the reserve cylinder to ensure that a sufficient amount of gas is available to complete the procedure.

Pressure Evaluation. The intraperitoneal pressure (more specifically, the pressure of the gas pocket in the region where the tip of the Verres needle is located) should be constantly monitored and visually displayed by a gauge or meter during insufflation. If the insufflating apparatus measures such pressure through the gas channel, the active flow of gas should be discontinued when one is reading the pressure to obtain the true intraperitoneal pressure. Otherwise, a falsely high pressure reading is obtained because the pressure measured reflects the result of gas flow multiplied by the resistance to the flow of gas. Thus, failure to eliminate the gas flow while measuring the intraperitoneal pressure gives erroneously increased readings.

Volume of Gas Insufflated. Although the volume of gas dispensed by the insufflating apparatus is not the exact amount of gas that enters the patient's abdomen, it provides the surgeon with a good index of how much gas was used as well as the reserve available in the small cylinder tank. If there is a discrepancy between the amount of gas used and the degree of abdominal distention obtained, it usually indicates some type of gas leakage (see Chapter 13).

Shut-off Valves. Safety valves which can be closed instantly for interrupting the flow of gas are an indispensable safety feature. When the insufflation switch is turned off, no flow of gas should occur. Additional flow control valves are located on the Verres needle and the laparoscopic trocar sleeve. They permit the surgeon to discontinue the flow of gas into the patient's abdomen as needed. Newer equipment is capable of automatic cessation of the flow of gas when a preestablished pressure limit is exceeded.

Manual-Automatic Insufflation. The more advanced insufflation equipment possesses a valve that allows the operator to reduce the inflow of gas from the standard flow of 1 liter per minute to a level that just replaces the amount of gas lost from the pneumoperitoneum on a continuous basis. Alternatively, it can be set to sustain intraperitoneal pressure at any level designated by the operator.

Distention Gases

As previously stated, creation of a pneumoperitoneum (gas compartment) is an essential preliminary step for laparoscopy. Different gases, ranging from room air to pure oxygen, have been used to distend the peritoneal cavity. Each gas has its own particular features, which make it preferable for one type of procedure, or which contraindicate it for others. Knowledge of the physical and chemical characteristics of every distending gas is essential for understanding their absorption and excretion rates as well as their respiratory and cardiovascular effects. The peritoneal irritation and discomfort that may be produced are important characteristics for a distending gas selected for a laparoscopy done under local or regional block anesthesia. When one expects to use electrical current for translaparoscopic surgery, the conductive and combustive properties of the gas should be taken into account to prevent unexpected and potentially serious complications (see Chapter 23). Characteristics of each gas will be described separately.

Carbon Dioxide. The general acceptance of carbon dioxide as a distention medium by gynecologic surgeons is due mainly to its safety. Carbon dioxide is highly soluble in blood and rapidly absorbed from the bloodstream, features which expedite its excretion. Humans can tolerate small amounts of carbon dioxide injected intravascularly without serious manifestations or consequences. In angiocardiography, intravascular carbon dioxide in doses as high as 7.5 ml per kilogram have been well tolerated. Nevertheless, cardiac arrhythmias are more commonly seen when carbon dioxide is used to produce the pneumoperitoneum than when other gases are used (see Chapter 9).

The rapid transperitoneal resorption of carbon dioxide is reflected in the increase of pCO_2 and the fall in pH. This is generally ameliorated but not completely corrected by controlled ventilation. Because carbon dioxide does not sustain combustion, it can be safely used in conjunction with electrosurgical procedures without the risk of an intra-abdominal explosion. Its use in patients who are awake is not recommended by some because it is highly irritating to the peritoneum, creating more discomfort than other gases (see Chapter 15).

Nitrous Oxide. Nitrous oxide is used principally for laparoscopy done under local anesthesia for diagnostic purposes. It is slightly less soluble in blood than carbon dioxide. Its reabsorption from closed cavities is slower than carbon dioxide. This creates a special problem because if it is inadvertently injected outside the peritoneal cavity, such as in cases of subcutaneous emphysema, the condition will persist longer than it ordinarily would (see Chapter 15).

Gynecologic laparoscopists have been reluctant to use nitrous oxide to create the pneumoperitoneum because of the hazards associated with the concomitant use of electrocautery. Nitrous oxide will support combustion and create the potential for an explosion to occur. This risk is magnified if the bowel has been inadvertently perforated. Hydrogen and methane are components of intestinal gas. When mixed with nitrous oxide, they produce a highly explosive mixture. Physicians performing diagnostic laparoscopy under local anesthesia prefer to use nitrous oxide because it causes less peritoneal irritation than carbon dioxide and thus produces less discomfort for the patient.[10]

Other Gases. Nitrogen and oxygen are only mentioned for completeness. It must be emphasized that they are potentially very dangerous because of the increased risk of producing a fatal gas embolism if inadvertently injected intravascularly. Therefore, they should never be used for the pneumoperitoneum.

The widespread popularity that laparoscopy has achieved has not been uniformly accompanied by the technological advantages it enjoys in the United States. In some less technologically developed countries, room air is still being pumped into the peritoneal cavity for the formation of a pneumoperitoneum. As will be described more in detail in Chapter 15, the use of room air should be discouraged because of the danger of fatal air embolization. Additionally, because not all the air insufflated for the peritoneal distention can be exsufflated (removed) at the end of the procedure, postoperative discomfort is increased in degree and prolonged in duration. Free air can be identified in the abdominal cavity in these cases for several weeks following the laparoscopic procedure.

TROCARS AND SHEATHS

The laparoscopic trocar and its sheath consist of an outer hollow cannula and an inner, solid-metal, sharp trocar used to pierce the abdominal wall tissue layers (Figure 1.6). The diameter of the outer cannula (or trocar sheath) is approximately 1 to 2 mm wider than the laparoscope it will house so as to permit the continuous insufflation of the distending gas while the laparoscope is in place. A Luer-lock connection is provided for attaching the gas tubing to the insufflating apparatus.

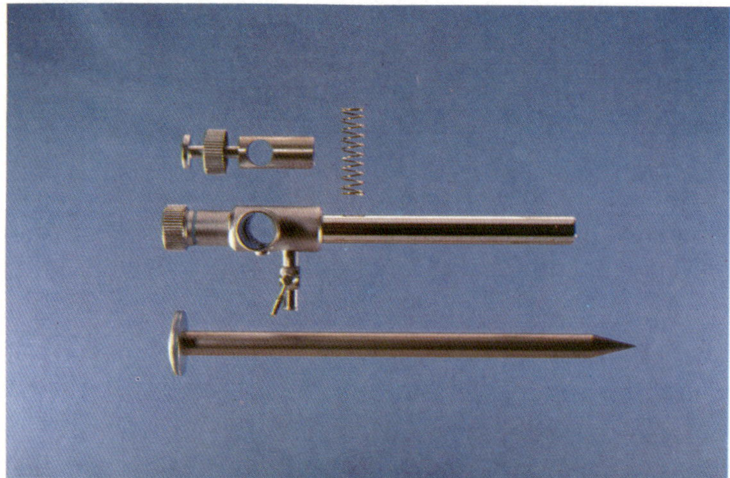

Figure 1.6 Unassembled sharp trocar and metal sleeve for single puncture laparoscope. Trumpet-like spring valve is shown outside its housing chamber.

Just above the gas connection, an automatic valve impedes the escape of intraperitoneal gas when the laparoscope is removed. Valve design variations are found among various models. The most commonly used type of valve is the trumpet-like spring which requires manual displacement before one can insert the laparoscope. A more modern ballspring automatic valve is available that allows the laparoscope to be inserted directly. The front end of the entering laparoscope merely displaces the obstructing element. This type of valve requires gentler handling of the entering laparoscope since the valve is displaced by the exposed forelying objective lens, a possible cause of lens damage.

A rubber gasket is fitted to the proximal end of the trocar sheath to hermetically seal off the periphery of the laparoscope, thus avoiding leakage of gas around it. Different sizes are available for each size trocar. At the distal end, the laparoscopic cannula is fenestrated laterally to allow the flow of insufflated gas to be diverted into the peritoneal cavity before reaching the objective lens. This avoids fogging the front lens by subjecting it to the cold gas (relative to the temperature within the peritoneal cavity) constantly being insufflated.

In an attempt to reduce the possibility of inadvertent electrical burns complicating the use of translaparoscopic electrosurgical instruments, it has been formally recommended that nonconductive laparoscopic cannulas be used. This is now known to be erroneous. Better understanding of the process of electrical capacitance as the cause of those burns (see Chapter 23), as well as how the trocar cannula serves to disperse heat, has made it appropriate to return to the use of all-metal sheaths for procedures in which electrosurgery is contemplated.

The solid metal trocar used to facilitate insertion of the laparoscopic cannula has a sharp point that protrudes from the end of its sheath. The point may be conical or pyramidal in shape (Figure 1.7). Experience has shown that the former requires less force to perforate the tissue layers of the abdominal wall.

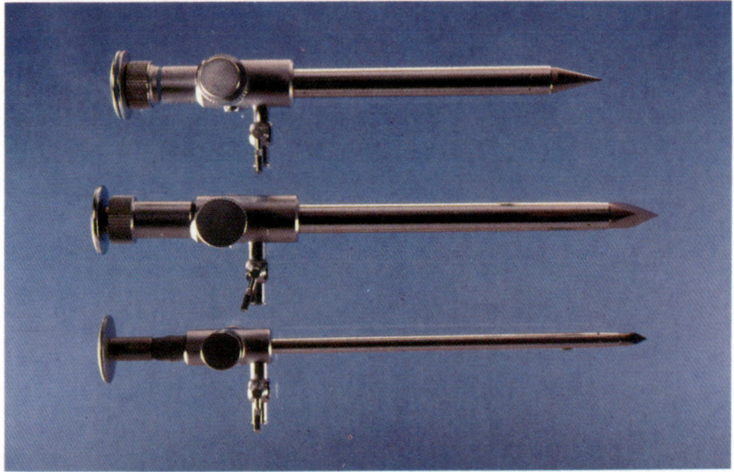

Figure 1.7 Various types of sharp laparoscopic trocars (from top down): 10 mm wide sharp conical trocar; 10 mm wide pyramidal shaped trocar; and 5 mm wide sharp pyramidal trocar.

Thus, one has more control over the penetrating thrust that takes place with the sudden loss of resistance experienced when the rectus fascia is traversed.

The auxiliary secondary puncture instrument consists of a simple, hollow cannula with an inner sharp trocar (Figure 1.8). It is available in different sizes to accommodate the various instruments that may have to be inserted through it. The sharp trocar is also available in a conical or pyramidal shape. The proximal end has a large collar that limits the depth to which the cannula can be inserted. A rubber gasket encircles the opening edge to prevent escape of gas around the instrument placed within it.

Although it is common practice to use a simple, hollow fiberglass cannula for the secondary puncture, one should give consideration to the use of a laparoscopic type trocar and sheath if one expects to do extensive operative proce-

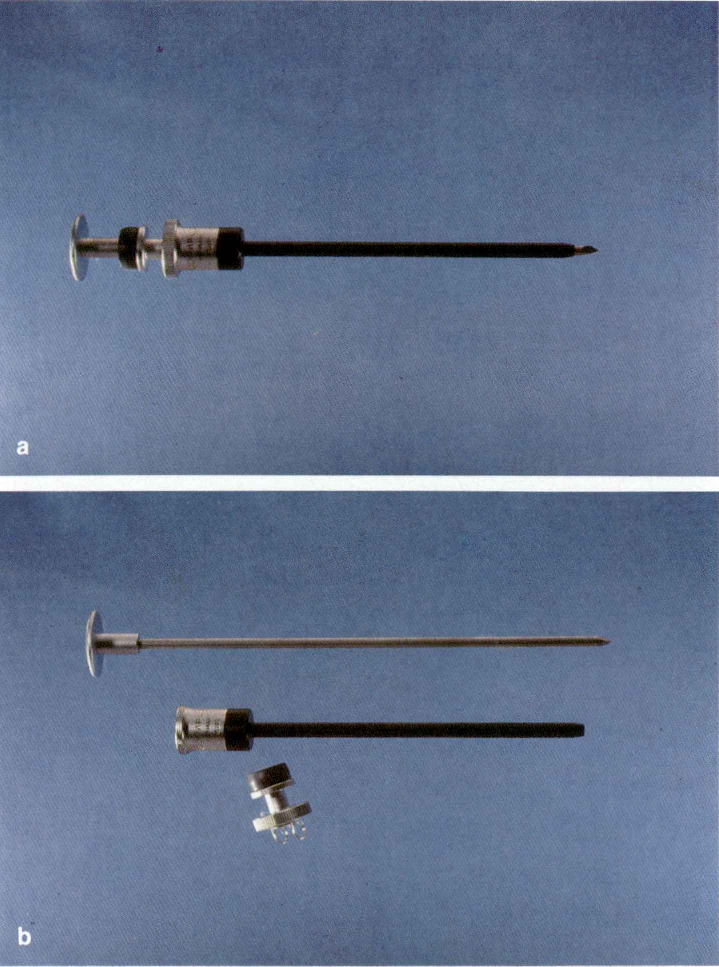

Figure 1.8 Ball-spring automatic valve 5 mm auxiliary trocar. The sharp pyramidal trocar is shown mounted *a*, and disassembled *b*. Conical sharp trocars can also be used for the auxiliary secondary puncture.

dures. The advantages this provides are twofold. First, it allows the attachment of an additional insufflating machine if rapid reinsufflation should be required in cases where the pneumoperitoneum is difficult to maintain due to a large gas leak or other cause. Second, it permits the introduction of the laparoscope through the inferiorly located cannula to provide a more panoramic view to encompass the upper abdomen and the anterior parietal abdominal wall. When a periumbilical site of entry is used, the usual penetration of the trocar sheath obstructs visualization of a portion of the wall (periumbilically) and of some intra-abdominal organs.

LAPAROSCOPE

The laparoscope is similar in construction to other endoscopes in common use. It consists of an optical system which conducts the light to illuminate the region to be explored. It has an optical system to return the image to be viewed or photographed. The illumination for the endoscope is generally conducted by way of optical glass fibers (fiberoptic bundles). The imaging portion and the mechanism by which the image is reflected to the observer determines the type of endoscope. If a bundle of aligned optical fibers is utilized to convey the image back to the operator, the resulting fiberscope has some inherent flexibility. If the images are obtained by a system of relay lenses, the optical transmission requires the endoscope to be of the rigid type. The number and size of the lenses interposed between the objective lens and the eyepiece lens distinguish the different varieties of rigid endoscopes (examples of which are the conventional and Hopkins-type laparoscope).[3] Flexible scopes are mainly used for thoracic or gastrointestinal visualization; these should be kept in mind as alternative instruments for laparoscopy. As a standard practice, gynecologic and urologic diagnostic and operative procedures utilize rigid laparoscopes.

The quality of a laparoscope is determined by the quality of the image it produces. Aspects to be considered when evaluating a scope are related to: (1) the image quality as related to color, contrast, resolution, and depth of focus, (2) the scope diameter, ranging from 2.3 mm to 12 mm, (3) the accessory channels for diagnostic and operative laparoscopes, and (4) the angle of view by the objective lens, namely straight, oblique, or foroblique (135°).

Image Quality

Color. If the color of the examined tissue is an important diagnostic consideration, a true impression is essential. Pale, pink, injected, or red coloration may signify very different kinds of disease states, for example. The color of the image one sees depends on the spectrum of the illuminating light and the spectrum of the transmitting optics.

Contrast. The greater the difference between the intensity of the image and that of the background, the greater the object contrast obtained.

Resolution. The ability of the optical system to separate two adjacent points in the resulting image is a measure of the power of resolution of that particular lens system. The greater the resolution and contrast, the clearer the image one will obtain.

Depth of Focus. Just as with a photographic camera, some endoscopes have a variable focus objective. Conventional laparoscopes are of the fixed focus type because variable focus objectives are difficult to use and troublesome to sterilize. In order to obtain a panoramic view, it has been necessary to compromise by sacrificing clarity at the periphery of the visual field. Newly developed optic systems, like the ones utilized to illustrate this book, have overcome this problem.

Laparoscope Diameter

Considerable progress in design and manufacture of optical systems has made it feasible to produce smaller diameter laparoscopes with little loss of image quality. Therefore, the choice of laparoscopic diameter is a matter of the laparoscopist's preference. Experience has shown that a 5 mm laparoscope achieves the desirable combination of good visualization while minimizing the size of the insertion wound. For extensive translaparoscopic surgical procedures, a 10 mm laparoscope is preferable (Figure 1.9). Its larger visual field provides a better panoramic view of the intraperitoneal organs. The larger insertion wound

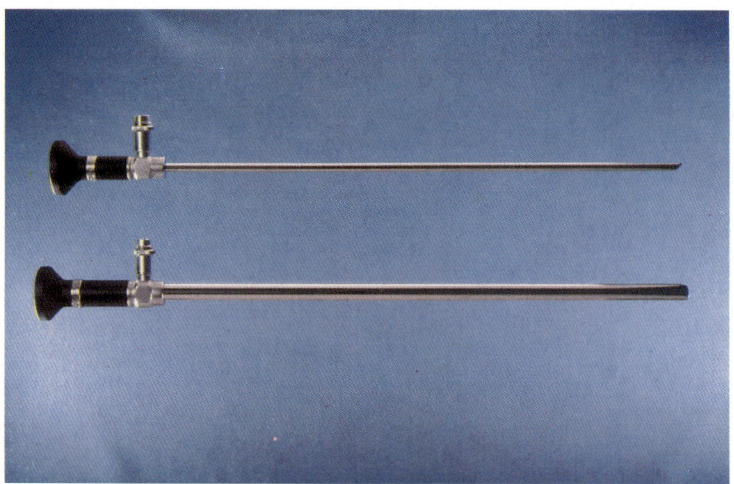

Figure 1.9 Olympus rigid laparoscopes: 5 and 10 mm diameter. Both instruments have a 0° angle of observation (180° from observer).

is of little esthetic significance. For "second-look" laparoscopy used as a means of follow-up after treatment for intra-abdominal malignancy, instruments as thin as 1.7 to 2.3 mm in external diameter are currently available.

Accessory Channels

Translaparoscopic surgery through a single trocar puncture laparoscope is made possible by the use of a larger diameter laparoscope to accommodate the operative instrument channel. There is still some controversy about whether electrosurgical procedures can be safely performed through an operative laparoscope.

The single puncture operative laparoscope was developed as a byproduct of the improvements made in the optical systems. When smaller diameter laparoscopes proved just as effective as the larger primitive instrument, the idea of using the leftover space as an instrument channel, thus avoiding the need for the auxiliary secondary puncture, gained in popularity. The acquired skills of some experienced operators allowed them to perform sophisticated procedures through the single puncture operative laparoscope. Nevertheless, the initial enthusiasm has since diminished as complications and technical limitations have become apparent.

Different types of operative laparoscopes available today range from those with a 12 mm diameter, which allows admittance of instruments through the accessory channel, up to those with a 7 mm diameter (for metal clip or silastic band applicators). The most commonly used instrument is 10 mm in outer diameter; it contains a 5 mm visual lens system and a 5 mm operative channel for utilizing thinner 5 mm instruments (Figure 1.10).

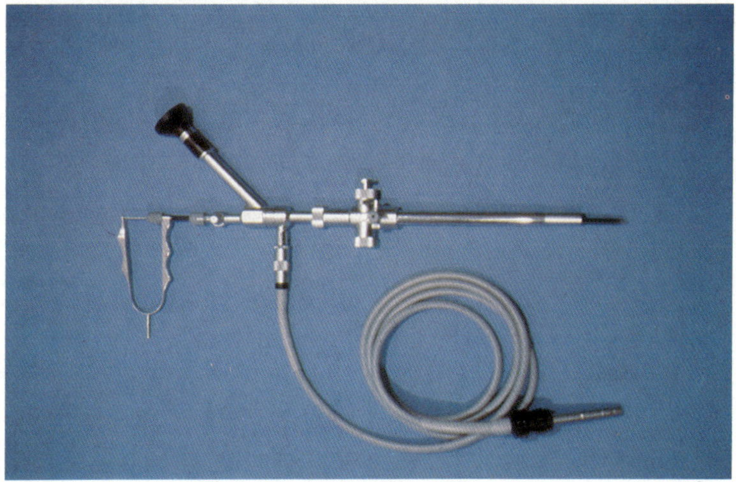

Figure 1.10 Single puncture operative laparoscope. A built-in instrument channel permits the insertion of auxiliary instruments.

Advantages attributed to the single puncture operative laparoscope range from the cosmetic single incision to the capability it offers for performing minor surgery (lysis of a single omental or peritoneal adhesion). If a single puncture operative laparoscope is available, it is advisable to use a 10 mm endoscope in most laparoscopies. The recommendation applies even when a 2 puncture technique is anticipated because it provides the operator with the flexibility to exchange the 10 mm laparoscope for an operative one and to acquire a third intraperitoneal instrument. This proves useful when fixation of the structure to be operated on is difficult.

Shortcomings of the operative laparoscope are mainly technical in nature and not easily resolved. They range from usual limitations of the operative field to limitation in mobility of the laparoscope during the operation. Attention given to the following conditions may prevent a complication or preclude the use of this type of laparoscope altogether.

Blind Spot in Visual Field. The instrument inserted in the accessory operating channel has to protrude from the lumen of the laparoscope to be visible to the operator. As seen in Figure 1.11, a portion of the area of vision beyond the instrument is obstructed by the instrument itself. The angle of view that cannot be visualized by the laparoscopist is determined by the objective lens used in that laparoscope. The wider the angle of view of the objective lens, the smaller the degree of visual interference by the accessory instrument's shaft. The importance of this obstructed part of the visual field is even greater when electrocautery is utilized because an intra-abdominal organ may come into contact with the electroinstrument and although hidden from the operator's view, it can receive the full impact of the energy applied to it (see Chapter 23).

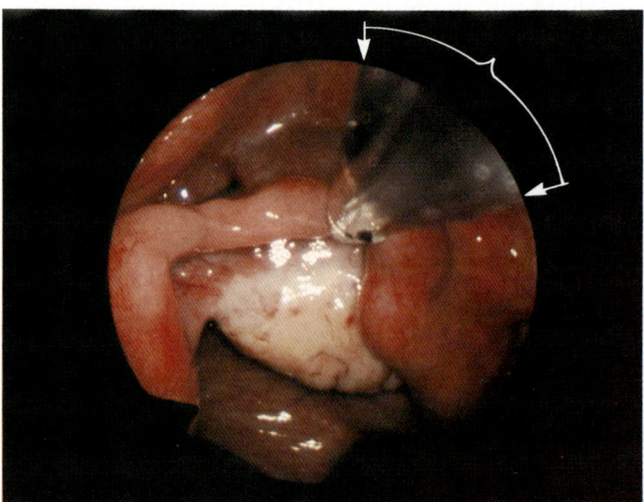

Figure 1.11 Blind spot in field of vision for a single puncture operative laparoscope with an instrument in place. The operator is not able to determine if an intraperitoneal organ is touching the back of the auxiliary instrument (arrows).

Inability to Mobilize Intestine. When a two puncture technique is utilized, it is a standard procedure to mobilize the small bowel out of the pelvis using a probe applied through the accessory puncture channel. It is essential to carry out this step under direct laparoscopic visualization to avoid injury to the intestine or any of the retroperitoneal vessels. The sweeping motion of the accessory probe should always be done under direct laparoscopic visualization.

When the single puncture operative laparoscope is used, the entire instrument is moved in a single motion. Therefore, in order to mobilize the intestine, the laparoscope has to be relocated from the pelvic visual field in order to move in conjunction with the accessory probe.

Fixed Visual Distance. The degree of protrusion of the accessory operative instrument is determined by the wide angle view of the objective lens as mentioned previously. It varies anywhere from 1.0 to 2.5 cm from the front end of the laparoscope. This protrusion is fixed and precludes a closer view of the tissue grasped by the operating forceps. This fixed instrument-to-objective distance also impedes the operator from mobilizing organs, such as the ovaries, and aids in visualizing their posterior aspects.

Inability to Independently Remove the Laparoscope. It is not unusual for the objective lens to become fogged or for the image to become blurred by secretions (blood, peritoneal, or ovarian cystic fluid) that smear the forward lens of the laparoscope. If such an event occurs while the accessory operative instrument is being used to manipulate tissue (fallopian tubes, bleeding vessel), it can create a problem of immense proportions. During double puncture laparoscopy, the laparoscope can be removed for cleaning purposes. Alternatively, it can be apposed to the uterus for a few moments to warm it up and thereby prevent fogging up of the lens. Neither of these maneuvers can be performed with the single puncture operative laparoscope. The laparoscope lens cannot be approximated to any structure because of the protrusion of the operating instrument and it cannot be removed from the abdomen without removing the accessory instrument at the same time; this requires the operator to release any tissue that the instrument is holding.

Angle of View by the Objective Lens

The field of vision through the laparoscope is related to its depth of focus and to the distance between the objective lens and the inspected object. The objective lens may provide either a straight 180° view or be angulated to give a lateral oblique field of view (see Figure 1.12).

TEACHING ACCESSORY

The descriptive adjective of "teaching" applied to the word accessory is perhaps its main shortcoming. Although the accessory is essential for teaching residents and students, it is no less important to an assistant who is required to aid in the laparoscopic surgery. One cannot expect consistently appropriate help from the assisting surgeon without him or her having visual access to the operative field. Moreover, at times, the lack of good visual surveillance by the assistant may invite complications. During procedures performed under local anesthesia, a flexible fiberoptic teaching attachment sometimes may allow even the patient to see and better understand the surgeon's explanations and objectives (Figure 1.13). This results in a more cooperative and informed patient.

For the image to be seen at both objectives—that is, at both the primary laparoscope and at the teaching accessory—a beam splitter divides the amount of light directed to each eyepiece. A 50:50 splitting of the image is available for surgical procedures. For photography, the division can be made 80:20 by a special accessory.

LIGHT SOURCE AND ILLUMINATION

In the past, a major obstacle to effective endoscopic procedures was the poor available light. There was just insufficient illumination delivered to the object under observation. Furthermore, the duration of the operation was limited by the heat produced by the power source. A major advance in the field of endoscopy was the advent of fiberoptic bundles capable of delivering high intensity cold light at a distance from the power supply. This not only allowed utilization of a more powerful light source, but at the same time, it permitted the laparoscopic procedure to be prolonged sufficiently to ensure that the required information would be obtained.

Power Source for Light. Conventional power sources include two 150-watt tungsten lamps powered by a dimming circuit, which allows the level of light intensity to be changed as needed. Newer quartz filament bulbs increase the potency of the light available for transmission. When documentation is desired by means of still photography or television, a more powerful light source can

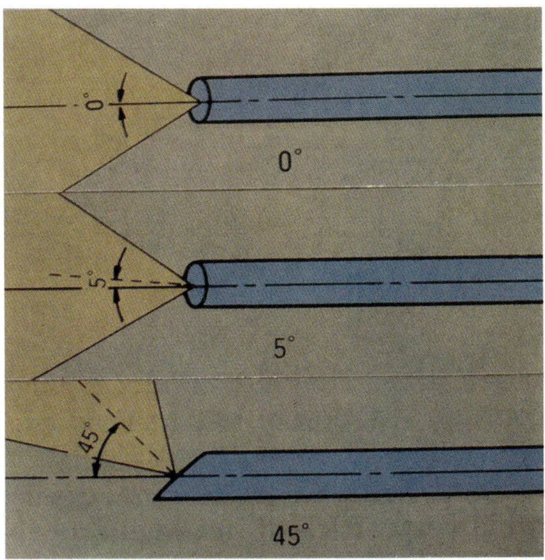

Figure 1.12 Visual angles of the most frequently used laparoscopes: (from top down) 0° angle view (180° from observer), 5° view (175° from observer), and 45° (135° from observer).

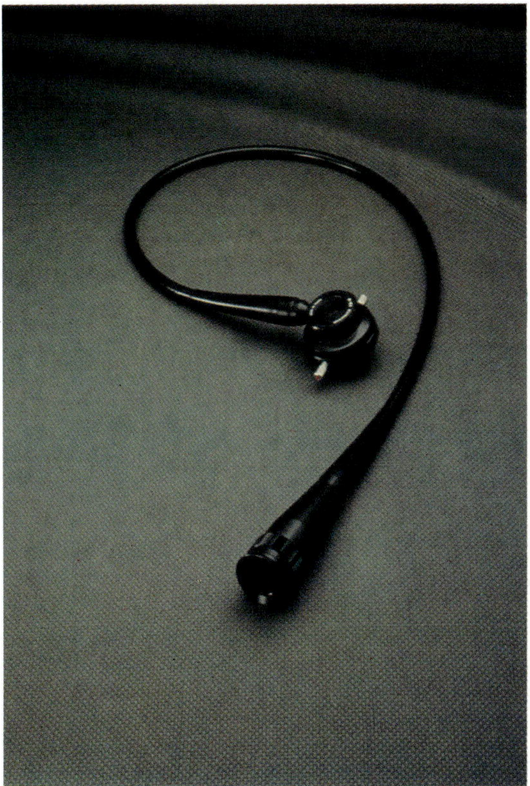

Figure 1.13 Flexible teaching attachment. Indispensable auxiliary instrument which provides concomitant visual access for the surgeon's assistant, student, or resident. In laparoscopies performed under local anesthesia, the patient can also be permitted to see the procedure by this means.

be provided by xenon lamps. These allow the operator to utilize small diameter laparoscopes (5 to 7 mm) and still to have sufficient illumination.

As newer power sources become available, it is useful to evaluate both the intensity of illumination and the refractory effect they have on the tissues. If they distort the color of the image that one obtains, they may prove unacceptable.

The power source for light has the capacity to produce some leakage current by the process of capacitance and inductive coupling. It is mandatory, therefore, to ground this equipment adequately to ensure there will be a path for the leakage current to escape.

Light Transmission. Fiberoptics have provided a means for adequate illumination at a distance from the heat produced by the power source. The development of this cold light technique should be considered one of the landmarks in the advancement of laparoscopy. Light entering the glass fiber refracts at the entry face and is transmitted by repeatedly reflecting off the glass rod walls until it reaches the distal end. Special construction of the bundle of fiberoptics results in little attenuation of the light intensity as the light travels the length of the light cord. Newer fluid-filled light transmission cords can be expected to conduct high intensity illumination with minimal color distortion due to their low refractive index and spectral content.

Miniaturization of endoscopic equipment requires the light to be concentrated and transmission to be carried by a small number of optic fibers. Laser illumination is capable of providing adequate illumination, but typical lasers produce monochromatic light that is not capable of offering the range of color information needed during a laparoscopic procedure.

AUXILIARY SURGICAL INSTRUMENTS

In addition to the telescopic lens, the availability of appropriate instrumentation may be decisive for successful laparoscopy. It would be just as imprudent to undertake a laparoscopic procedure without adequate instruments as it would be to perform a major abdominal surgical procedure under like conditions.

Advances in translaparoscopic surgery have prompted the development of a variety of operative instruments. Although a full description of them is beyond the scope of this book, there are some that should be part of the basic laparoscopic kit and that should be available before every laparoscopy. Instruments for laparoscopic surgery are divided into those that are electrical in nature and those that are not. In addition, the electrical instruments are further divided into monopolar and bipolar, according to the kind of electrogenerator and design of circuitry they employ.

Grasping Forceps. A two-bladed, nontoothed grasping forceps is required for mobilizing intra-abdominal organs. It facilitates the complete visual evaluation of pelvic and abdominal structures. The forceps should provide a smooth but firm grasp of the fine intraperitoneal structures and produce minimal surgical trauma. Some are designed with special curvatures to permit one to grasp the round ligament or fallopian tubes without causing a crush injury. This instrument should be able to conduct electrical current so as to enable one to coagulate small bleeding points encountered during the procedure.

Probe. Usually of metallic composition, the probe is used to help mobilize the intraperitoneal structures with minimal trauma. The intraperitoneal or distal portion of this instrument is graduated in centimeters to allow accurate measurement of the organ or structure being evaluated. Inconsistent magnification by the lens system is inherent in the design of the laparoscope, and makes calibration of the probe indispensable for use in diagnostic procedures.

Hollow Cannula. A hollow metal insulated cannula is essential to permit the laparoscopist to aspirate intraperitoneal fluid collections for analysis or therapy. It can also be used as a probe. This cannula should have a Luer-lock proximal connecting port for attaching a syringe. It should also have a shut-off valve so that one can disconnect the syringe from the cannula without escape of intraperitoneal gas and deflation of the pneumoperitoneum. This instrument should also be capable of connection to the electrogenerator for coagulating a bleeding site on contact. An example of how this instrument can help avoid the need for major surgery is the case of a bleeding corpus luteum cyst. The cannula can simultaneously aspirate the hemoperitoneum and coagulate the bleeding vessel if it is clearly identified.

Electrosurgical Scissors. The need to divide adhesions during a laparoscopy may require translaparoscopic scissors. The cutting blades of some scissors are sharp enough to obviate the need for cutting current to sever the tissue. Because intraperitoneal adhesions are often vascularized—and the blood vessel may not always be seen when the adhesion is placed on tension—electrocoagulation is always recommended before one divides them.

While the instruments listed above are the minimum required for a laparoscopic procedure, a whole array of additional equipment has been developed. One should consider acquiring some of them if the needs of the individual operator and institution warrant it.

POWER GENERATORS

It is common practice for a laparoscopist to utilize the power generator that is also available for other surgical procedures. While this may be acceptable, some generator units used for general surgery or urology will produce an excessive amount of energy output far beyond that needed to carry out translaparoscopic surgery.[4] It is imperative, therefore, to know the particular specifications of any unit that is being used. The specifications, which are important for the laparoscopic surgeon, are: (1) type of generator, (2) output circuitry, (3) output waveforms, (4) output voltage, (5) output power, (6) unit control setting, (7) activation indicators, and (8) power switch control.

Type of Generator. Low frequency current cannot be utilized for electrosurgery because it causes muscular stimulation and violent contractions. The electrosurgical generator transforms low frequency current from 50 to 60 cps into high frequency current of approximately 1,000 cps. The latter can be used in human surgery. Different methods of producing high frequency current are the basis for the diverse types of generators, including spark-gap, vacuum tube, and solid state circuitry.

Spark-gap generators are mainly used for fulguration procedures. They produce a frequency current of approximately 750 kilohertz. These devices are considered high-output voltage generators. Such units have been used preferentially for coagulation and hemostasis of bleeding points. Their main disadvantage is the tendency for the current to jump to adjacent areas causing damage to neighboring tissues.

Vacuum tube generators produce an undamped type of wave mainly with cutting properties and little tissue coagulating effect. These solid state electronic devices develop a high frequency current in the range of 500 to 5,000 kilohertz and have a low output voltage that diminishes the tendency for the current to jump, although not eliminating it completely. Different wavelengths and frequencies produce the several types of currents required for different procedures. Whenever possible, low peak voltage generators should be used.

Output Circuitry. The essence of safe electrosurgery is to be able to control the flow of current to the patient and back to the generator along a preestablished circuit. Any deviation from the planned pathway results in current taking inappropriate routes to dissipate. This enhances the potential for tissue to be inadvertently burned. The two kinds of systems presently used are either grounded or isolated.

In the grounded system, the electrosurgical instrument is the active electrode. It delivers the electrical current to the surgical site. A plate attached to the patient collects the current as it leaves the patient, returning it back to the generator to complete the circuit. In the isolated system, the current delivered to the patient is returned to the generator through an ungrounded plate. Thus, the circuit created is isolated from the ground and the generating current. In the latter, the generator is completely isolated and thus safer. Nevertheless, this is only true in low power units; current leakage occurs when high-frequency, high-wattage generators are used.

Output Waveforms. The shape of the voltage wave characterizes the type of current supplied through the electrosurgical instrument. High voltage peaks producing long and infrequent sparks serve as a coagulating or fulgurating current. This is mainly a highly damped current producing cellular dehydration. Low voltage peaks forming very short sparks constitute the cutting current. Intense heat is generated within the tissues to which this current is applied. This literally makes the cells explode, and thus allows the cutting through of tissues. The combination of these waveforms creates the blend current which has both cutting and coagulating properties at the same time.

Output Voltage. Knowledge of the maximum peak-to-peak voltage is important in regard to the type of tissue involved. The greater the tissue resistance, the higher the voltage required to accomplish the task. When the voltage is applied to tissues, power is produced. The power is measured in watts. Power generators have their own unit control setting for each type of current. The laparoscopic surgeon must be familiar with the unit being used in order for him or her to appreciate the amount of energy applied to the treated tissues.

Activation Indicators. Generators have a variety of methods to indicate that current is being delivered through the surgical instrument. In some, different pitches of noise distinguish one type of current from another. Light indicators produce a visual signal in others. Because laparoscopy is usually performed in a darkened operating room with the power generator at some distance from the operator's field of view, it is preferable to have some type of audible signal. In this way, the surgeon knows at all times if current is being delivered through the active electrode of the electroinstrument.

Power Switch Control. Most units in current use for translaparoscopic surgery are the type that have a foot-pedal switch. Newer models are being developed that place the activating switch on the handle of the electroinstrument. This type of unit should provide more accurate control of the flow of current.

OPEN LAPAROSCOPY INSTRUMENTATION

Performance of open laparoscopy requires special instrumentation.[5] With the exception of the Hasson blunt trocar cannula all other instruments are commonly found in most operating rooms. These consist of: (a) surgical knife with a No. 15 blade; (b) one pair of Addison toothed forceps; (c) several straight hemostats and Kelly forceps clamps; (d) absorbable suture material (chromic catgut, polyglycolic acid) on a 5/8 curved needle; and (e) two narrow retractors.

Hasson Cannula. This instrument is designed to be inserted into the peritoneal cavity under direct vision. Its major differences from the standard sharp laparoscope trocar previously described consist of: (a) blunt obturator trocar; (b) a cone shaped sleeve; and (c) suture holding devices (Figure 1.14).

The blunt obturator serves as a guiding rod and pushes away intraperitoneal organs coming in contact with the cannula. Because its insertion follows sharp division of the abdominal wall planes by incision, the risk of trauma is minimal.

The cone shaped sleeve is mounted on the cannula casing and slides over it to adjust for different thicknesses of the abdominal wall. The main function of the sleeve is to obliterate the fascial opening and thereby help maintain the

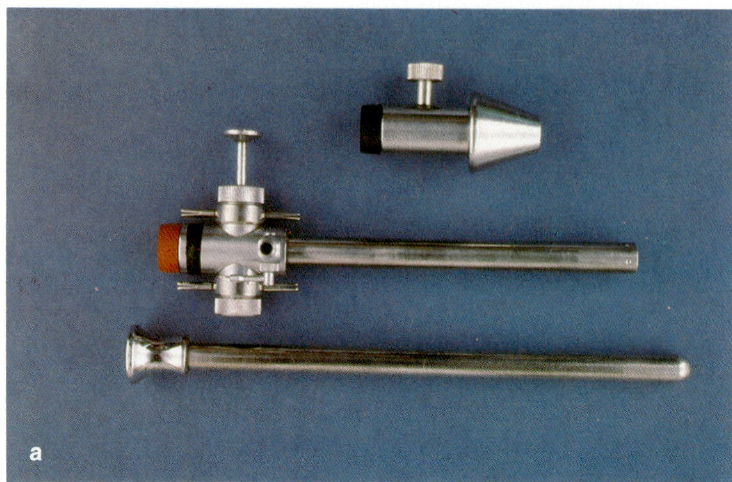

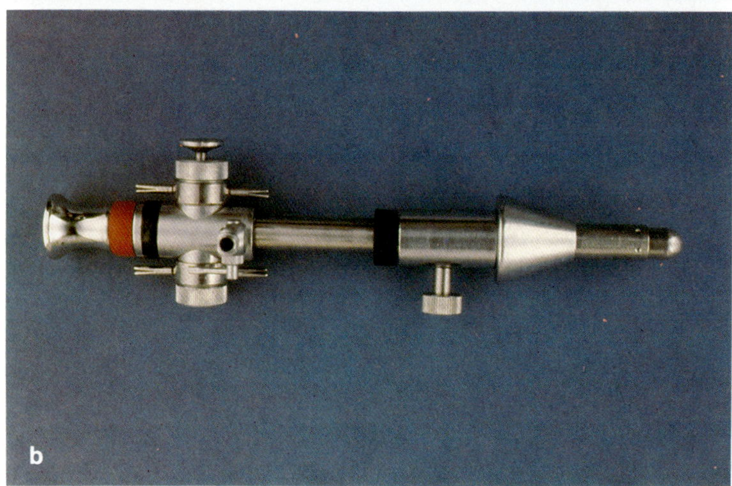

Figure 1.14 *a*. Hasson cannula. Components of unassembled instrument (from top down): blunt obturator trocar, trocar sleeve with the suture holding devices on either side of the trumpet-like valve, and cone shaped sleeve which obliterates fascial opening. *b*. Assembled cannula. Cone shaped sleeve can be slid up and down the trocar sleeve to adjust for the thickness of the abdominal wall.

pneumoperitoneum. Its final position on the cannula must be set prior to the attachment of the anchoring sutures.

The suture holding devices are located on each side of the trocar sleeve. Fascial stitches are wrapped around them under tension to hold the cannula firmly in place. Anchoring the sutures creates a gas seal between the fascial opening and the cone shaped sleeve.

CARE OF EQUIPMENT

Just as for all other surgical instruments, the components of the laparoscopy set should be cared for by knowledgeable personnel. To maximize the useful life of the instruments, they have to be thoroughly cleaned and properly stored between procedures. They must be handled with care during use. It is a wise investment for the laparoscopist to spend some time explaining the care of each instrument in detail to the supporting team. Everyone must understand the importance of a well maintained set.

All instruments used during a laparoscopy should be soaked and washed immediately upon the completion of the surgical procedure. With the exception of the laparoscope and the fiberoptic light cord, all other instruments have to be thoroughly cleansed and dismantled into their primary components. Each piece should be handled individually. Special brushes are available for dealing with the instrument channels.

Most fiberoptic illuminated endoscopes and their accessories can be gas sterilized or cold disinfected (see Chapter 21). Despite some manufacturers' recommendations that their equipment can be steam autoclaved, experience has shown that autoclaving the lens and fiberoptics will shorten the lifespan of these instruments.

Special metal trays with cloth partitions are useful to minimize collisions between these delicate instruments. This avoids scratching the lenses and bending the brittle fiberoptic bundles. When heat sterilization is used, one should remove all rubber sealing cups from the trocar sleeves. This will prevent the extreme heat applied to the metal from melting the rubber material.

General rules applicable to handling the laparoscopic equipment can be summarized as follows:

Do not steam autoclave or boil any instrument containing fiberoptics or a lens system.

Do not use solvent solutions, other than alcohol or acetone, to clean the instruments.

Do not use any corrosive agent as a germicide.

Do not leave instruments soaking in sterilizing solutions for prolonged periods of time (longer than 30 minutes).

Do not use clamps or forceps to affix the instruments to the sterile field drapes.

Handle instruments individually. Do not pile them together. This will prevent heavy instruments from damaging the delicate fiberoptic fibers.

Metal stopcocks on the Verres needle, the laparoscopic trocar sleeve, and the biopsy forceps pivots should be periodically lubricated to ensure their free movement. Fiberoptic cables should be stored extended if possible, or in their own casing. Acute bending of the light conducting fiberoptic cord produces fiber breakage. This is not easily seen with the naked eye, but it will adversely affect the transmission of light.

References

1. Corson SL. Two new laparoscopic instruments: Bipolar sterilizing forceps and uterine manipulator. Am J Obstet Gynecol 1976; 124:434-436.
2. Dingfelder JR. Direct laparoscopic trocar insertion without prior pneumoperitoneum. J Reprod Med 1978; 21:45-47.
3. Epstein M. Endoscopy: Developments in optical instrumentation. Science 1980; 210:280-285.
4. Esposito JM. The laparoscopist and electrosurgery. Am J Obstet Gynecol 1976; 126:633-637.
5. Hasson HM. Open laparoscopy: A report of 150 cases. J Reprod Med 1974; 12:234-238.
6. Hasson HM. A modified ballooned uterine elevator cannula. J Reprod Med 1980; 25:72-74.
7. Morgan HR. Laparoscopy: Induction of pneumoperitoneum via transfundal puncture. Obstet Gynecol 1979; 54:260-261.
8. Neely MR, McWilliams R, Makhlouf HA. Laparoscopy: Routine pneumoperitoneum via the posterior fornix. Obstet Gynecol 1975; 45:459-460.
9. Scott JW. A new uterine manipulator for use at laparoscopy. Am J Obstet Gynecol 1983; 147:458-459.
10. Sharp JR, Pierson WP, Brady CE. Comparison of CO_2 and N_2O-induced discomfort during peritoneoscopy under local anesthesia. Gastroenterology 1982; 82:453-456.
11. Valtchev KL, Papsin FR. A new uterine mobilizer for laparoscopy: Its use in 518 patients. Am J Obstet Gynecol 1977; 127:738-740.

2 TECHNIQUE

The technical details of laparoscopy have been described by a number of physicians in different ways. Despite the many reported variations, some basic principles are indispensable for carrying out the procedure with minimal morbidity. Although the incidence of complications from a laparoscopic operation is low, when they occur they can be very serious. The knowlege of basic anatomy and instrumentation is imperative for performing a safe laparoscopy.

It is a tribute to the usefulness of laparoscopy as a basic diagnostic and/or operative procedure that there have been many modifications and innovations added since it was first popularized as a standard gynecologic procedure. In this chapter, the standard single and double puncture closed laparoscopic technique will be described in detail along with the alternative open laparoscopic method.

ANATOMY

Knowledge of the anatomic landmarks is essential before undertaking a laparoscopic procedure. A review of the anatomy of the anterior abdominal wall and its variations is valuable even for surgeons who regularly perform major abdominal operations. The umbilicus and its relationship to auxiliary puncture sites should be familiar to the laparoscopist not only for preventing iatrogenic morbidity, but also for identifying and correcting an abnormal condition when it arises.

Muscle and Fasciae. The anterolateral abdominal musculature and its corresponding investing fascia are illustrated in Figure 2.1. For all practical purposes, the midline raphe is considered a single layer. The planes of the abdominal wall gain importance when trocar insertion sites are to be made laterally to the linea alba. Two layers of fascia will be traversed when puncturing above the semilunar line of Douglas, whereas only a single fascial stratum is encountered when entering below that line.

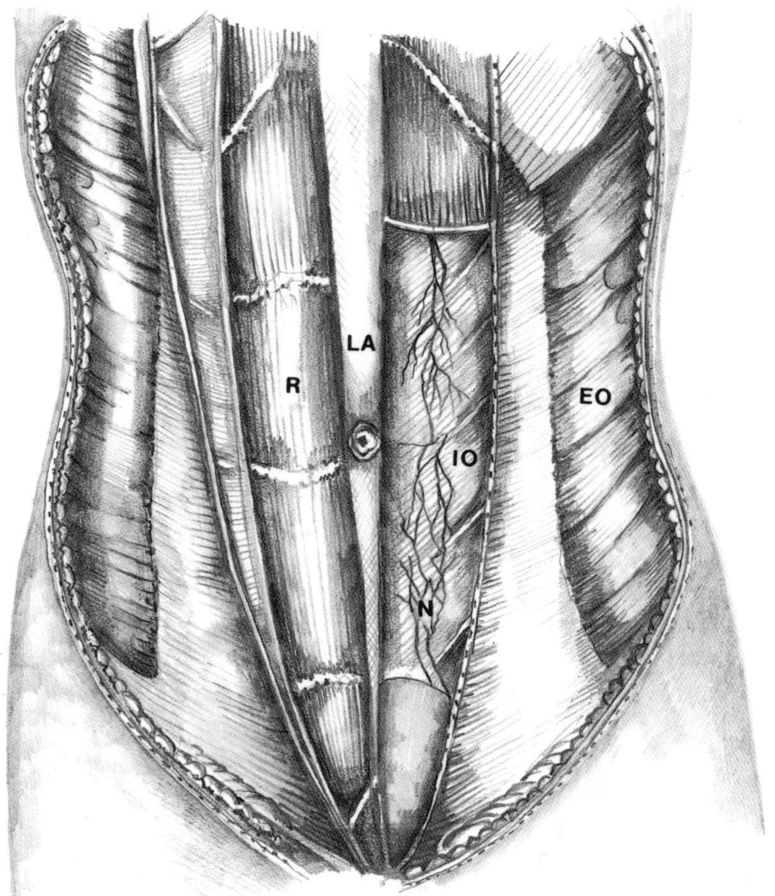

Figure 2.1 Muscles of the anterior abdominal wall. Illustration shows the rectus muscle (R), the external oblique (EO) and the internal oblique (IO). Their aponeurotic covering becomes a single layer at the medial raphe (linea alba) (LA). Innervation (N) to the anterior abdominal wall is shown on the left (patient's).

Vessels. The superficial epigastric artery arises from the femoral artery about 1 cm below the inguinal ligament. It ascends in the subcutaneous tissue of the anterior abdominal wall, lateral to the rectus muscle, until it reaches the level of the umbilicus.

The inferior epigastric artery arises from the external iliac artery just above the inguinal ligament. After traversing the transversalis fascia, it ascends posterior to the rectus muscle parallel to the semilunar line. It divides into several branches that anastomose with the terminal branches of the superior epigastric artery, a subdivision of the internal thoracic artery. These arteries are accompanied by their corresponding veins; they divide to nurture the surrounding muscles (Figure 2.2).

The lower margin of the umbilicus provides the most optimum location for inserting the primary laparoscopic trocar. At the level of the umbilicus, the skin of the anterior abdominal wall is attached to the fascial layer and anterior parietal peritoneum without any intervening subcutaneous fat or muscular tissue (Figures 2.3 and 2.4). In reality, the umbilicus presents a ring-like structure devoid of true fascia. Therefore, the navel may be considered a type of congenital abdominal wall hernia. The fibrous tissue found at the lower pole represents the remnants of the obliterated umbilical vessels and the upper end of the urachus drawn together (Figure 2.5). Patients in whom an evident umbilical hernia is diagnosed and those whose entire linea alba is weakened by diastasis of the rectus muscle have no fibrous tissue in this area. As a consequence, little resistance is encountered when a sharp instrument is used to penetrate here.

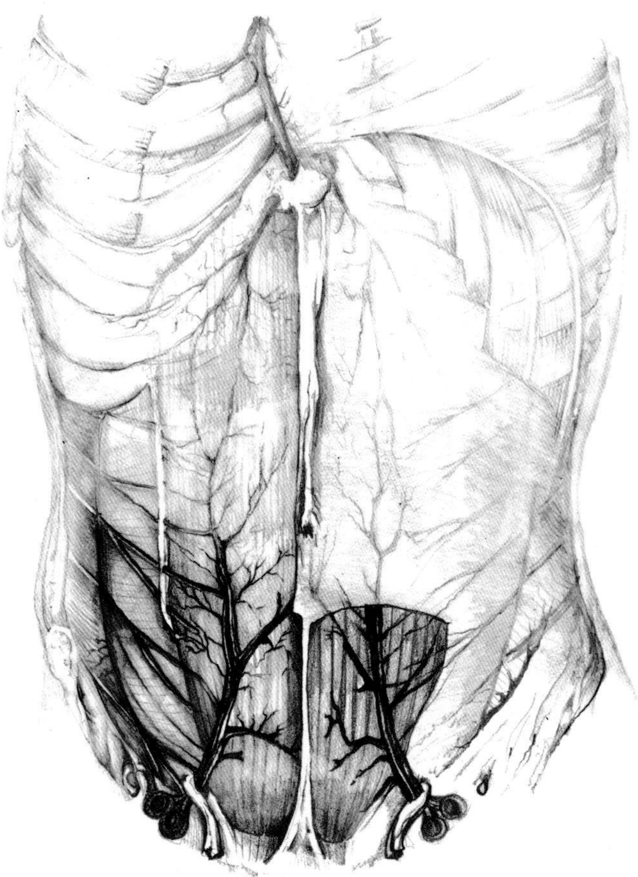

Figure 2.2 Vessels of the anterior abdominal wall (posterior view) with the posterior rectus sheath intact (left). The inferior epigastric vessels are shown communicating with the superior epigastric ones. Vascularization to the umbilicus is also depicted.

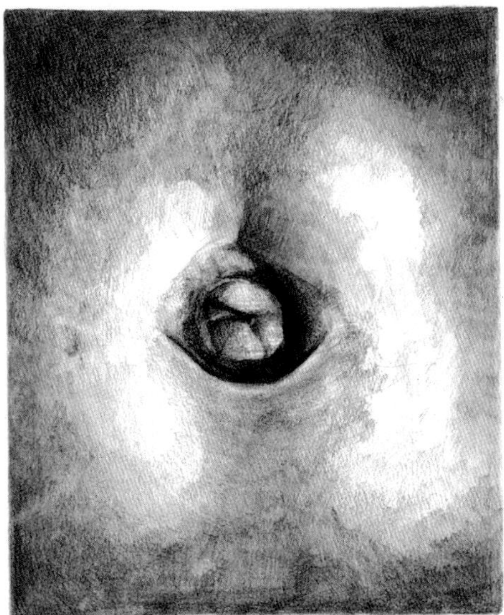

Figure 2.3 Frontal view of umbilicus. An incision placed in the inferior fold produces a cosmetically hidden scar.

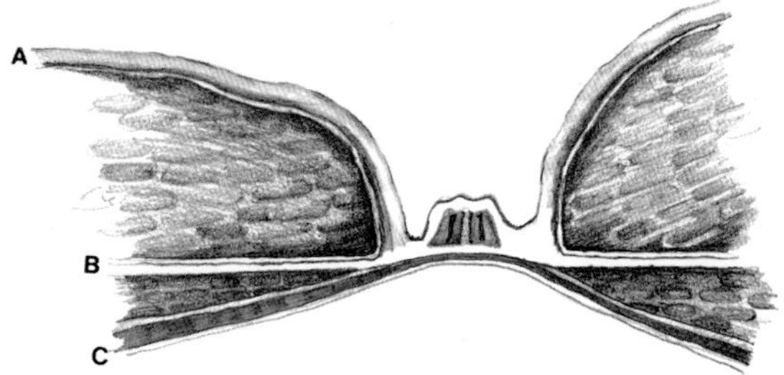

Figure 2.4 Coronal section of the umbilicus and periumbilical region. All layers of tissue are confluent at the umbilicus thus presenting the thinnest depth on the anterior abdominal wall. Skin (A), fascia (B) and anterior parietal peritoneum (C) form a single plane at this level.

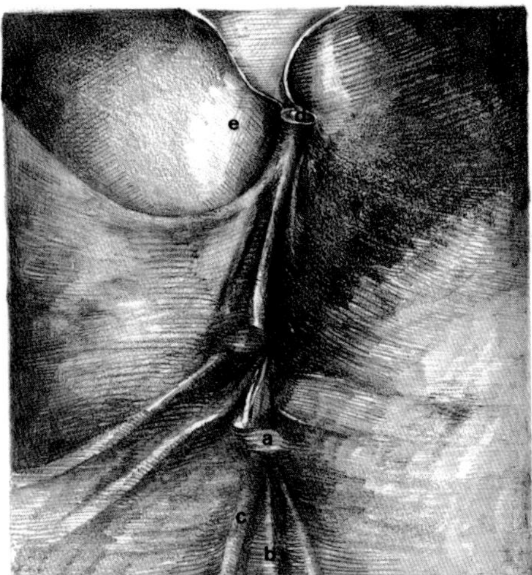

Figure 2.5 Posterior view of the anterior abdominal wall. (a) umbilicus; (b) urachus; (c) obliterated umbilical arteries; (d) obliterated umbilical vein; (e) suspensory hepatic ligament.

If the midline avascular linea alba is utilized for an additional entry into the peritoneal cavity, no other organ or vascular structure should be encountered within the abdominal wall susceptible to injury. The only exception is a patent urachus or urachal cyst (see Chapter 19). By contrast, when one chooses a lateral lower quadrant site to enter the abdominal cavity, the location of the superficial and deep inferior epigastric vessels should be identified first. As seen in Figure 2.2, the deep inferior epigastric vessels are usually located posteriorly to the belly of the rectus muscle. The rectus muscle is well developed and is extremely vascular, making identification of the vessels by transillumination difficult and sometimes impossible.

POSITIONING AND PREPARING THE PATIENT

Although placing the patient on the operating table is usually carried out by ancillary personnel, it is the surgeon's responsibility to guide this aspect of the preparation and to ensure precise positioning prior to the operation. Even though laparoscopy is usually a short procedure, peripheral nerve injuries may result from lack of attention to proper intraoperative positioning (Chapter 24).

The semilithotomy position is most commonly used for laparoscopy, with hanging stirrups holding the legs in a 45 ° incline. We have found this to be a particularly uncomfortable arrangement for both surgeon and assistant. This problem becomes more evident when operating on a woman who is either tall or short; in both cases, the patient's knees interfere with one's ability to get close to the operative site (Figure 2.6). The use of knee support stirrups corrects the matter by relocating the patient's legs away from the abdomen and separating them sufficiently to provide access to the vaginal instruments for uterine manipulation (Figure 2.7).

When placing the patient on the operating table, one should take care to make the perineum protrude over the lower edge sufficiently so that the uterine instruments can be moved almost vertically. Enhancing the natural lordosis of the patient's vertebral column should be prevented by avoiding excessive pro-

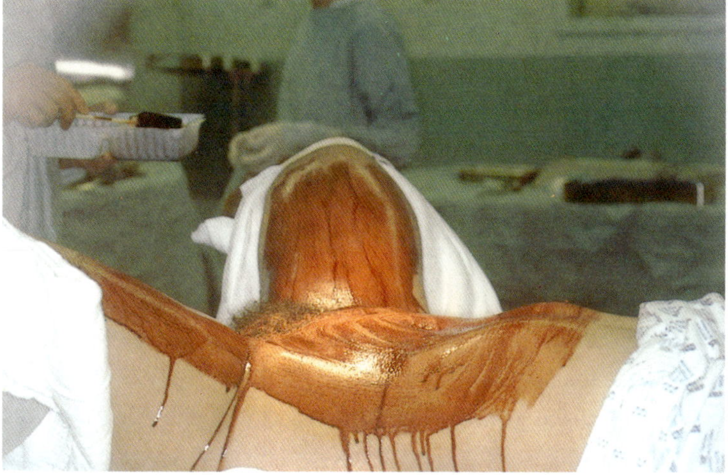

Figure 2.6 Semilithotomy position with legs in hanging stirrups. In the short or tall woman as well as the very obese subject, the knees can interfere with the surgeon's ability to get close to the operative site.

trusion of the buttocks beyond the lower end of the operating room table. Proper positioning allows some leeway for the usual cephalad displacement which takes place when the patient is moved into the Trendelenburg position. Ability to manipulate the uterus properly is sometimes a decisive factor for successfully carrying out a planned laparoscopic procedure.

After adequate positioning of the patient has been accomplished, the vaginal and abdominal surgical fields are prepared separately as sterile fields with antiseptic solutions. Particular attention is directed to cleansing the umbilical fossa thoroughly. This is necessary because it often contains a collection of lint and sebaceous secretions. The carbon dioxide rubber tubing for gas insufflation and the flexible fiberoptic light bundle must be long enough so that undue tension is not placed on the instruments, especially after they are attached to the intraperitoneal instruments. One has to be especially alert to bending the light conduction cord sharply; if this occurs, it fractures the fiberoptic fibers. Broken light conducting fibers usually go unnoticed until one realizes that the amount of intraperitoneal illumination is insufficient for the procedure (see Chapter 12).

The insufflating machine, light source, and electrical power generators, if used, are placed directly opposite the primary surgeon within the operator's visual field. In this way, he or she does not have to turn away from the surgical field in order to see the instrument controls.

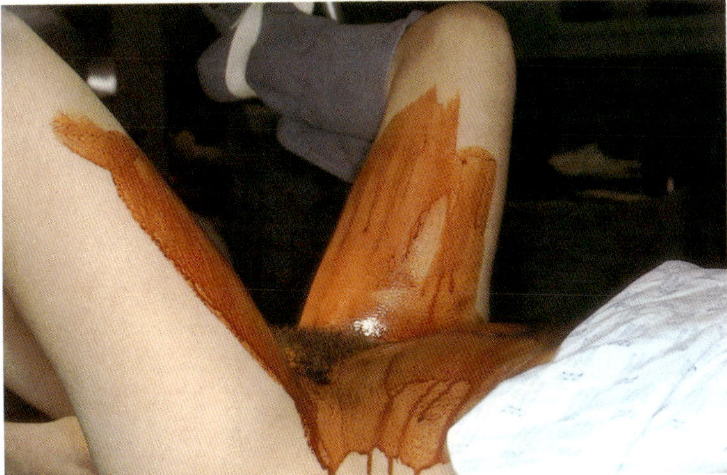

Figure 2.7 Knee support stirrups allow access to the vaginal instruments while keeping the legs at a 30° angle with the horizontal. This provides sufficient room for the surgeon and the assistant.

VAGINAL PROCEDURES

To ensure that the urinary bladder is empty, catheterization of the bladder should precede any vaginal or operative manipulation. A simple straight catheter is used for this purpose with appropriate sterile precautions. A bladder containing 100 cc or more of urine can be injured during a suprapubic puncture. It may also obstruct clear visualization of the anterior uterine wall and its peritoneal fold (Figure 2.8).

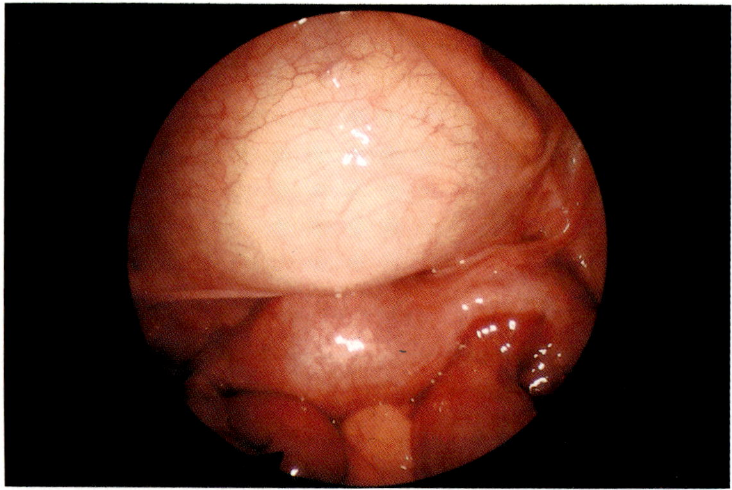

Figure 2.8 Failure to catheterize the bladder prior to laparoscopy increases the risk of injury to that organ. Bladder depicted in the photograph contained 100 cc of urine.

Bimanual pelvic examination is a prerequisite for this procedure. It must be done before any instruments are inserted. The position of the uterus is ascertained precisely to avoid complications from inserting the uterine elevator. If an additional nonlaparoscopic surgical procedure is indicated, it is preferably deferred until after the abdominal procedure; alternatively, such procedures (including cervical dilatation and uterine curettage) may be done under laparoscopic visual control. Retrograde transtubal flow of blood or endometrial cells may give rise to misdiagnosis at the time of laparoscopy (Figure 2.9).

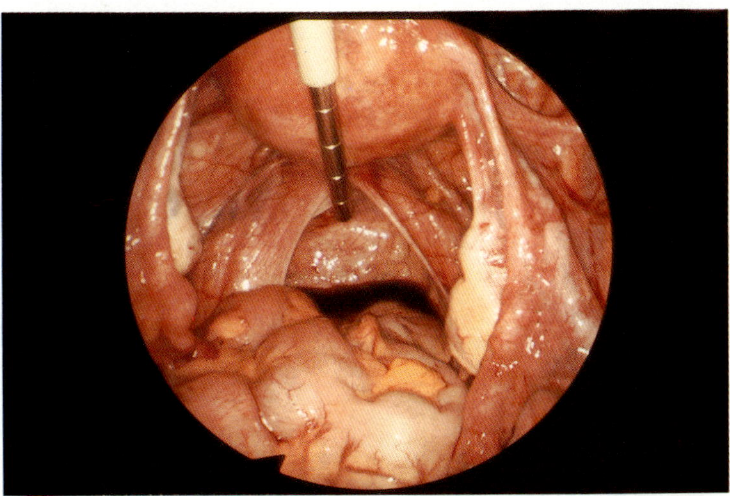

Figure 2.9 Retrograde transtubal flow of blood. Collection of blood in the pouch of Douglas seen at laparoscopy following a uterine curettage. Similar findings can be seen at laparoscopy during menses or immediately postmenstrual.

A weighted speculum or special Graves speculum is inserted in the vagina to visualize the cervix. If a Graves speculum is selected for a laparoscopic procedure, it ought to be possible to remove it with the uterine instruments in place. If a single toothed tenaculum is used as a component of the instrument complex for uterine manipulation, it must be firmly applied to the anterior or posterior cervical lip, including adequate amounts of cervical stroma. Application of the tenaculum transversely avoids slippage and tearing. To establish the correct direction of the cervical canal, its relationship to the axis of the uterine corpus, and the uterine depth, one should sound the uterus gently before inserting the uterine elevator.

If verification of tubal patency is one of the goals of the laparoscopic procedure, a properly fitting acorn tip is paramount. The hermetic seal this provides at the exocervix avoids any spilling of the solution that is to be injected under pressure into the uterine cavity. The uterine manipulator is firmly affixed to the cervical tenaculum (Figure 2.10). Excessive tension should be avoided to prevent the cervix from tearing when the uterine instrument is moved.

The vaginal weighted speculum or special Graves speculum should be removed so as not to interfere with the free motion of the uterine instruments. The instruments protruding from the vagina are draped in a sterile fashion so

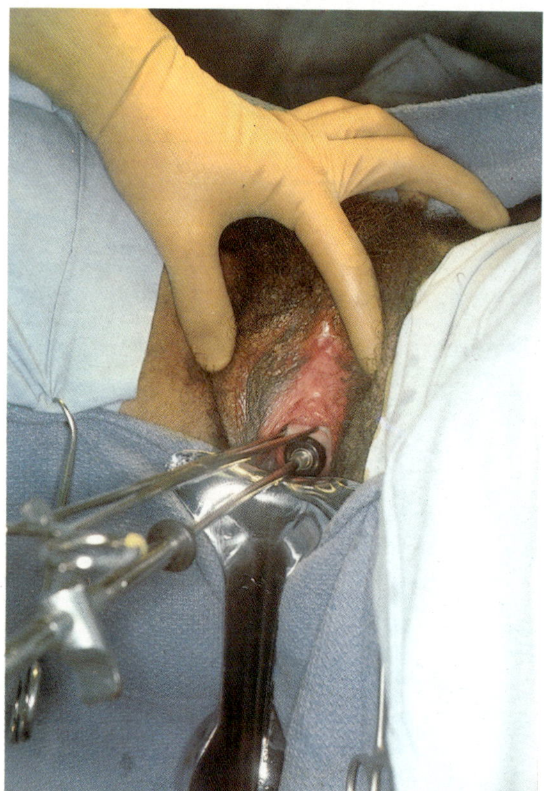

Figure 2.10 Cohen patent cannula attached to tenaculum applied to cervix. Intrauterine forward aspect of the acorn tip is affixed to the cannula in the direction of the uterine position (anterior for anteverted or anteflexed and posterior for retroverted or retroflexed).

that they can be manipulated during the abdominal part of the procedure without contamination. Gloves should be changed before proceeding to the abdominal portion of the operation.

PNEUMOPERITONEUM

The establishment of an adequate intraperitoneal gas compartment or pneumoperitoneum is fundamental for the adequate visualization of the abdomino-pelvic organs as well as for the performance of any operative procedure during laparoscopy. While most laparoscopists establish the pneumoperitoneum before inserting trocar and laparoscope, insufflation of gas may also follow the insertion of these instruments.[1,2] Diverse gases such as carbon dioxide, nitrous oxide, and room air (see Chapter 1) and various routes of administration (transabdominal, transfundal, or by way of the posterior vaginal fornix) have their proponents.[7,8] We prefer to establish a suitable pneumoperitoneum prior to the insertion of the laparoscope trocar using carbon dioxide for insufflation transabdominally; this is the currently accepted standard.

The Verres needle is inserted through a small incision in the lower border of the umbilicus. Attention to detail is essential. The needle must be sharp and the spring stylet checked for proper functioning. The blunt-ended inner hollow needle protrudes from the sharply bevelled outer sleeve. This permits one to verify the penetration of the abdominal wall tissue planes by its upward displacement as each tissue plane is traversed.

The abdominal wall is manually elevated to offer resistance to the insertion of the Verres needle. Elevating the subumbilical anterior abdominal wall also increases the distance between the posterior face of the umbilicus and the sacral promontory over which the major retroperitoneal vessels run. This maneuver is carried out alone by the operator or with the help of an assistant (Figure 2.11).

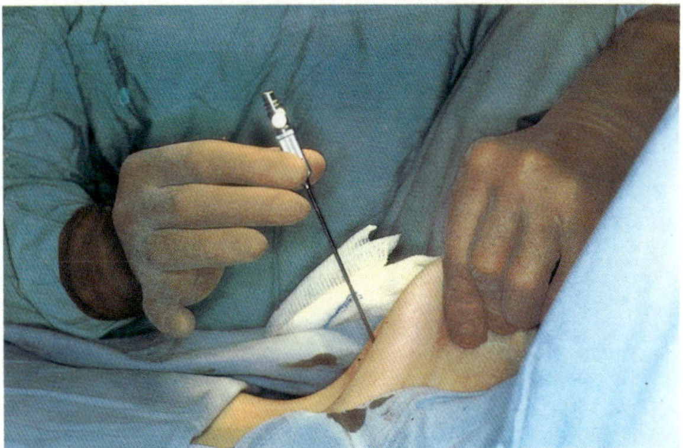

Figure 2.11 Insertion of Verres needle. A 60° angle aiming towards an imaginary point located anterior to the hollow of the sacrum is the proper direction of insertion. Manual elevation of the anterior abdominal wall makes the Verres needle pierce the fascia layer at right angles.

Direction of thrust of the insufflating needle is extremely important. The needle must penetrate the abdominal wall at a right angle aiming toward an imaginary point located at the uterine fundus. This is accomplished by elevating the abdominal wall accordingly. Two upward displacements of the inner needle can be appreciated, first as it perforates the rectus fascia and second when it pierces the peritoneal layer (Figure 2.12).

The proper placement of the insufflating needle is the most important step for successfully producing a pneumoperitoneum free of complications. Several tests have been proposed to verify the correct intraperitoneal position of the Verres needle.[6] These include saline drop aspiration; use of low insufflating pressure; percussion of abdominal tympany; observation of the fluctuation of the pressure gauge needle with inspiratory and expiratory diaphragmatic motions; loss of liver dullness on percussion of the right upper abdominal quadrant; and injection of small amounts of normal saline through the insufflating needle with immediate reaspiration.

None of these tests is entirely accurate, except for the saline instillation-aspiration method. Shortcomings of the aforementioned tests are factual. A single drop of saline placed on the distal end of the needle can be aspirated by the negative pressure created by lifting the anterior abdominal wall. A low insufflation pressure reading can be obtained if the tip of the Verres needle is located in any distensible organ, such as intestine or the urinary bladder. A tympanitic sensation can be obtained by percussing any gas-filled chamber, including a subcutaneous emphysema or a distended stomach. Fluctuation of the intra-abdominal pressure gauge reading will occur from diaphragmatic excursions. A properitoneal subfascial accumulation of insufflated gas reflects such changes in intra-abdominal pressure even though it is extraperitoneal in location. The loss of liver dullness on percussion is a late sign requiring a large amount of gas to be insufflated before it can be elicited. An overdistended stomach can be similarly misleading. Percussion is more valuable as a confirmatory sign of intraperitoneal gas insufflation than as an index of proper initial placement of the needle (Figure 2.13).

Injection of 5 to 10 ml normal saline intraperitoneally cannot be reaspirated because it is dispersed (Figures 2.14). If placed extraperitoneally, however, it forms a sequestered fluid collection so that it can be recovered by applying negative pressure with a syringe. Aspiration is important because it helps rule out injury to important structures. If the needle has been placed intravascularly, blood is aspirated; if intraintestinal, intestinal fluid or fecal material is recovered; if in the urinary bladder, urine is obtained (see Chapter 15).

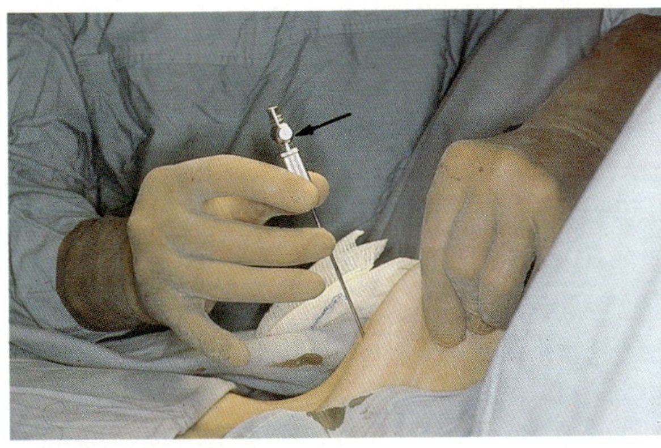

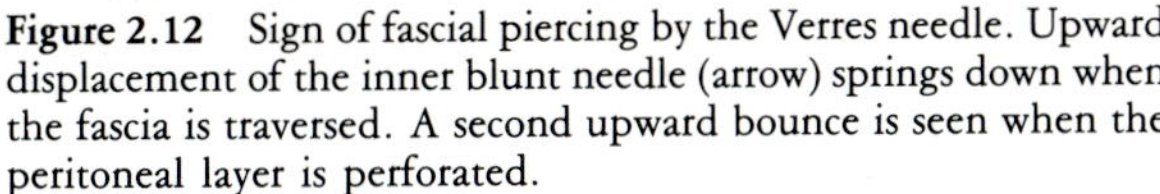

Figure 2.12 Sign of fascial piercing by the Verres needle. Upward displacement of the inner blunt needle (arrow) springs down when the fascia is traversed. A second upward bounce is seen when the peritoneal layer is perforated.

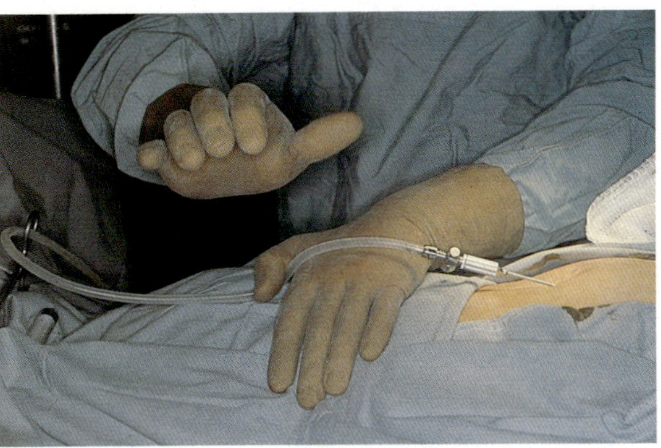

Figure 2.13 Loss of liver dullness on percussion of the right subdiaphragmatic area confirms the intraperitoneal insufflation of the distending gas. This is rather a late sign since more than 1 L of gas has to be insufflated to elicit this sign.

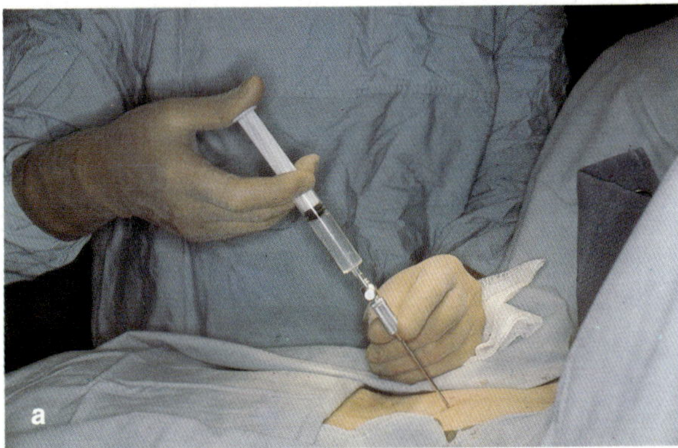

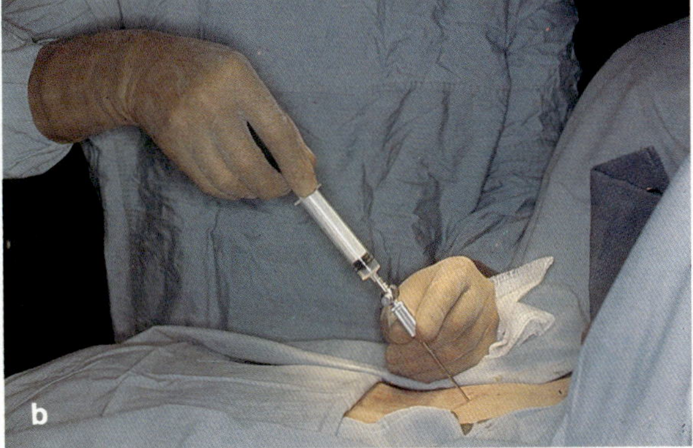

Figure 2.14 Test for proper needle placement. Normal saline solution 5–10 cc is injected through the Verres needle *a*. If it enters the peritoneal cavity, it cannot be reaspirated, *b* because it disperses between the loops of bowel. If the saline is reaspirated, it signifies that the tip of the Verres needle is in a closed cavity or newly formed space (subcutaneous, properitoneal).

No gas ought to be insufflated before the proper location of the Verres needle is verified. The total volume of gas instilled varies according to the size of the patient and the distensibility of the abdominal wall. At the usual insufflation flow rate of 1 L of gas per minute, the intra-abdominal pressure must not exceed 20 mm Hg. If a fast flow insufflation rate (3 L per minute) is used, the pressure may rise as high as 30 to 35 mm Hg. To obtain a true reading of the intra-abdominal pressure, the flow of gas from the insufflating machine should be shut off while keeping the Verres needle and tubing channel open.

Use of the automatic insufflator (see Chapter 1) to maintain the pneumoperitoneum reduces the danger of overinsufflation and averts complications (Chapter 15). Nevertheless, it is mandatory for the surgeon to maintain a close watch on the intra-abdominal pressure readings.

Failure to achieve and maintain a suitable pneumoperitoneum is the most common source of procedural failure (Chapter 13). It gives rise to an inordinate number of complications (Chapter 15). Most abdomino-pelvic injuries occur at the time of needle insertion for establishing the pneumoperitoneum.

PRIMARY TROCAR INSERTION

The insertion of the laparoscopic trocar is termed a blind procedure because the surgeon cannot see the site of entry into the abdominal cavity. It is a maneuver that relies completely on the operator maintaining adequate control of the perforating instrument. A special sequence of sensations is perceived as each layer of the anterior abdominal wall is traversed. Knowledge of the anatomical landmarks and their mutual relationships (see pp. 28-31) is paramount if complications are to be avoided.

Successful insertion of the laparoscopic trocar depends on a number of factors: 1. There must be an adequate skin incision. 2. The instrument has to be in good working condition. 3. It must be advanced in the proper direction. 4. Coordination between resistance and insertion force is important. 5. The operator should ensure control over the depth of insertion.

Size of Skin Incision. Prior to the insertion of the laparoscopic trocar, the skin has to be incised to accommodate the trocar sleeve.[3] Too small an incision increases the friction and resistance to the penetration of the trocar. It makes this step more difficult and increases the potential of undesirably deep penetration of the sharp trocar once the abdominal wall resistance is overcome.

The incision can be sharply enlarged with a small blade (No. 11 or No. 15). The skin is placed under traction with single toothed skin hooks. Alternatively, my preference is to place the skin under tension by moving the Verres needle laterally prior to its removal (Figure 2.15).

Condition of Instrument. The degree of force needed to perforate the different planes of the anterior abdominal wall is directly proportional to the size of trocar utilized and inversely related to its sharpness. The smaller laparoscopes in current use, usually 5 mm in diameter, require much less force for trocar insertion than the older 10 to 12 mm laparoscopes. The smaller size also makes it easier to maintain the sharp end of the inserting trocar. The sharper point further reduces the pressure needed for piercing the fascial layer. The choice between the conical shaped trocar and the pyramidal shaped one is a matter of personal preference. The conical tip appears to require a smaller thrusting force and less rotational motion to perforate the rectus fascia.

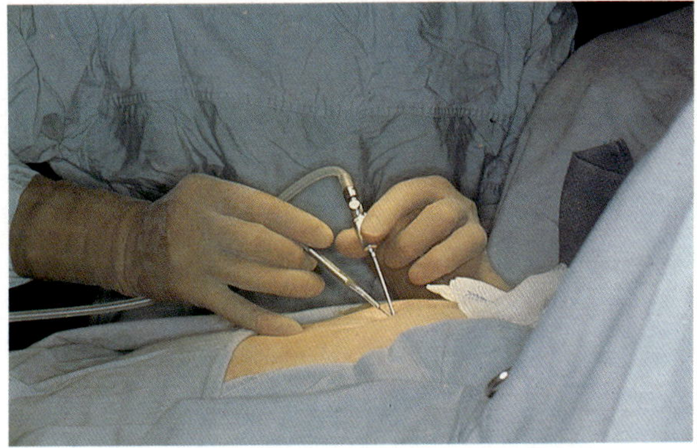

Figure 2.15 Lateral movement of the Verres needle places the skin under tension, facilitating sharp extension of the incision to accommodate the laparoscopic trocar. This maneuver obviates the use of skin hooks.

Trocar Direction. To fully comprehend the importance of the direction for insertion, the major anatomic landmarks and their relationships must be known. The umbilicus is located at the level of the third and fourth lumbar vertebrae. The abdominal aorta usually bifurcates between the fourth and fifth lumbar vertebral body in patients who are in the supine position. Thus, the aorta is directly below the point of insertion. Under these conditions, the proper direction for the laparoscopic trocar is a 60° angle with respect to the abdominal wall plane. It should point to the hollow of the sacrum (Figure 2.16).

Elevation of the lower extremities to place the patient in the semilithotomy position plus the Trendelenburg position change the interrelationship of these important structures somewhat. Elevating the legs rotates the pelvis and moves the anterior wall of the sacrum into a more horizontal plane. Additionally, the Trendelenburg position raises the pelvis and causes an anterocephalad rotation of the lower end of the abdominal aorta, thereby bringing the anterior wall of the aorta closer to the plane of the umbilicus. To prevent damaging the major retroperitoneal vessels, it is essential to take these changed anatomical relationships into account and to correct the penetrating angle of the trocar. Caution should also be exercised to assure that no deviation from the midline takes place. This avoids possible injury to the common iliac vessels (see Chapter 17).

Coordination of Resistance and Insertion Forces. Whereas some resistance to the trocar penetration can be expected from the distention of the anterior abdominal wall by the pneumoperitoneum, some additional mechanical support is still required to avoid indenting the abdominal wall that can endanger the retroperitoneal structures. Additional mechanical support is usually provided by the surgeon by manually elevating the anterior abdominal wall subumbilically.

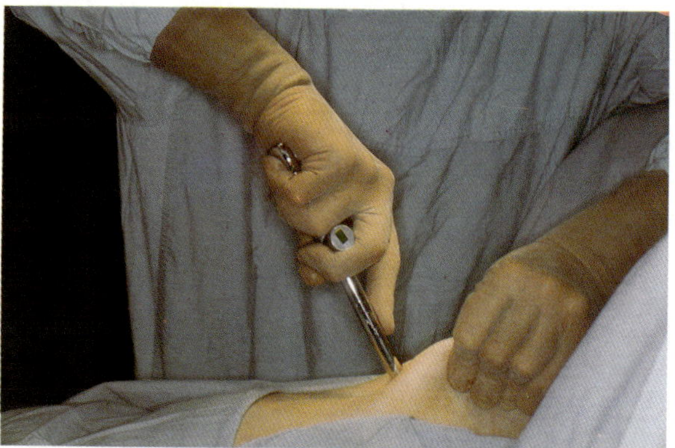

Figure 2.16 Direction of laparoscopic trocar insertion is a 60° angle from the horizontal, pointing towards the hollow of the sacrum. Concomitant elevation of the subumbilical abdominal wall makes this step of the procedure safer.

Laparoscopy as currently practiced is generally accepted to be a one operator procedure. Nevertheless, in well staffed hospitals, an assistant is usually available. Even when such help is available, it should not be used for the procedure of elevating the abdominal wall. Uneven elevation yields unequal resistance which may cause deviation of the perforating trocar. This increases the likelihood of injury to structures in the lateral pelvic walls (see Chapter 17). If the operator is simultaneously applying pressure on the laparoscopic trocar and elevating the subumbilical abdominal wall, there is less risk of incoordination (see Figure 2.16). Possible inadvertent damage of intraperitoneal and retroperitoneal structures is thereby greatly diminished.

Depth Control. If a straight perpendicular entry approach is used at the level of the umbilicus, the thickness of the abdominal wall transversed is usually no more than 1 to 2 cm. A Z-form of penetration enters through the skin incision and courses more caudally to perforate fascia and peritoneum. The thickness of the abdominal wall in this area is between 3 and 4 cm in normal adults and in obese patients it can even be double this depth.

After clinically deciding the approximate depth of penetration, one lifts the abdominal wall to offer additional resistance to inserting the instrument. The trocar and its sleeve is grasped by the operator with the index finger extended to the point of maximal planned penetration (Figure 2.17). The right hand is used by right handed surgeons. The extended finger acts to prevent the sharp trocar tip from thrusting too deeply and coming in contact with any intra-abdominal or retroperitoneal structure. The trocar is rotated in a semicir-

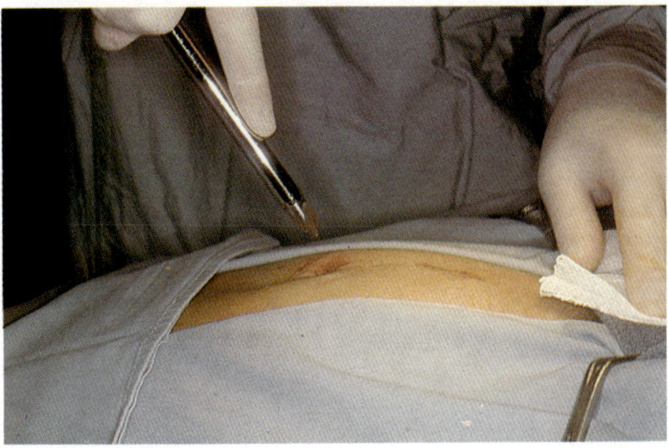

Figure 2.17 Extended index finger marks the point of maximal planned penetration of the laparoscopic trocar.

cular fashion on its long axis while controlled, firm, downward pressure is being applied (Figure 2.18). Sudden loss of resistance, usually accompanied by an echophonic popping sound, indicates that the linea alba has been traversed. With only the peritoneal layer preventing entrance into the pneumoperitoneal compartment, the force applied to the trocar is relaxed at once. The trocar is then introduced into the abdomen by gentle rotation. The correct position of the trocar and sleeve is confirmed by the free escape of intraperitoneal gas when the sharp trocar is removed. This part of the procedure is particularly hazardous, as previously stated. The complications associated with it will be discussed in detail in Chapter 16.

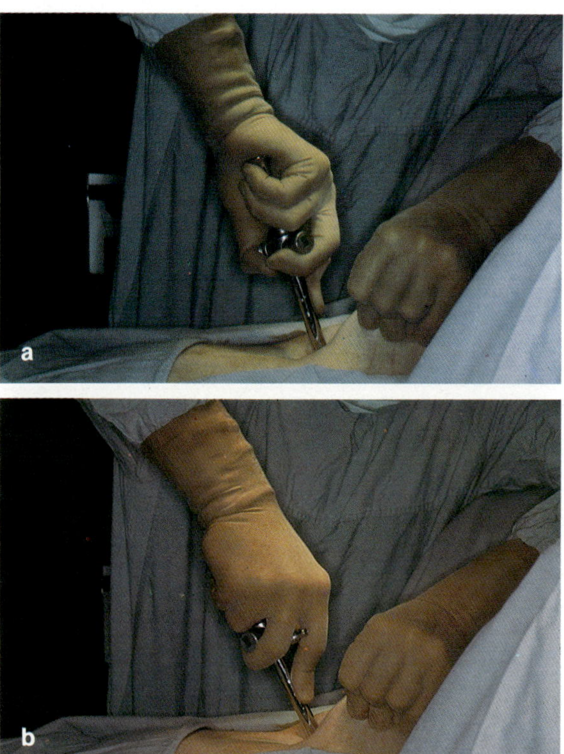

Figure 2.18 Semicircular motion is applied to the laparoscopic trocar to perforate the fascial layer of the abdominal wall: *a*. pronation; *b*. supination. The correct position of the trocar is confirmed by the free escape of intraperitoneal gas when the sharp trocar is removed.

SECONDARY TROCAR PUNCTURE

Nearly 90 percent of laparoscopic procedures require the insertion of a second trocar. In diagnostic procedures, a separate puncture site for use of additional instruments allows better manipulation of the intra-abdominal organs so that they will be under direct vision at all times. Moreover, the approach does not limit the observer to a single visual plane. This contrasts with the constraints inherent in the single puncture operative laparoscope. For a more in-depth comparative analysis, the choice of instruments is detailed in Chapter 1.

Selection of entry site and attention to proper technique are no less important for inserting the secondary trocar than for the primary laparoscopic trocar. A fair number of complications have been reported to occur at this stage of the procedure.

The insertion of the accessory instrument trocar in the midline utilizes the avascular linea alba to avoid injuring subfascial vessels (Figure 2.19). Visual control of the entry site for the auxiliary trocar should always be utilized, recognizing that transillumination of the abdominal wall only provides visualization of the superficial subcutaneous venous circulation. Control of the direction and depth of thrust is essential to prevent deviation from the midline and possible

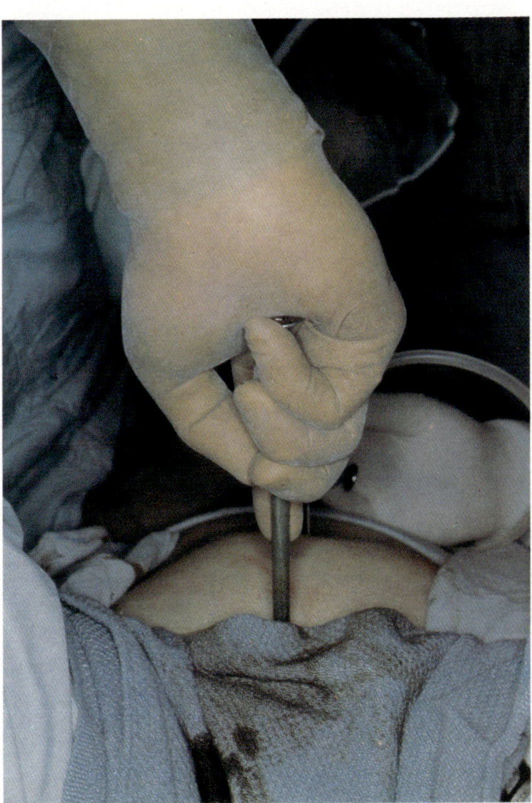

Figure 2.19 Secondary auxiliary puncture. Technique of insertion is similar to the one employed for the insertion of the laparoscopic trocar. Control of depth and direction is essential.

injury to intra-abdominal or retroperitoneal structures. The abdominal wall is lifted to offer appropriate resistance to the force required to perforate the fascial layer. Whenever possible, perforation of the peritoneal layer should be accomplished by rotation of the sharp trocar rather than by applying direct forceful pressure.

It is also important to attempt to insert the secondary trocar suprapubically at a reasonable distance from the entry site of the laparoscopic trocar (Figure 2.20. This permits instruments inserted into the two channels to move freely and independently. Misdirecting the secondary trocar puncture causes inserted instruments to collide intraperitoneally, thereby limiting their usefulness.

Direct visualization of the site of entry of the second trocar by way of the laparoscope at the first site is recommended. This technique is a simple way for assessing correct placement. Instruments inserted through correctly placed openings have the full range of movement required of them.

In the course of a prolonged and difficult translaparoscopic surgical procedure, there may be loss of adequate pneumoperitoneum due to gas leakage. This makes the operation more difficult and at times dangerous. A well tested and helpful preventive measure involves use of a small laparoscopic trocar sleeve (5 mm) for the secondary puncture to serve for supplementary insufflation. The

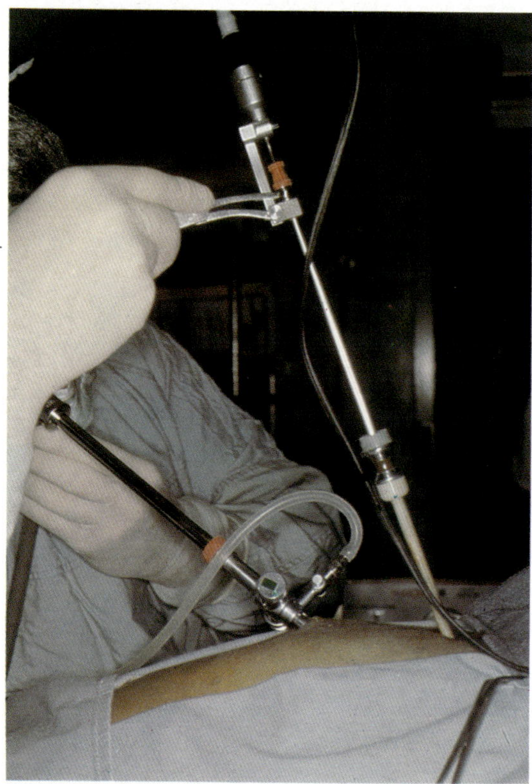

Figure 2.20 Appropriate distance between primary and secondary trocars. Misdirecting the secondary trocar will cause instruments to collide intraperitoneally.

insufflating channel, which the trocar possesses, allows one to attach a second insufflating machine to reform the pneumoperitoneum rapidly as needed.

AUXILIARY PUNCTURES

Many gynecologic laparoscopists believe that most laparoscopic procedures should be limited to a two puncture entry technique, using a primary puncture for the laparoscope and a secondary puncture for an accessory instrument or probe. At times, attempts to follow such guidelines make the procedure difficult and add unnecessary operative time and risk. Some of the procedures, which may benefit from a third auxiliary puncture, are ovarian biopsy, lysis of adhesions, and aspiration of a cyst. In all of them, fixation of the structure to be operated on greatly facilitates the operation. The following alternative steps can be utilized to improve the translaparoscopic operative capabilities while minimizing the technical difficulties usually encountered.

One can employ an operative laparoscope and supplement it with a secondary puncture. In such instances, the secondary puncture is for the instrument required to stabilize the structure to be operated upon. This accomplished, the instrument channel of the operative laparoscope is used to carry out the actual surgery.

A third puncture can be utilized for fluid aspiration. When a mobile cyst is in need of aspiration, the secondary puncture can be used to immobilize it (Figure 2.21). At the same time, a long 14 to 20 gauge needle is inserted at a third site under direct vision for the aspiration. This technique is currently being used for ovum harvest from graafian follicles in connection with in vitro fertilization.

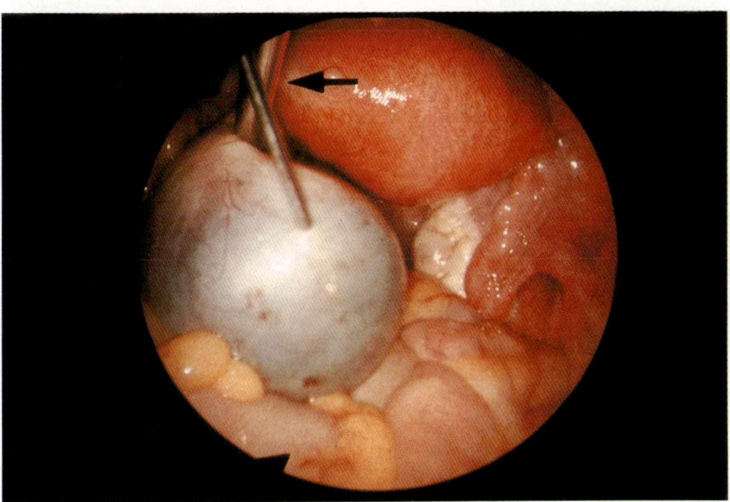

Figure 2.21 Auxiliary puncture required to aspirate an ovarian cyst. The solid metal probe (arrow) inserted through the secondary puncture is used to immobilize the ovary thus offering the aspirating needle a firm plane to puncture.

A third puncture may also serve for surgical instruments. When a biopsy or lysis of adhesions is required, additional 5 mm accessory trocar punctures are used as deemed necessary. Care should be exercised when inserting this additional operative channel. It has to be of sufficient internal diameter to allow the removal of the excised tissue through its lumen (Figure 2.22). In case of translaparoscopic salpingectomy or extirpation of an ectopic pregnancy, the removal of the specimen in toto enhances the accuracy of the pathologic diagnosis.

If the surgeon anticipates having to perform adnexal surgery through the laparoscope, the secondary trocar insertion should not be done in the midline suprapubically, but rather in the lower lateral abdominal quadrant. The third puncture is made in the contralateral quadrant. This technique facilitates both stabilization of the adnexa and performance of the surgical steps. Additional sites for abdominal punctures that may be required for abdomino-pelvic surgery are depicted in Figure 2.23.

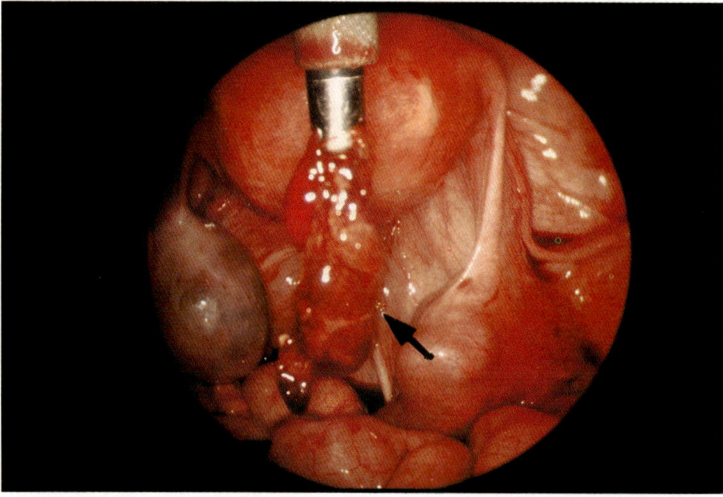

Figure 2.22 The auxiliary trocar sleeve has to be of sufficient internal diameter to allow the removal of tissue through its lumen. An ectopic pregnancy sac (arrow) is being aspirated through the secondary puncture.

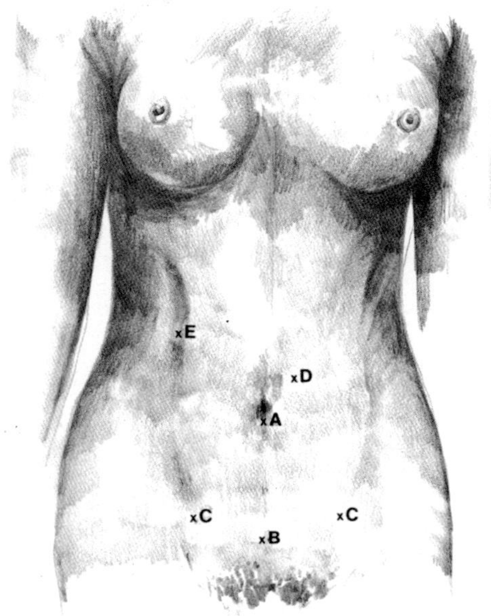

Figure 2.23 Additional sites for abdominal punctures (Verres needle or trocar). Subumbilical (A); suprapubic (B); low paramedian, (C); supraumbilical paramedian (D); subhepatic (E). A and D are safe points for Verres needle insertion. C, D and E are areas for insertion of the secondary trocar under direct visualization.

ALTERNATIVE METHOD FOR ABDOMINAL ENDOSCOPY (OPEN LAPAROSCOPY)

Complications resulting from the conventional technique of insufflating the distending gas for the creation of pneumoperitoneum (closed technique) have created the need to search for alternative ways of entering the abdominal cavity. One of the methods which has gained recognized acceptance is open laparoscopy as described by Hasson in 1974.[4,5] The main advantage attributed to it is that the peritoneal cavity is entered under continuous visual surveillance. The original description of this method consisted of six initial steps and one final step which differed from the usual way of performing laparoscopy:

Incise skin and expose fascia.
Lift fascia.
Incise the fascia and place sutures.
Expose and enter the peritoneum.
Insert cannula in the peritoneal gap.
Fix the sutures and insufflate the abdomen. The final step consisted of closing the incision in layers.

Detailed Technique of Open Laparoscopy

Incise Skin and Expose Fascia. A subumbilical elliptical 1.5 to 2.0 cm incision is made through the skin (Figure 2.24). The subcutaneous tissue is dissected to expose the fascial tissue.

Lift the Fascia. The exposed fascia should be lifted to separate the abdominal wall from bowel and omentum. Due to the inclined direction of the fascial layer, two Kocher clamps or toothed forceps are utilized to immobilize the area to be incised (Figure 2.25).

Incise the Fascia and Place Sutures. An incision smaller in diameter than the trocar sleeve is made (approximately 5 mm) and enlarged by blunt stretching with a hemostat. Because the original entry is enlarged bluntly, a better fit is assured for the laparoscopic trocar sleeve, minimizing the possibility of gas leakage at the insertion site. Both edges of the fascial incision are tagged with an independent suture of sufficient tensile strength to sustain the tension required to keep the laparoscope cannula in place (Figure 2.26).

Expose and Enter the Peritoneum. The peritoneal surface is dissected clear of properitoneal tissue and a blunt entry into the peritoneal cavity with a hemostat clamp is achieved. As is described later, this step does not completely eliminate the possibility of injuring a loop of bowel adherent to the undersurface of the parietal peritoneum at the entry site, but it does reduce it considerably.

Insert Cannula in the Peritoneal Gap. The conical shaped stopper is adjusted to the desired depth according to the thickness of the abdominal wall. The cannula should insert tightly, any incision excess being obliterated by the conical stopper (Figures 2.27 and 2.28).

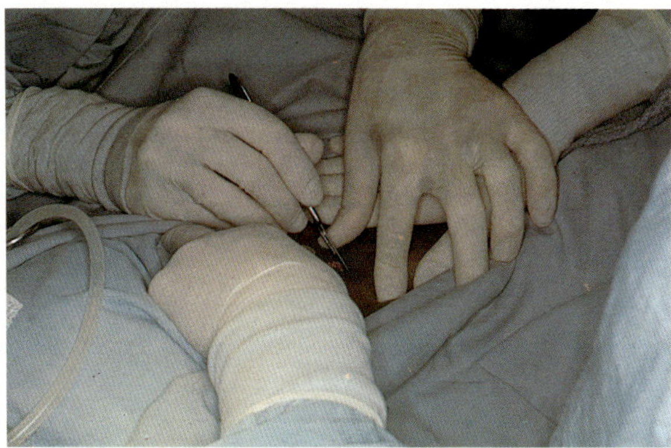

Figure 2.24 Open laparoscopy. Semilunar subumbilical skin incision (1.5 to 2.0 cm) is made with a small blade.

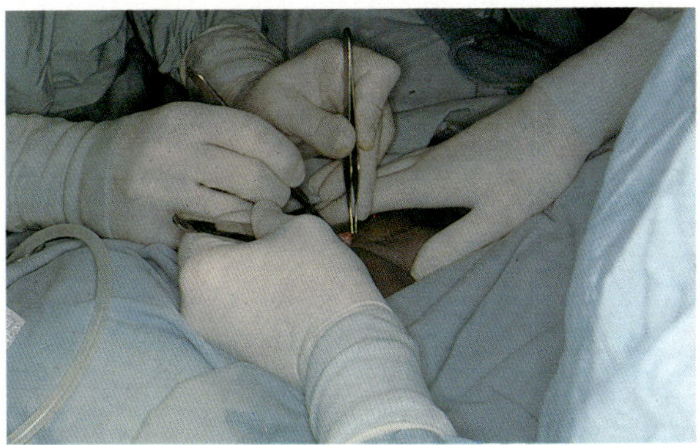

Figure 2.25 Open laparoscopy. Sharp dissection of the fascia. Fascia is lifted with two toothed forceps and 5 mm incision made.

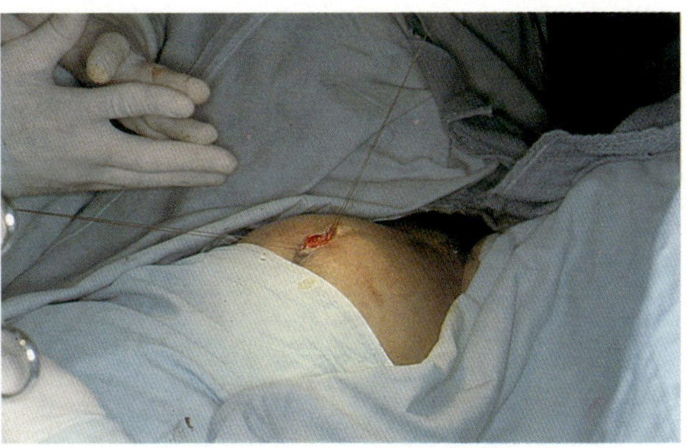

Figure 2.26 Open laparoscopy. Both edges of the fascial incision are tagged with a suture of sufficient tensile strength. This suture keeps the Hasson cannula in place.

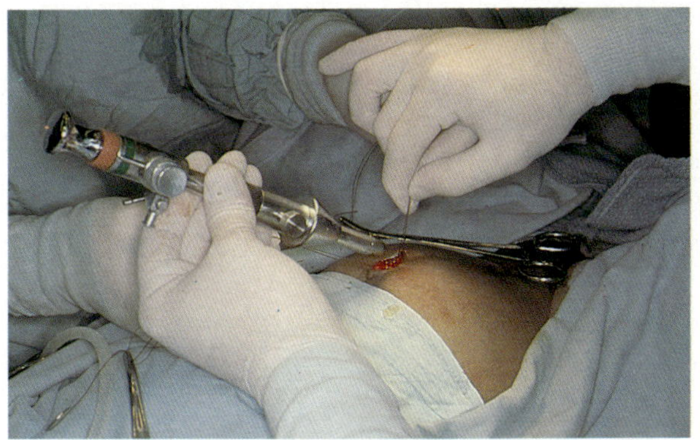

Figure 2.27 Open laparoscopy. Properitoneal tissue is bluntly separated. Hemostat clamp is used to pierce the peritoneum. The conical shaped stopper is adjusted to the desired depth according to the thickness of the abdominal wall.

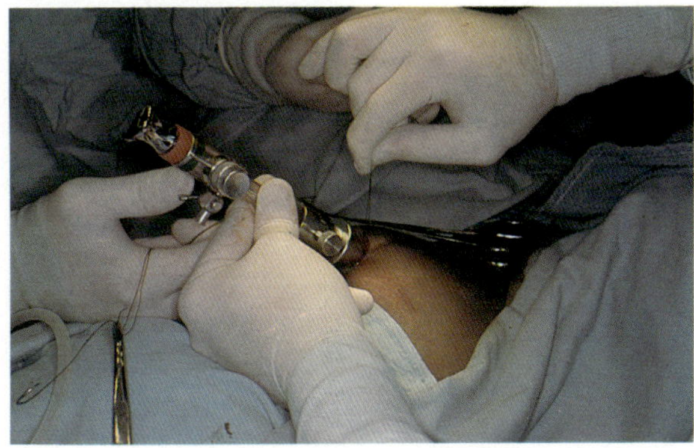

Figure 2.28 Open laparoscopy. Insertion of the Hasson cannula with its blunt trocar.

Fix the Sutures and Insufflate the Abdomen. With the laparoscope cannula fixed in place, the tagging sutures are affixed to the suture holders firmly apposing the cannula's cone against the fascia in an attempt to produce an airtight seal. The tubing from the insufflator is attached to the cannula and gas is dispensed at the regular rate of 1 L per minute or at the fast flow of 3 L per minute (Figure 2.29).

When in doubt about the presence of intraperitoneal abnormalities, the laparoscope can be inserted while the distending gas is being insufflated thereby allowing visualization of the formation of the pneumoperitoneum (Figure 2.30). This maneuver allows one to minimize the amount of gas insufflated to the volume just sufficient to permit a thorough inspection.

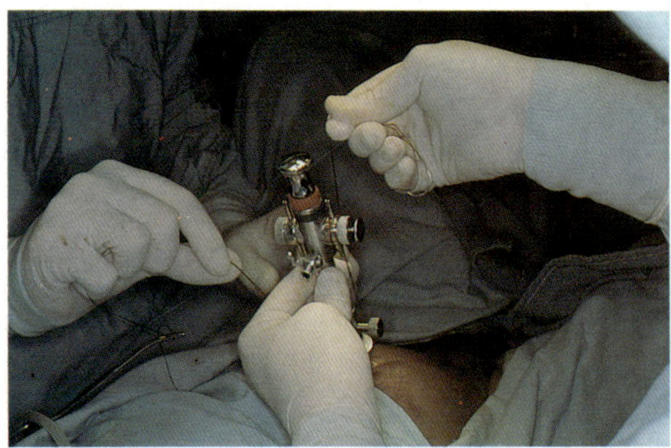

Figure 2.29 Open laparoscopy. Affixing fascial stitches to the Hasson cannula suture holding device.

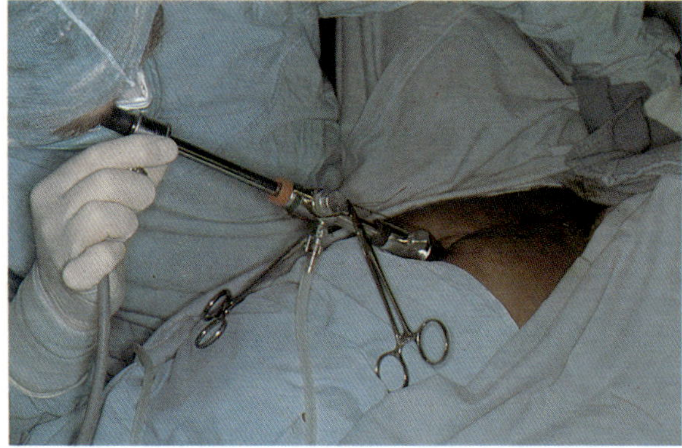

Figure 2.30 Open laparoscopy. Insufflation of distending gas under direct laparoscopic visualization.

At the conclusion of the laparoscopic procedure, following the removal of all the instruments, the several layers of the abdominal wall should be independently reapproximated (Figure 2.31).

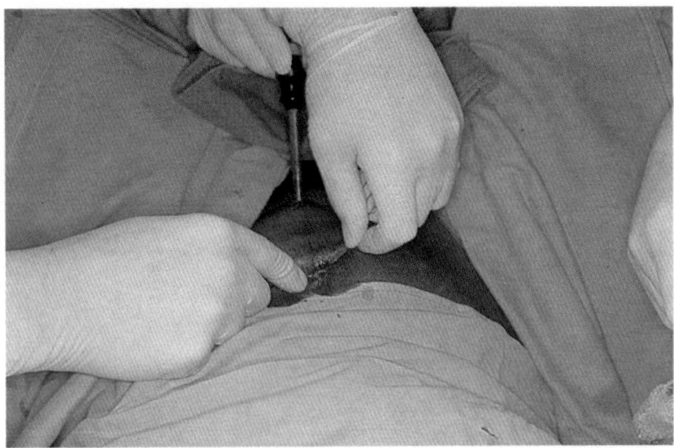

Figure 2.31 Open laparoscopy. Abdominal wall layers are approximated with the transfascial stitches previously used to hold the Hasson cannula in place.

References

1. Copeland C, Wing R, Hulka JF. Direct trocar insertion at laparoscopy: An evaluation. Obstet Gynecol 1983; 62:655-658.
2. Dingfelder JR. Direct laparoscopic trocar insertion without prior pneumoperitoneum. J Reprod Med 1978; 21:45-47.
3. Driscoll GL, Tyler JP, Simpson P. Closure of laparoscopy incisions. Clin Reprod Fertil 1982; 1:241-242.
4. Hasson HM. Open laparoscopy: A report of 150 cases. J Reprod Med 1974; 12:234-238.
5. Hasson HM. Open laparoscopy vs. closed laparoscopy: A comparison of complication rates. Adv Plann Parent 1978; 13:41-50.
6. Lacey CG. Laparoscopy: A clinical sign for intraperitoneal needle placement. Obstet Gynecol 1976; 47:625-627.
7. Morgan HR. Laparoscopy: Induction of pneumoperitoneum via transfundal puncture. Obstet Gynecol 1979; 54:260-261.
8. Neely MR, McWilliams R, Makhlouf HA. Laparoscopy: Routine pneumoperitoneum via the posterior fornix. Obstet Gynecol 1975; 45:459-460.

3 DIAGNOSTIC LAPAROSCOPY

Indications for laparoscopy in gynecology have multiplied as experience with this technique has accumulated. Although limited to operative procedures a decade ago, the main role of laparoscopy at the present time is for diagnosis. Its ability to elucidate the cause of acute or chronic pelvic pain, to rule out the existence of an ectopic gestation, and to evaluate a pelvic mass preoperatively is irreplaceable in the current practice of gynecology.

Utilization of laparoscopy for evaluation and follow-up of female infertility has enhanced the reproductive endocrinologist's ability to diagnose and treat patients by nonsurgical means. Entities such as minimal endometriosis, unruptured luteinized follicle, and congenital abnormalities of the reproductive organs are easily diagnosed translaparoscopically. Without doubt, the possibility of excluding tubal and peritubal disease suspected on the basis of hysterosalpingography has improved the quality of care provided to this population of patients.

The indications for laparoscopy will be dealt with separately in several chapters in this text, but it is understood that the division is arbitrary. It was done for didactic purposes. This chapter on diagnostic laparoscopy will limit itself to the nonoperative applications of this technique. Subsequent chapters will detail its operative applications.

PELVIC PAIN

Pelvic pain is one of the most common symptoms which triggers an interdisciplinary consultation or referral to the gynecologist. It is often accompanied by nonspecific physical signs. It can be acute or chronic in nature. Definitive diagnosis often requires some type of exploration of the abdominal cavity. Acute pelvic pain poses an urgent diagnostic problem and should be addressed accordingly. By contrast, the diagnosis of chronic pelvic pain tends to be delayed over prolonged periods of time to the detriment of timely and appropriate therapy.

Laparoscopy has been shown to be useful in corroborating or refuting the presence of a suspected clinical condition.[11] It is equally valuable in this regard for patients presenting with acute and chronic pelvic pain. With the exception of cases in which a laparoscopy is contraindicated or in which there is a clearly defined acute surgical abdomen, laparoscopy should always precede (or substitute for) a laparotomy for the diagnosis of pelvic pain. Among the long list of conditions that present with acute pelvic pain and that are amenable to investigation and confirmation by laparoscopy are acute pelvic inflammatory disease, twisted ovarian cyst, ruptured corpus luteum with or without active bleeding, retrograde menstrual bleeding, ovulation bleeding, and ectopic pregnancy. Entities most commonly found during a laparoscopic evaluation of chronic pelvic pain are endometriosis, chronic pelvic inflammatory changes (including hydrosalpinx, periovarian and peritubal adhesions), and persistent corpus luteum cyst.

Poor correlation has been reported between the clinical diagnosis based on history, pelvic examination, and laparoscopic findings in patients presenting with acute pelvic pain. Anteby et al were able to avoid laparotomy in 145 of 223 patients (65 percent) presenting with acute abdominal pain by means of preliminary diagnostic laparoscopy.[1] More recently, Cunanan et al reviewed 1,194 consecutive patients who had a diagnostic laparoscopy for pelvic pain.[4] Among 749 patients with a normal pelvic examination prior to laparoscopy, 63 percent (479) had abnormal pelvic findings visualized endoscopically. In those 445 patients who had an abnormal pelvic examination prior to laparoscopy, 17.5 percent (78) actually had a normal pelvis. For these patients the planned surgery proved unnecessary. The high yield of unexpected pathological conditions encountered in patients presenting with pelvic pain and normal pelvic examination verifies the critical importance of laparoscopy for the diagnosis of this condition.

Laparoscopy need not to be limited to the adult gynecologic patient. Pelvic and low abdominal pain in the teenager presents a constant challenge to the gynecologist treating adolescents. It is often difficult to distinguish functional derangements from organic disorders. In the past, prolonged symptomatic treatment was common without prior adequate diagnostic evaluation.

Kleinhaus et al laparoscopically investigated 50 girls aged 12 to 18 years old who presented with abdominopelvic pain that required hospitalization.[10] His results were similar to those encountered in the adult female population. Laparoscopy established a diagnosis in 28 of them. In 32 who had a specific preoperative diagnosis suspected, the diagnosis was proved incorrect by laparoscopy in 15. Laparotomy was avoided in 18 instances. Goldstein et al evaluated 140 adolescents who presented with chronic pelvic pain by laparoscopy.[7] He reported a surprisingly high incidence of endometriosis (47 percent); the youngest patient with this condition was 10.5 years old. Only 18 percent of patients revealed no pathologic findings to explain their presenting complaint.

The tendency to ascribe any complaint of pelvic pain in a sexually active teenager to pelvic inflammatory disease is inappropriate. One must be aware that abnormalities similar to those found in the adult population can also be present in postpuberal adolescents, and laparoscopy offers the opportunity to make an early diagnosis. Expeditious treatment of conditions such as endometriosis not only provides relief of symptoms but may also help preserve the reproductive potential of these youngsters.

PELVIC MASS

Finding a pelvic mass on a routine gynecologic examination presents a diagnostic challenge as to its site of origin and nature. A discussion of diagnosis and pathophysiology of pelvic masses is beyond the scope of this book. Nevertheless, the important role of laparoscopy as a diagnostic and/or therapeutic tool in a patient with a pelvic mass requires further elaboration.

Some pelvic masses are amenable to positive roentgenographic identification. A pelvic kidney, for example, can be identified by means of an intravenous pyelogram. A dermoid cyst of the ovary may reveal characteristic contents, such as a tooth or calcifications. In these instances, surgical intervention may be prevented or indicated solely on the preoperative evaluation.

In most cases, pelvic sonography provides confirmation of the presence of a mass in the pelvis and gives information as to its structural composition (solid or cystic). At times, a pelvic sonogram may also identify the organ from which the mass originates. Technological advances in ultrasonography now allow one to measure the dimensions accurately and to determine the anatomical site of such masses (Figure 3.1).

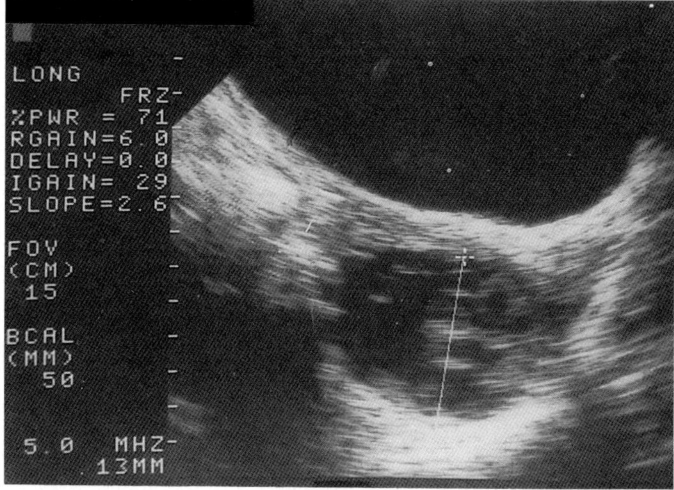

Figure 3.1 Pelvic ultrasonogram demonstrating cystic mass with intracavitary echoes posterior to the uterus. The site of origin of the mass cannot be ascertained by this study. The patient had a clinically palpable adnexal mass (see Figure 3.3).

Laparoscopy for the evaluation of a pelvic mass offers advantages not replicated by any other diagnostic modality except exploratory laparotomy. Its benefits include specific information on the existence of the mass, its exact site of origin, the spatial relationship to adjacent organs, and differentiation between functional and organic origin.

Confirmatory Evidence. Clinical confirmation of the existence of a pelvic mass is sometimes difficult if not altogether impossible. Pelvic pain or discomfort may not permit one to perform a complete and satisfactory bimanual examination. Obesity may hinder the palpation of a suspected mass or preclude its reasonable evaluation. It may not be possible to do a thorough pelvic examination in young women with no prior sexual experience. In all these instances, laparoscopy offers the operating surgeon confirmatory evidence of the existence of the suspected pelvic mass. Far more important is the fact that such confirmation helps avoid unnecessary laparotomy which may have far-reaching implications in the future for these patients.

Site of Origin. Knowledge about the precise site of origin of a pelvic mass, when established prior to corrective surgery, helps the surgeon plan the surgery and counsel the patient appropriately. Differentiation between a large hydrosalpinx and an ovarian cyst can only be made by direct visualization in most instances (Figures 3.2 and 3.3). Identification of a tubal rather than an ovarian disorder may require the utilization of microsurgical techniques not otherwise

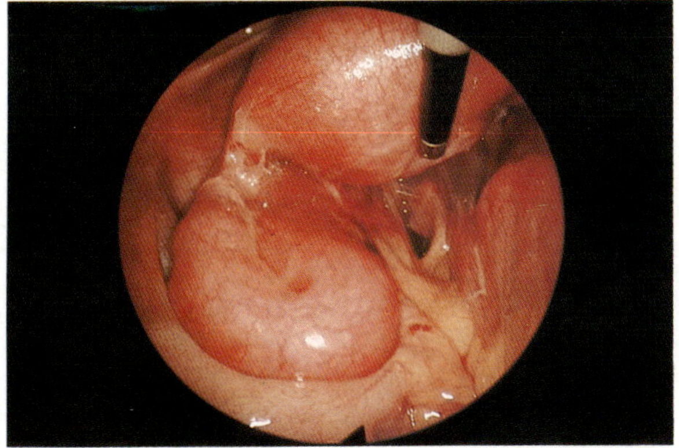

Figure 3.2 Pyosalpinx, left. The uterus is displaced anteriorly by the secondary probe. The distended pyosalpinx is curved in on itself giving the impression of a large single mass on bimanual examination. A multiloculated cystic mass had been reported by ultrasonography.

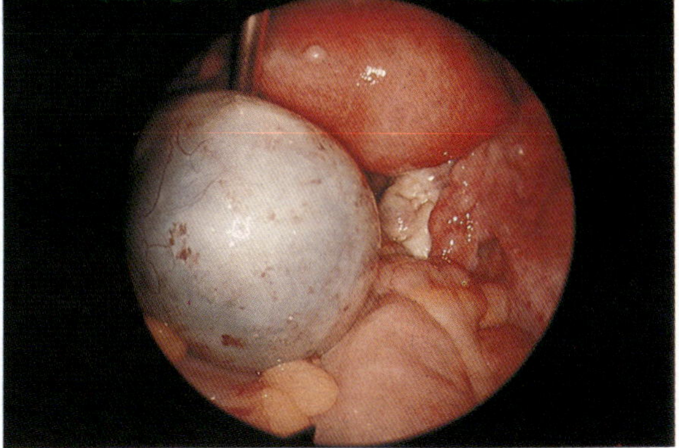

Figure 3.3 Ovarian cyst, left, seen on laparoscopic evaluation of the mass shown ultrasonographically in Figure 3.1. The cyst has a smooth capsule with no adhesions to any adjacent structure. The benign nature of this ovarian lesion, which proved to be a corpus luteum cyst, was confirmed by translaparoscopic needle aspiration.

commonly employed by the general gynecologic surgeon. Appropriate referral motivated by these findings at laparoscopy may prove essential for preserving the reproductive capability of these patients. Masses occupying the pouch of Douglas may or may not be adherent to adjacent organs (uterus, rectum, ureter). Suspected involvement of the rectosigmoid by the cul-de-sac mass requires special preoperative evaluation (barium enema, sigmoidoscopy) and preparation (bowel preparation, enema) as well as the collaboration of a general surgeon at the time of laparotomy (Figure 3.4). This may change the anticipated surgical approach. No less important to the planning of a major surgical procedure is the explanation to the patient of the nature of the disorder. The extent of the intended plan of management and the expected consequences, which may result from the surgical procedure, ought to be shared with the patient preoperatively. The need for consultation and collaboration with other physicians should also be shared with the patient.

Relationship to Adjacent Organs. Most pelvic masses originate from the adnexal structures (fallopian tubes, ovaries) or affect them by apposition. Lately, much progress has been made in the area of conservative surgery of the adnexa. The use of microsurgical techniques for that purpose requires specialized training. It is not acceptable at the present time to perform extirpative surgery (salpingectomy, salpingoophorectomy) in young patients for the unexpected finding of an hydrosalpinx or fimbrial occlusion at the time of laparotomy (Figures 3.5 and 3.6). It is, therefore, advantageous to know in advance if special skills will be needed at the anticipated laparotomy.

Laparoscopy offers the additional benefit of helping to determine the extent of surgery likely to be required. This may prove critical when counseling a young patient with respect to her future reproductive potential. Prior knowledge of bowel involvement in the pelvic mass (Figures 3.7 and 3.8) alters preoperative management by ensuring that the patient is prepared for surgery (by bowel preparation). Moreover, it may prove necessary and wise for the surgeon to call in a consultant if the need for specialized surgical expertise can be expected.

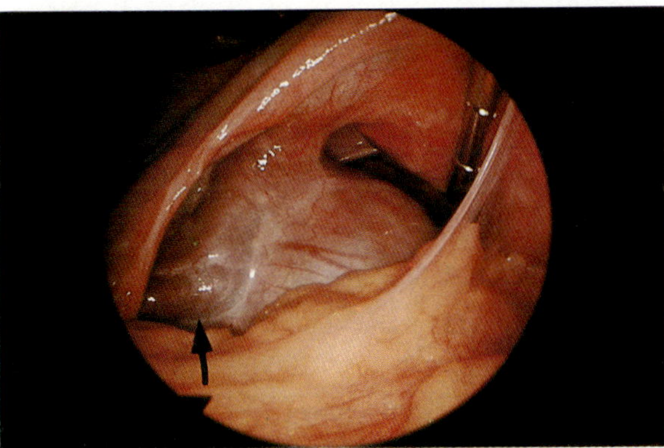

Figure 3.4 Ovarian cyst, left, partially occluded by adherent bowel. Inability to mobilize the mass with the secondary probe confirms the presence of fixed adhesions deep in the pelvis. Note the venous stasis in a dilated ovarian vein in the infundibulopelvic ligament (arrow).

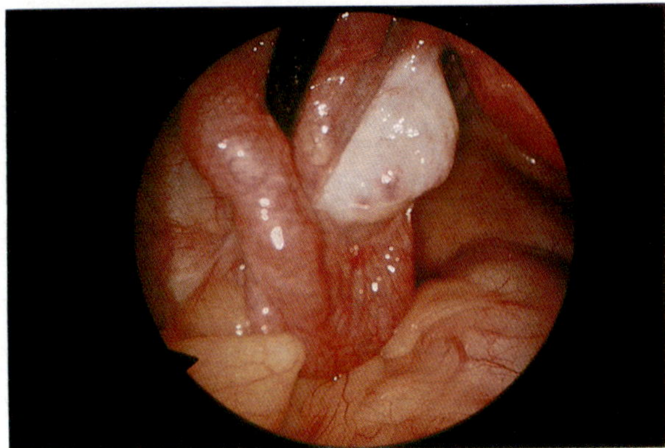

Figure 3.5 Hydrosalpinx, left, with obliterated fimbria adherent to the posterior undersurface of the ovary. Presurgical counseling must anticipate salpingostomy and salpingoplasty.

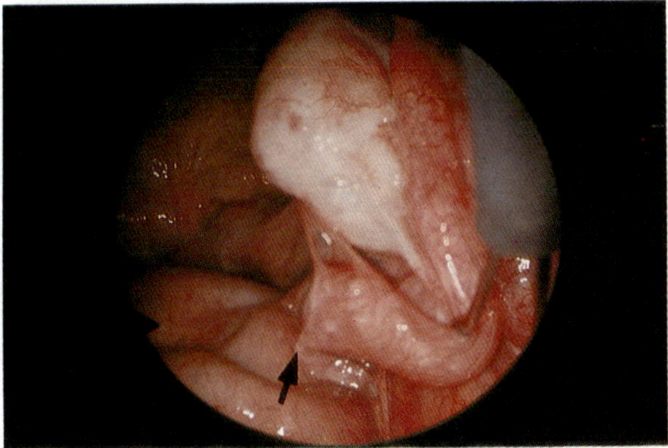

Figure 3.6 Tubo-ovarian adhesions. Use of the atraumatic accessory forceps helps disclose many of these adhesions. Adhesions are also present between bowel and the obstructed fimbrial end of the tube (arrow).

Functional Condition Versus Organic Disease. Ovarian enlargements in the young female are commonly functional in origin. If diagnosed as such, they are amenable to translaparoscopic aspiration and cyst wall biopsy. They are usually nonrecurrent. In other instances, if an adnexal mass is felt in a patient with prolonged amenorrhea or during the early stages of pregnancy, the laparoscopic diagnosis of an enlarged corpus luteum may avert an unnecessary laparotomy (Figure 3.9).

For cosmetic reasons, a low transverse incision is usually used in surgery of the adnexa in young women. A malignancy may be found on laparoscopic exploration in this group of patients, albeit infrequently. The transverse incision could be preempted under these circumstances in favor of a midline one. This would allow the surgeon to explore the upper abdomen more thoroughly. Controversy still exists about the routine use of laparoscopy for clinical staging of cancer in patients who are suspected of harboring an ovarian malignancy.

It is with no hesitation that experienced laparoscopists recommend the routine use of laparoscopy prior to performing a laparotomy. With the exceptions noted, in which a firm diagnosis can be established by noninvasive techniques or in which the laparoscopy itself is contraindicated, this practice is often beneficial for the patient and surgeon alike. Better planning of the type of surgery and a better informed and more intelligently counseled patient are important advantages.

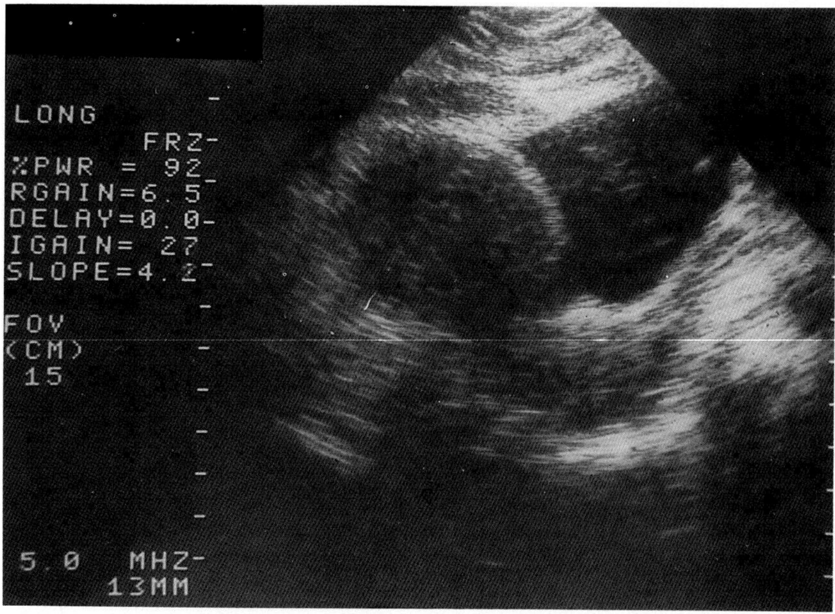

Figure 3.7 Ultrasonogram of a patient with a palpable left adnexal mass. A 4.5 × 4.5 cm mass with numerous internal echoes is seen, consistent with a benign teratoma of the ovary.

PELVIC INFECTION

The diagnosis of acute salpingitis has conventionally been based on clinical considerations. Pelvic inflammatory disease (PID) has become a catch-all term to designate the condition in women presenting with unexplained pelvic pain. It is often in error. At times, a purulent discharge lends evidence to support such a diagnosis without distinction between cervicitis, endometritis, salpingitis or salpingo-oophoritis as the source of the exudate. Once the diagnosis of PID is made, it carries other implications. A woman so stigmatized usually receives multiple antibiotic treatments without further work-up. It is not unusual to perform a major surgical procedure in these cases and find little evidence to support the presumptive preoperative diagnosis of chronic PID.

In the early 1960s, Jacobson and Westrom advocated the routine use of laparoscopy to make the diagnosis of acute pelvic inflammatory disease objectively.[8] They reported 905 laparoscopies in cases with a clinical diagnosis of acute

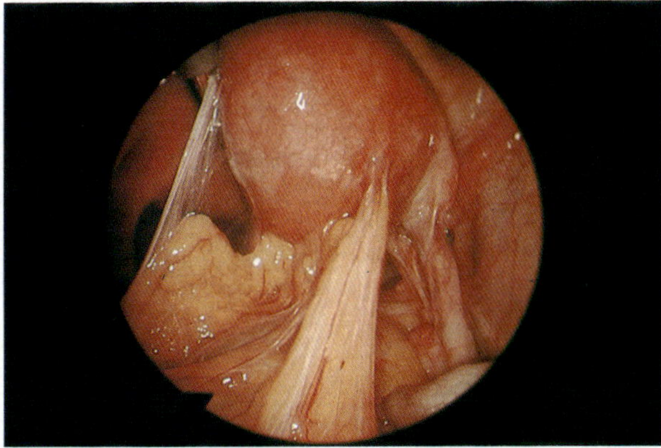

Figure 3.8 Laparoscopic evaluation of the adnexal mass diagnosed sonographically and depicted in Figure 3.7. Only multiple omental and bowel adhesions are visualized. Posterior cul-de-sac is obliterated and utero-sigmoidal adhesions are suspected. Bowel preparation prior to extensive surgical dissection is recommended.

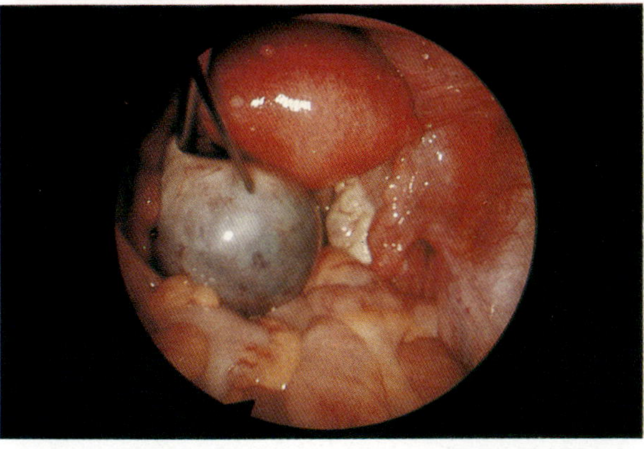

Figure 3.9 Corpus luteum cyst, left. Functional origin is confirmed by aspiration of straw colored fluid at laparoscopy.

salpingitis based on the usual signs and symptoms, including acute pelvic pain, abnormal vaginal discharge, fever, menstrual irregularities, and marked tenderness of the pelvic organs on bimanual examination. The preoperative diagnosis of PID was confirmed by laparoscopy in less than 65 percent of the cases; 23 percent of patients had normal pelvic organs without evidence of inflammation; and 12 percent had conditions unrelated to pelvic infection.

This recommendation by Jacobson and Westrom for routine use of laparoscopy in suspected cases of acute salpingitis was not widely adopted for several reasons. First, PID is a disease that mainly affects young sexually active women; therefore, no surgical intervention was deemed needed unless complications, such as pyosalpinx or tubo-ovarian abscess, arose. Second, the cause and effect relationship between acute salpingitis (even mild in nature) and infertility was not confirmed until the middle to late 1970s. Finally, gynecologic laparoscopy was not routinely practiced in the United States by gynecologists until the decade of the 1970s when it first gained popularity as an operative tool for sterilization procedures. Even then, gynecologists did not readily accept the challenge to their clinical judgement.

The current epidemic of sexually transmitted diseases has been paralleled by a concomitant increase of acute salpingitis. Even mild degrees of tubal infection may affect the future fertility potential in these patients by the formation of pelvic adhesions and tubal obstruction.[3] An accurate early diagnosis would assure timely therapy to prevent residual sequelae (Figure 3.10).

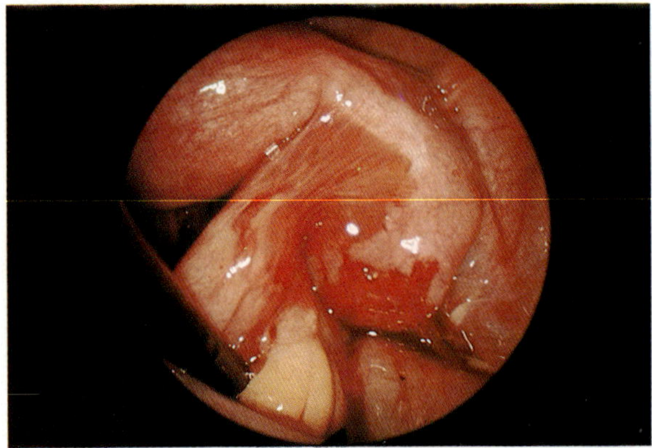

Figure 3.10 Acute salpingitis, right. Bowel and omentum are adherent to the infected tube, representing the early walling off process. Note the edema and hyperemia of the tissues.

Appropriate treatment of acute salpingitis requires not only confirmation of the clinical diagnosis but also the microbiologic identification of the offending organism. Attempts to obtain peritoneal fluid for bacteriologic study by culdocentesis have not proved to be satisfactorily accurate. Laparoscopy has been suggested as the most reliable method to make a correct diagnosis as well as to facilitate the process of sampling material for bacteriologic culture. Sweet compared laparoscopically obtained specimens (tubal and peritoneal fluid) with peritoneal fluid obtained via culdocentesis in patients with acute salpingitis.[17] He concluded that direct culture from the fallopian tubes may be necessary to determine the microbiologic etiology and pathogenesis of acute salpingitis.[18]

Laparoscopy also allows one to obtain an uncontaminated specimen for evaluation. This is essential for the culture to reflect accurately what is occurring in and around the fallopian tubes. It also provides the ideal method of fluid collection for anaerobic cultures and serologic studies (Figure 3.11).

When laparoscopy is used for evaluation and/or follow-up of patients with pelvic infection, it should also include the evaluation of the entire abdominal cavity. Acute appendicitis as the primary source of a pelvic infectious process must be excluded. Lymphatic reabsorption of intraperitoneal exudate occurs mainly in the right subphrenic region. The observation of perihepatic adhesions suggests that the pelvic process is of a recurrent nature rather than a primary

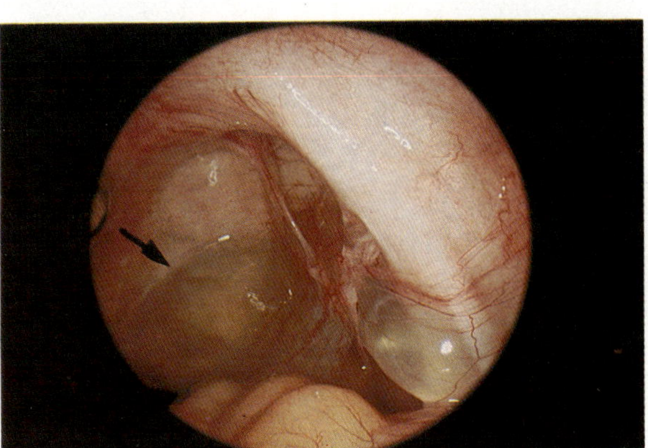

Figure 3.11 Fluid for bacteriologic evaluation can be obtained in a woman with pelvic inflammatory disease without contamination at the time of laparoscopy. Needle aspiration is used to collect a sample from an area of loculated fluid accumulation (arrow).

one. Visualization of the upper abdomen may also demonstrate the subdiaphragmatic adhesions characteristic of the Fitz-Hugh-Curtis syndrome (Figures 3.12 and 3.13). Semchyshyn reviewed 124 patients treated for pelvic inflammatory disease.[16] In 15 cases, Fitz-Hugh-Curtis syndrome was suspected clinically (right upper quadrant pain in conjunction with abdominal pain, fever, chills and tender adnexa). In 14 of these patients, perihepatic adhesions were confirmed during gynecologic surgery.

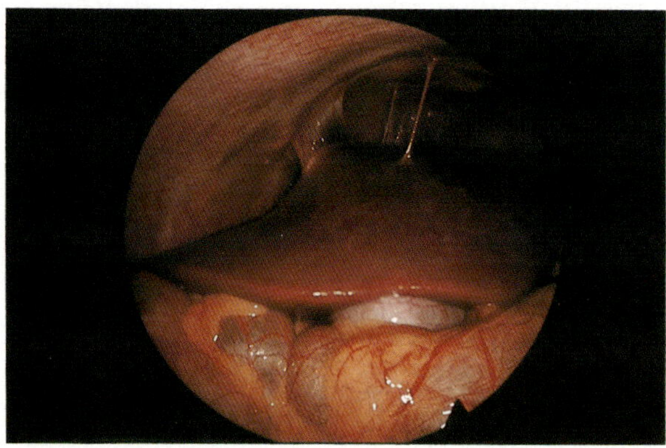

Figure 3.12 Subdiaphragmatic perihepatic adhesions characteristic of the Fitz-Hugh-Curtis syndrome. When these adhesions are present, a recurrent infectious process is more likely than a primary acute one.

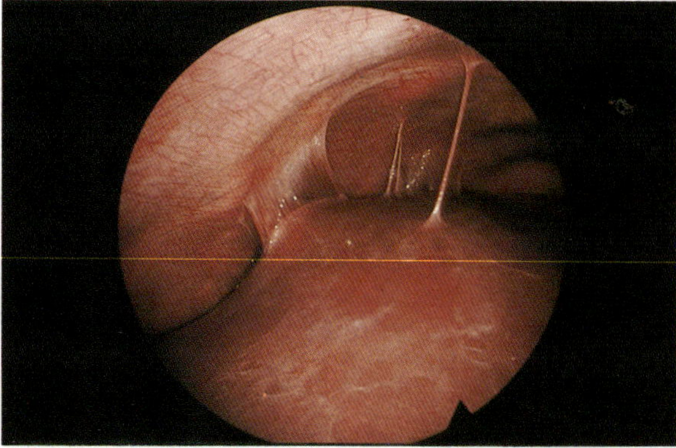

Figure 3.13 Thick fibrotic band between the liver capsule and the undersurface of the diaphragm. Tension and distortion of the liver capsule may be the cause of right upper quadrant abdominal pain.

ECTOPIC PREGNANCY

In the past, the diagnosis of ectopic pregnancy was usually made at a late stage after the development of serious symptoms. Severe abdominopelvic pain, hypotension, and shoulder pain were common signs pointing toward the diagnosis. Ectopic pregnancy still remains the leading cause of maternal death. In the past, early diagnosis was limited to cases in which the surgeon had a high degree of suspicion because the patient presented with a history of amenorrhea, unilateral pelvic pain and adnexal mass. Even then, the diagnosis was usually made only after a catastrophic event, such as tubal rupture, had occurred. The condition was already so advanced that salvaging the affected fallopian tube was not feasible.

The poor results of late care made early diagnosis an important objective. The practice of intervening at the earliest possible stage prompted many surgeons to perform superfluous exploratory laparotomy in undiagnosed cases. Since many other gynecologic conditions mimic the symptom pattern of ectopic pregnancy, it was not unusual for unnecessary major surgical procedures to be performed. Advent of the very sensitive and specific radioimmunoassay technique of measuring the beta-subunit of human chorionic gonadotropin (hCG) made it possible to diagnose pregnancy at a very early stage. While identifying the presence of hCG at very low levels in the serum, this test left the location of its source unknown. Low serum levels suggested abnormal implantation, but it was found that more than half the tubal pregnancies will produce normal amounts of hCG until the time they rupture through the site of implantation.

Attempts to diagnose tubal gestation by direct endoscopic visualization of the pelvis were first made transvaginally through the posterior fornix (culdoscopy). Mastery of this technique required extensive training and it did not become popular in the United States. Acceptability was minimized by the need to place the patient in the genupectoral (knee-chest) position, thus increasing her discomfort. Administration of a general anesthesia was another limiting factor. Although the technique of laparoscopy dates back to the early 1900s, it was not until the popularization of translaparoscopic sterilization that it became an integral part of the gynecologist's armamentarium. At the present time, one of the main indications for laparoscopy is exclusion of an ectopic pregnancy. Positive identification of eccyesis at an early stage not only prevents later occurrence of catastrophic events, but it also allows one the opportunity to preserve the affected tube. Details of translaparoscopic treatment of ectopic pregnancy will be discussed in the chapter on operative laparoscopy (see Chapter 4).

At the present time, in the absence of signs of an acute surgical abdomen, one cannot justify undertaking an exploratory laparotomy to rule out an ectopic pregnancy. Laparoscopy is able to confirm or rule out an extrauterine gestation reliably in most instances (Figures 3.14 to 3.17). If there are contraindications to the use of the closed technique, open laparoscopy with a small-to-moderate pneumoperitoneum is usually sufficient to establish the correct diagnosis and completely eliminate unnecessary major surgery.

Recent improvements in diagnostic pelvic ultrasonography allow the identification of an intrauterine gestation (amniotic sac ring) as early as 5 to 6 weeks from the last menstrual period. The rarity of concurrent intrauterine and ectop-

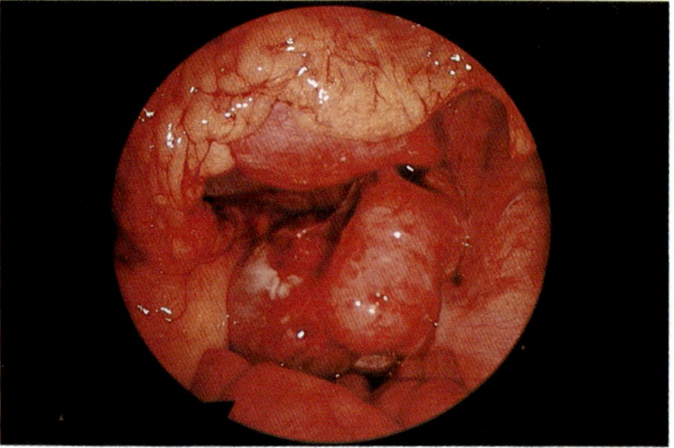

Figure 3.14 Advanced ectopic pregnancy (9½ weeks from last menstrual period), right tube. Peritubal adhesions are the result of a previously confirmed history of recurrent pelvic inflammatory disease. Left fallopian tube is absent having been surgically removed for a prior ectopic pregnancy.

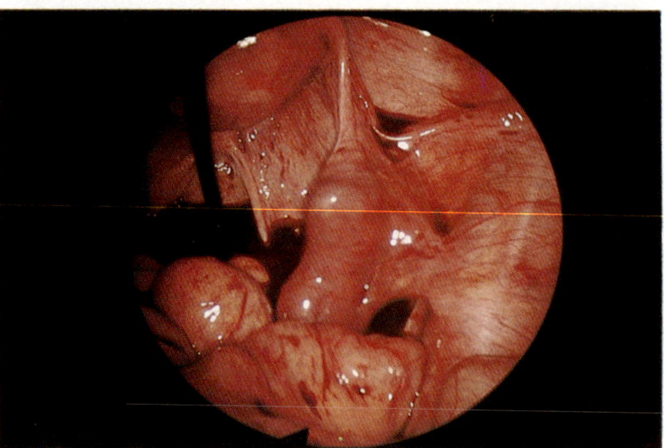

Figure 3.15 Ectopic pregnancy, right, with hemoperitoneum resulting from transfimbrial bleeding. At laparotomy, a segmental resection was performed. Tubal reanastomosis could be attempted in the future, if necessary.

ic gestation (1 in 10,000 cases of ectopic pregnancy) makes this combined condition very unlikely. Thus, the sonographic appearance of a well-defined intrauterine gestational sac makes it unnecessary to do a laparoscopy to exclude an ectopic gestation. This is extremely important in women who wish to preserve their pregnancy (if it is implanted in the uterus), particularly since the teratogenic effects of a general anesthesia at such an early stage of gestation are essentially unknown at present.

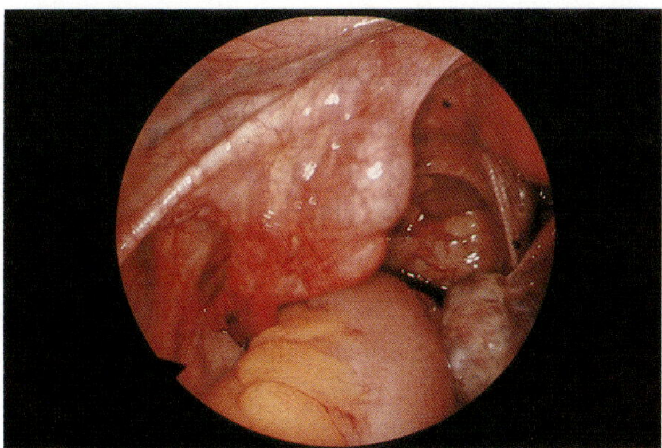

Figure 3.16 Ectopic pregnancy, left, early (6 weeks from last menstrual period) and unruptured. Diagnosis at this stage makes salpingotomy more feasible.

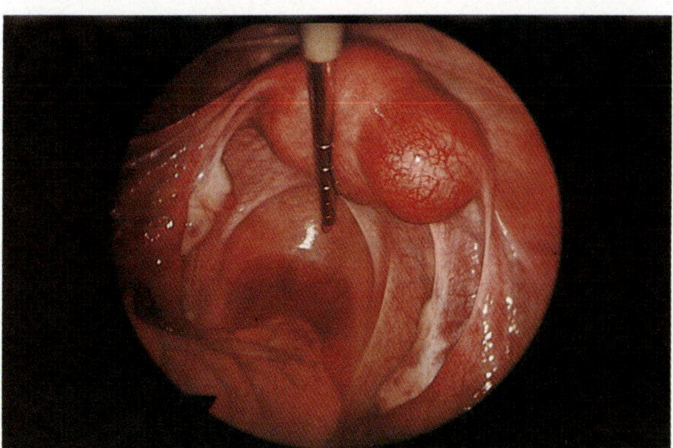

Figure 3.17 Cornual pregnancy, unruptured, right. No ultrasonographic evidence of an intrauterine gestation in a patient with high values of circulating human chorionic gonadotropin prompted the diagnostic laparoscopy. Early diagnosis is desired because of the characteristic premature rupture of this type of eccyesis.

Thus, the prerequisites for a laparoscopy to rule out ectopic gestation must include a positive pregnancy test (serum or urine) and the absence of an intrauterine gestation by sonogram (Figure 3.18). The appropriate time to perform the laparoscopic evaluation depends on the patient's symptoms. Caution should be exercised not to undertake diagnostic laparoscopy too early in the pregnancy because one then risks missing an eccyesis because the tube may not yet be sufficiently distended for it to be recognized. Tubal distortion is usually evident in gestations of more than 6 weeks' duration from the last menstrual period.

LAPAROSCOPY IN INFERTILITY

Evaluation, management, and follow-up of the infertile woman is perhaps the most common use for diagnostic laparoscopy at present. At first, it was used to assess peritubal and periovarian adhesions. It has since grown in use to become an indispensable tool for the infertility specialist. In this section, our discussion is limited to the diagnostic use of laparoscopy in the infertile population, whereas translaparoscopic surgical procedures are detailed in the section on operative laparoscopy.

Timing of the laparoscopic evaluation of an infertile woman remains controversial.[12] Those who advocate performing it during the proliferative phase of the cycle claim that the risk of pregnancy is nonexistent and the size of the tubal lumen maximal because it is not reduced by secretory changes affecting the mucosa. Additionally, when dilation and curettage for evaluation of uter-

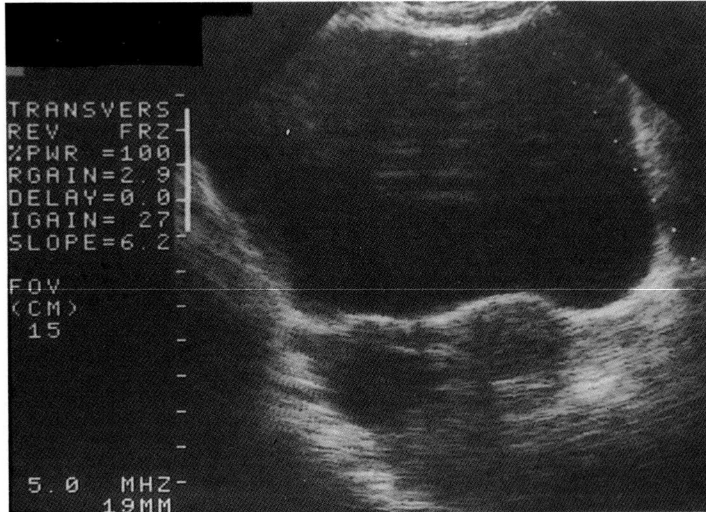

Figure 3.18 Ultrasonogram of a patient who was later found to have a right ectopic pregnancy. Although the extrauterine site cannot be seen, absence of an intrauterine gestational sac in conjunction with a positive pregnancy test is highly suggestive of ectopic pregnancy, warranting diagnostic laparoscopy.

ine factors is required, the first half of the cycle is the appropriate time. To the contrary, those preferring laparoscopy during the secretory phase maintain that they are able to evaluate the adequacy of the corpus luteum function better by visualizing the ovarian stigma at the corpus hemorrhagicum, confirming that ovulation has occurred.

With rapidly growing experience, newer indications for the use of laparoscopy in infertility are continuously being added to those currently accepted. At present, they include evaluation of tubal patency, external anatomic configuration of the fallopian tubes, tubo-ovarian spatial relationship, ovarian morphology, normality of ovarian function (corpus luteum), integrity of the posterior cul-de-sac, and the presence of endometriosis, genital tract anomalies, and salpingitis; it is also used for second-look postoperative follow-up.

Tubal Patency. Hysterosalpingography (HSG) remains the primary diagnostic procedure for evaluating tubal patency in the initial stages of the infertility work-up. Nevertheless, there are instances in which failure to show free spillage of the contrast material into the peritoneal cavity gives a false impression of obstruction.[6] This finding is not always a sign of tubal occlusion. It may be caused by cornual spasm of unknown etiology. Apparent unilateral tubal occlusion, based on failure of dye to pass, can also result from the escape of dye via the path of least resistance, namely the contralateral open tube.

Direct translaparoscopic visualization of the perfusion of indigo carmine solution overcomes the aforementioned problems. Evaluation of the quality of dye spillage at the fimbrial end (free flow, slow drip) may reveal degrees of fimbrial phimosis or obstruction (Figures 3.19 and 3.20). In other cases, laparosco-

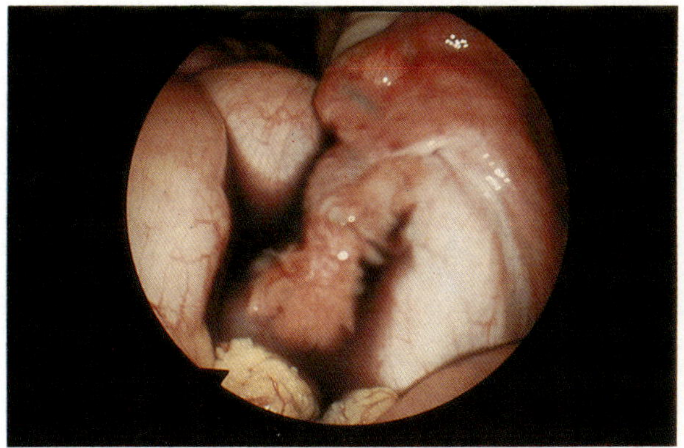

Figure 3.19 Dye spillage at the fimbrial end confirms tubal patency. Free flow of indigo carmine is seen from the right fimbria.

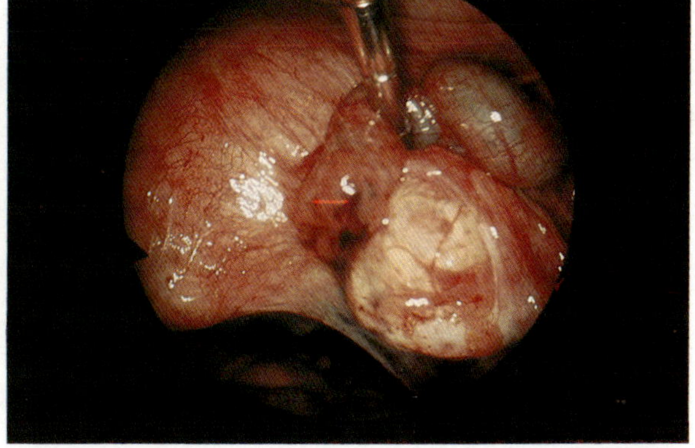

Figure 3.20 Small amount of indigo carmine is seen spilling from the fimbrial end of the left tube. Prefimbrial tubal obstruction (fimbrial phimosis) is the most likely cause. Tubal distention is seen proximal to the site of obstruction at the right of the metal probe.

py may demonstrate that cornual obstruction demonstrated by HSG is actually only distal tubal obstruction (Figure 3.21). Knowledge of such conditions is essential to help plan the surgical procedure adequately and counsel the patient appropriately.

External Anatomic Configuration. Evaluation of the configuration of the fallopian tubes is an integral component of the basic infertility work-up. Distortion of the normal contour by external compression (by a cornual or intraligamentous fibroid, for example) is not readily diagnosed except by direct endoscopic visualization (Figure 3.22). The isthmic portion of the tube can be evaluated for the characteristic nodularity found in salpingitis isthmica nodosa.

In patients presenting with true cornual or midtubal blockage, laparoscopic evaluation of the distal portion of the tube is essential. Success of the surgical repair depends heavily on the normal configuration of the remaining portion of the tube (Figure 3.23). The fimbrial end can be effectively evaluated by means of laparoscopy.

Recent advances in gynecologic microsurgical techniques have improved the success rate of tubal reanastomosis procedures. Fertilization following the reanastomosis depends not only on adequate tubal patency but on the normal function of the reconstructed tube. Normality of tubal function is directly related to the length of the tube. Preoperative evaluation of the remaining unaffected segments of the fallopian tubes is imperative before a major microsurgical procedure is undertaken (Figure 3.24).

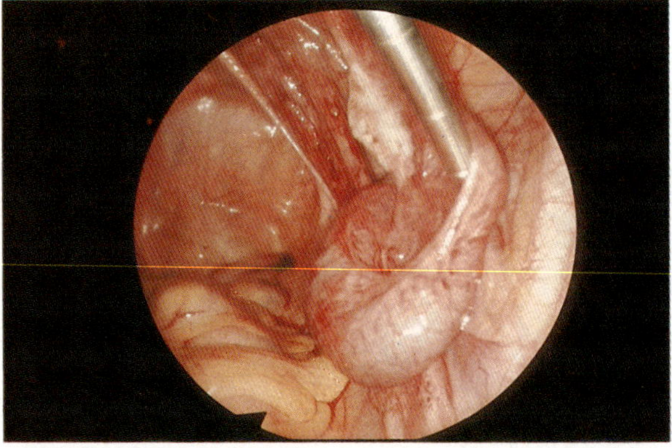

Figure 3.21 Indigo carmine fills the entire length of the right fallopian tube but no dye spills from the fimbrial end. This confirms that the tubal obstruction is fimbrial rather than cornual as reported by the hysterosalpingogram in this case.

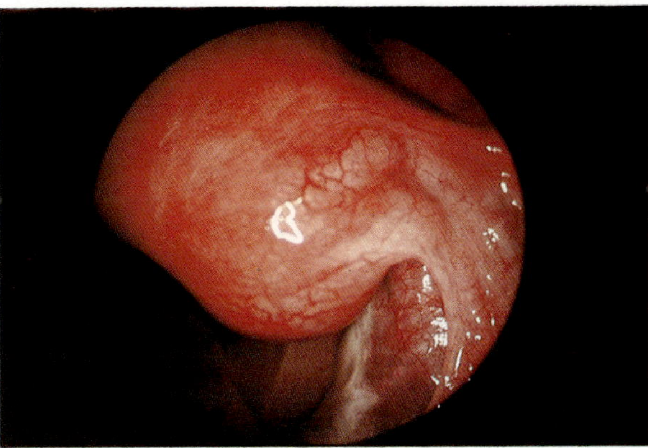

Figure 3.22 Right cornual fibromyoma distorts proximal third of the fallopian tube. Tubal reimplantation may be required following myomectomy.

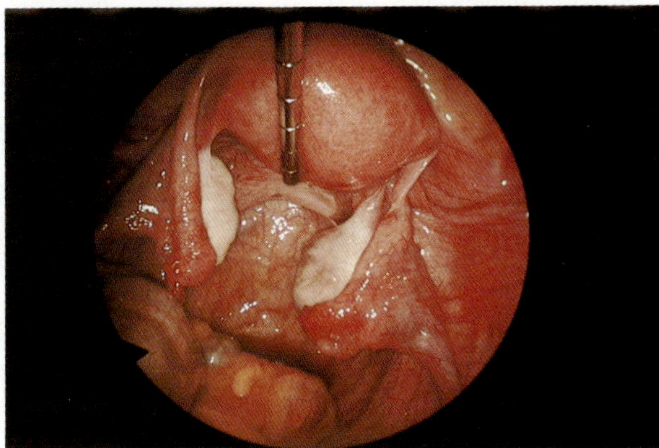

Figure 3.23 Bilateral cornual obstruction. The external appearance of the distal portion of both fallopian tubes is normal.

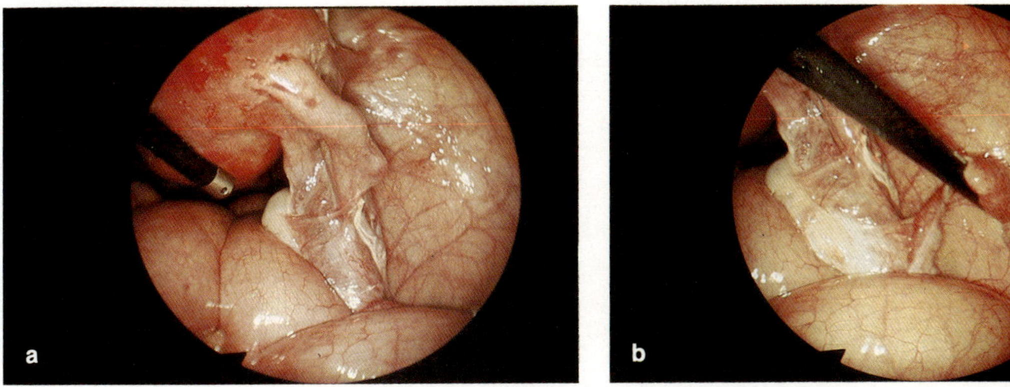

Figure 3.24 Laparoscopic evaluation for tubal reanastomosis following a sterilization procedure. *a.* Proximal remnant of right fallopian tube measures 3 cm in length; this should prove adequate for attempted reanastomosis. *b.* Distal segment (fimbrial) of right tube is less than 2 cm in length; the large lumen and inadequate extent of this segment makes reanastomosis suboptimal.

Tubo-Ovarian Spatial Relationship. At the time of ovulation, the fimbrial end of the tube normally apposes the follicular pole of the ovary to accomplish ovum pickup. It has been suggested that ovum pickup by the fimbria may also occur from the posterior cul-de-sac. In order for the tube to be able to function in this way, there must be a normal tubo-ovarian spatial relationship. Direct laparoscopic visualization of the adnexal areas provides an accurate evaluation of the fimbria ovarica, its relationship with the ipsilateral ovary, and its mobility (Figures 3.25 to 3.27). Factors limiting tubal mobility and/or free access of the fimbria to the expelled ovum may underlie the infertility condition. Preoperative evaluation by means of laparoscopy is important in this regard since it helps the surgeon plan the appropriate therapeutic modality to be used.

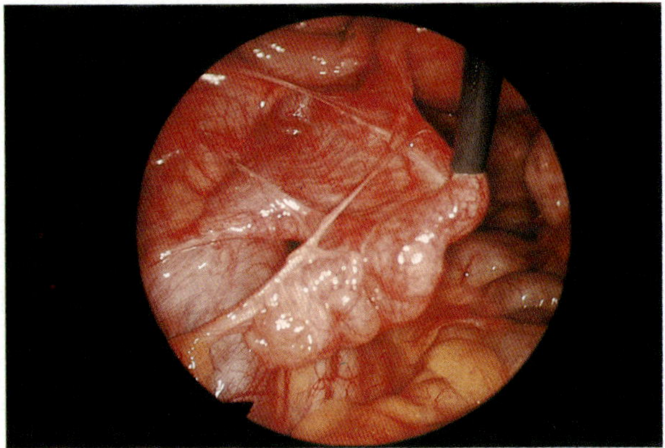

Figure 3.25 Multiple peritubal adhesions to the left fallopian tube. Ancillary cannula is displacing the uterus forward. Adhesions between the left isthmic, ampullary, and fimbrial portion of the tube and the lateral pelvic wall maintain the tube fixed in an extended position away from the ipsilateral ovary. This precludes normal ovum pickup.

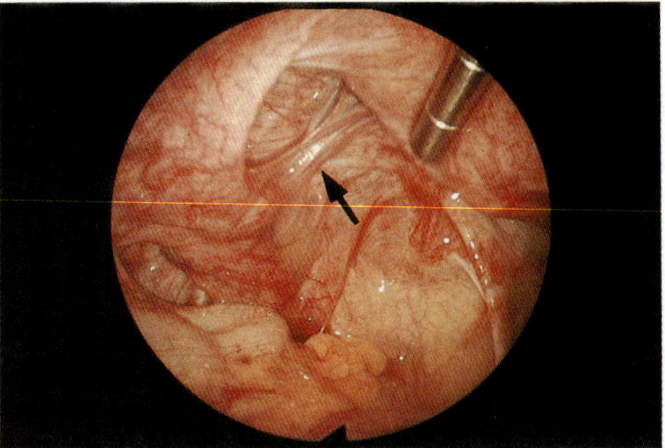

Figure 3.26 Tubo-uterine adhesion. Filmy adhesion (arrow) inhibits free mobility of the tubal fimbria required for ovum pickup. In this case, the adhesion also covered the fimbrial end adding an obstructive barrier to the already abnormal tubal function.

Ovarian Morphology. Objective evaluation of the external morphologic aspects of the ovaries obtained at the time of laparoscopy yields important information. Overall size of the ovaries, appearance of their external capsule, and correlation with the stage of the menstrual cycle at the time the procedure is being performed may prove essential diagnostic information. A laparoscopic evaluation that does not provide a detailed description of the ovarian morphology must be considered incomplete.

One can accurately measure the size of the ovaries by means of a graduated probe introduced by way of a second puncture (Figure 3.28). Small ovaries (less than 2 cm in largest diameter) in women of reproductive age should raise the suspicion of dysfunction or premature menopause. In contrast, large ovaries

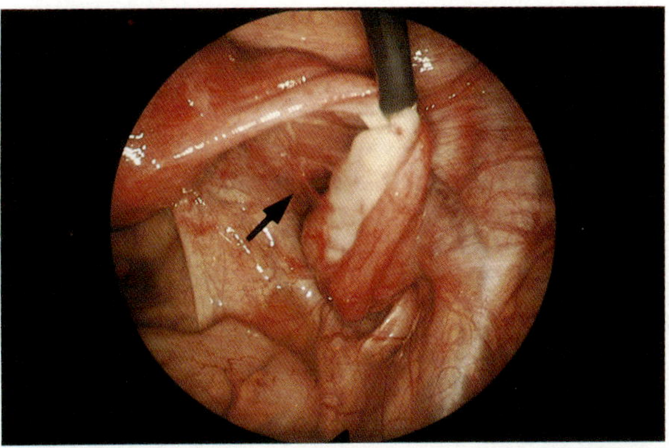

Figure 3.27 Utero-ovarian adhesion. Filmy adhesion between the ovary and the posterior wall of the uterus keeps the ovary in a fixed position. Distal pole of the ovary is covered by an adhesion also precluding normal fimbrio-ovarian apposition.

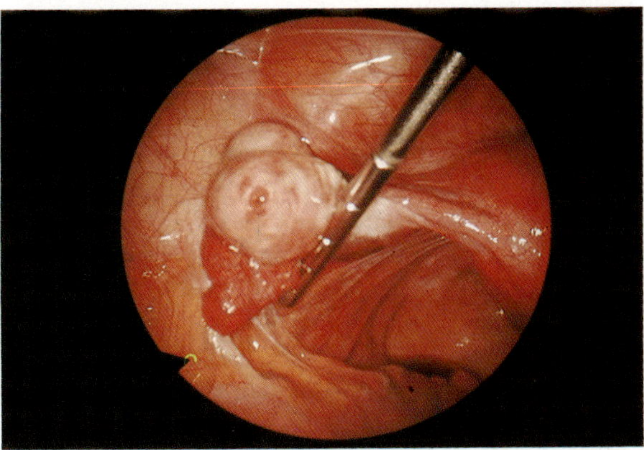

Figure 3.28 Graduated solid metal probe enables the operator to measure any abdomino-pelvic mass accurately. This slightly enlarged luteal phase ovary measured 5 × 4 × 4 cm in size.

(more than 4 cm in largest dimension) in a postmenopausal patient should prompt a more in-depth evaluation to rule out the possibility of a malignancy (Figure 3.29). Delicate elongated ovaries, fibrotic in appearance, are characteristic of streak ovaries. This entity may or may not be accompanied by concurrent congenital genitourinary abnormalities.

Serious ovulation disorders may be associated with ovaries that appear normal. Nevertheless, it is not unusual to find characteristic abnormalities of the ovarian capsule in the course of the evaluation of an infertile woman. Large, smooth, pearly-white multicystic ovaries are pathognomonic of the Stein-Leventhal syndrome (Figure 3.30). Similarly, small ovaries with a thickened capsule may also be encountered in women with the polycystic ovarian syndrome.

Anovulation may be strongly suspected if a laparoscopy performed during the proliferative phase fails to identify follicular enlargement with thinning of the ovarian capsule. This diagnosis is likely if there is no corpus luteum found

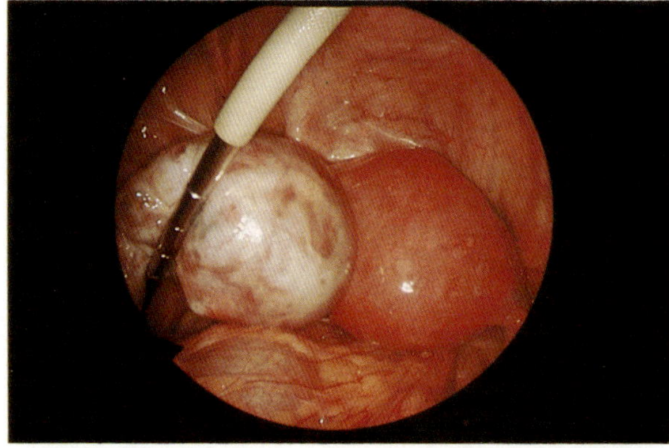

Figure 3.29 Ovarian enlargement in a perimenopausal woman. Smooth capsule without adhesions to any adjacent organ suggested a benign condition. Pathological evaluation of the specimen obtained at laparotomy showed it to be a benign corpus luteum cyst.

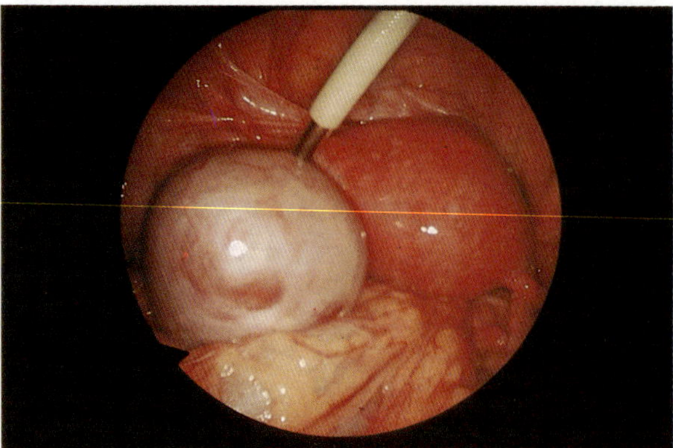

Figure 3.30 Multicystic ovary, left. Laparoscopy offers confirmatory evidence of polycystic ovary syndrome diagnosed by hormone assay. The ovary is 1.5 times the size of the uterine corpus and characteristically smooth and pearly white.

at a laparoscopy performed during the secretory phase of the cycle. Morphologic evaluation of the ovaries should not be limited to laparoscopies performed for infertility. Incidental findings of dysmorphic ovaries are always important laparoscopic observations (Figure 3.31).

Ovarian Function. Elevation of basal body temperature in the second half of the menstrual cycle and biopsy identification of secretory endometrium are evidence of progesterone secretion by the ovary. Until recently, endogenous production of progesterone was considered proof that ovulation had occurred. In 1970, Jones et al described the luteinized unruptured follicle (LUF) as a frequent cause of infertility.[9] The luteinized follicle is believed to contain the entrapped ovum, even though it secretes progesterone.

The site of ovulation usually leaves an opening on the corpus hemorrhagicum called the stigma of ovulation (Figure 3.32). Failure to identify the stigma laparoscopically was considered diagnostic of LUF. More recent studies showed

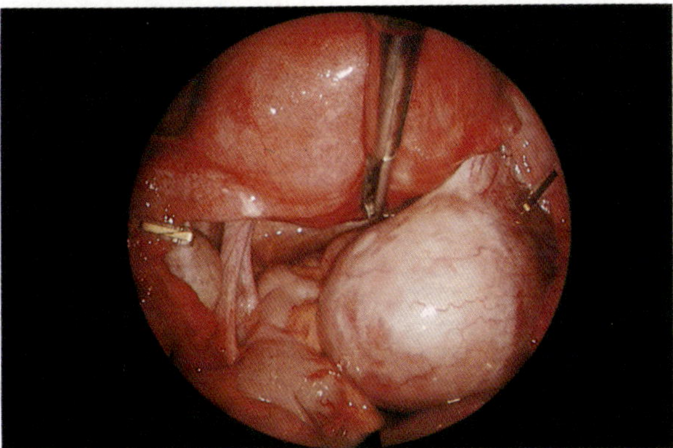

Figure 3.31 Right ovarian cyst encountered incidentally at the time of a sterilization procedure. Hormonal suppression therapy caused it to regress, confirming its benign nature (corpus luteum cyst).

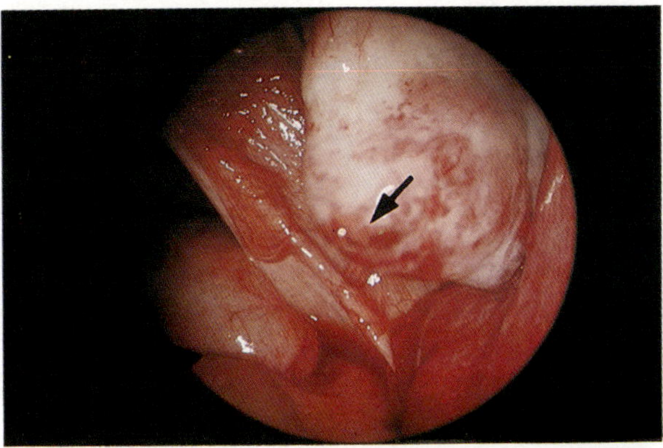

Figure 3.32 Stigma of ovulation, showing site of ovulation (arrow) as seen within 72 to 96 hours following oocyte expulsion.

that the presence of the ovulatory stigma is related to the timing of the laparoscopy. Reepithelialization of the follicular opening may occur as early as 4 to 5 days following ovulation (Figure 3.33). One would have to perform a laparoscopy within the first 3 days after ovulation to establish the presence of the stigma. This precludes the concomitant use of dye pertubation to check for tubal patency because it may wash out an intratubal fertilized ovum.

Posterior Cul-de-Sac. Integrity of the pouch of Douglas is believed to be an important factor in fertility. Albeit unconfirmed, the posterior cul-de-sac is thought by some to be the primary site of ovum pickup by the fallopian tube. Evidence to support this contention is found in the recovery of unfertilized ova by translaparoscopic aspiration of cul-de-sac fluid. It is essential, therefore, that a thorough evaluation of the pouch of Douglas be part of the laparoscopic evaluation for infertility (Figures 3.34 and 3.35).

Because it is the most caudal point of the peritoneal cavity, any fluid or secretion within the peritoneal cavity tends to accumulate in the posterior cul-de-sac. Clear peritoneal fluid, blood, fibrinous and/or purulent secretions can

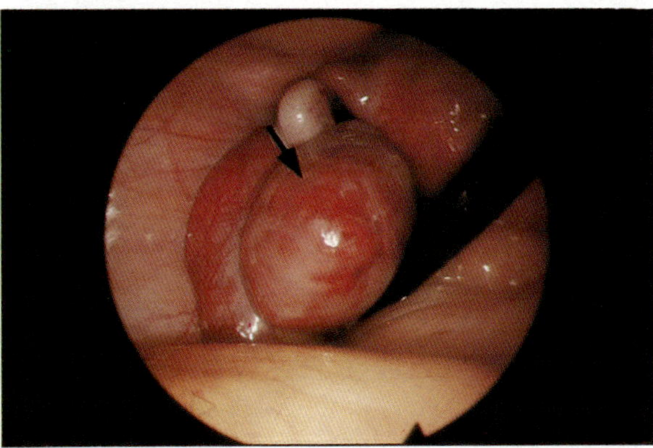

Figure 3.33 Corpus luteum one week following ovulation. No evidence of the stigma of ovulation is seen at the probable site of oocyte expulsion (arrow). Complete reepithelialization may occur as early as 4 to 5 days following ovulation.

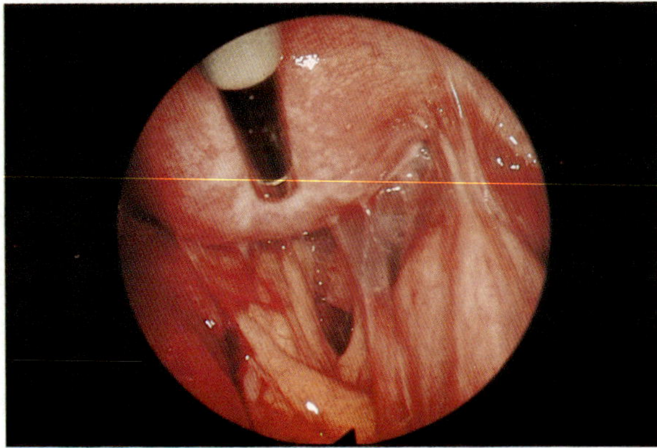

Figure 3.34 Sigmoid-uterine and small bowel-to-uterus adhesions obliterate the pouch of Douglas. Integrity of the posterior cul-de-sac is believed to be required for ovum pickup by the fallopian tube.

be encountered in the pouch of Douglas. Aspiration for evaluation by Gram stain and appropriate culture aids in the identification of the nature of the fluid found (Figure 3.36).

Endometriosis. The increased incidence of endometriosis in an infertile population strongly suggests a cause and effect relationship. Lack of correlation between the degree of endometriosis and the severity of the associated infertility underlies the controversy surrounding the choice of appropriate mode of therapy for endometriosis. Notwithstanding the discrepant opinions concerning treatment, it is universally agreed that verification of the existence of ectopic endometrial implants is critical before any form of treatment is begun. Recently, the American Fertility Society adopted a staging classification of endometriosis based on the evaluation of size and location of the endometriotic lesions.[20] The presence of adhesions increases the severity of the process.

Before the advent of laparoscopy in modern gynecology, endometriosis was usually diagnosed at the time of laparotomy. Consequently, unless considered inoperable, the treatment consisted of surgical excision and/or electrofulguration. The use of diagnostic laparoscopy to confirm the presence of the disease with simultaneous staging of the severity has changed this considerably. It has allowed implementation of regimens consisting of medical treatment alone. Additionally, it offers the possibility of combining medical and surgical forms of treatment. For example, danocrine or oral contraceptives can be given for various lengths of time prior to surgery. Presurgical management may help reduce the severity of the disease as well as technically facilitate surgical extirpation.

When endometriosis is found at the time of a diagnostic laparoscopy, one should follow a methodical evaluation program. A second auxiliary puncture is indicated to allow mobilization of the abdominopelvic structures. Fluid or

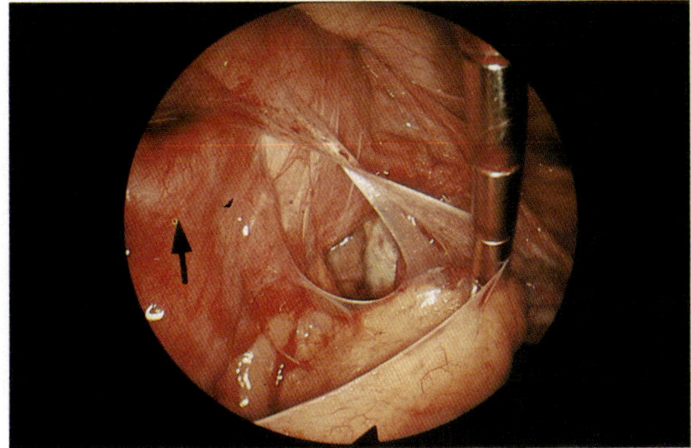

Figure 3.35 Multiple adhesions distort the configuration of the posterior cul-de-sac. A normal ovary can be seen below the adhesions. Obliteration of the pouch of Douglas is usually the consequence of recurrent inflammatory disease. Left pyosalpinx is seen (arrow) adherent to the uterine fundus.

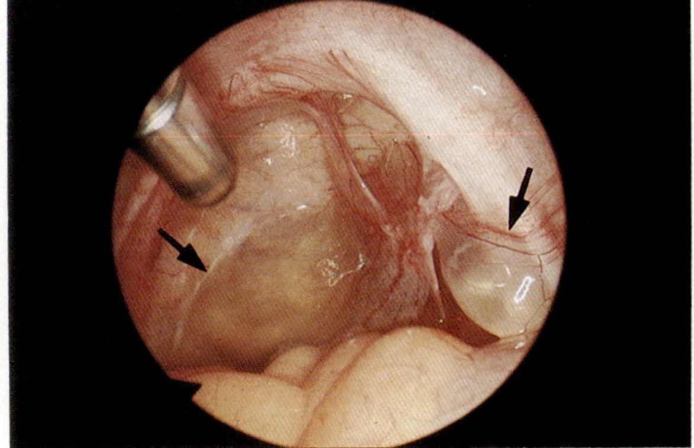

Figure 3.36 Accumulation of fibrinous material in the posterior cul-de-sac is not unusual in association with pelvic infections. Aspiration for evaluation by Gram stain and appropriate culture will aid in identifying the nature of the fluid.

blood accumulated in the posterior cul-de-sac ought to be aspirated using a hollow aspiration cannula through the accessory puncture sleeve (Figures 3.37). Transcervical pertubation with dye solutions (methylene blue or indigo carmine) should be left as the last step in the diagnostic laparoscopy. Although probably innocuous, large amounts of dye solution accumulating in the pouch of Douglas are best evacuated by aspiration. The use of a probe introduced through the accessory puncture allows the laparoscopist to mobilize the ovaries so as to visualize their undersurface. Fixation of the ovaries to the posterior surface of the broad ligament by small endometriotic foci is not unusual.

Even though endometriosis is more often found in the most dependent areas of the pelvis (pouch of Douglas, uterosacral ligaments) than elsewhere, this distribution does not preclude its concomitant presence in other areas. The anterior cul-de-sac is also a common site of endometriotic implants. When endometriosis is found in scattered foci seeding the peritoneal surface, it is important to evaluate all its locations with respect to possible impact on important abdominopelvic structures (e.g., ureter, iliac artery and vein) (Figures 3.38 to 3.43).

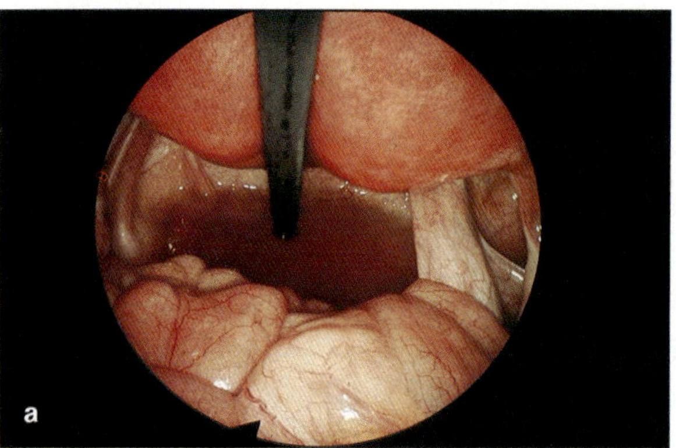

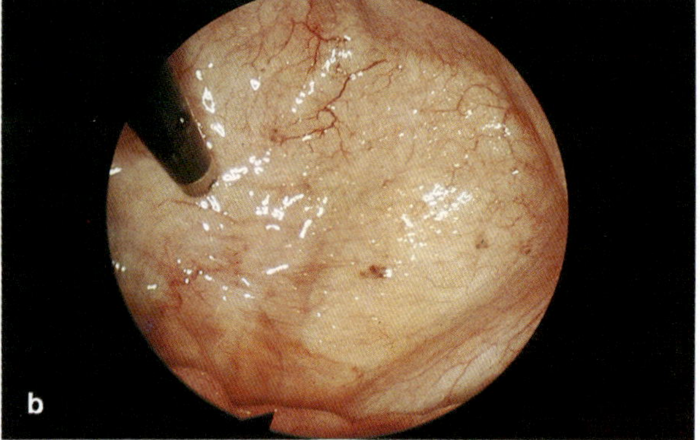

Figure 3.37 Aspiration of cul-de-sac fluid. Fluid or blood accumulated in the pouch of Douglas should always be removed by means of a hollow cannula. *a*. 50 cc of blood-tinged peritoneal fluid is seen in the posterior cul-de-sac. No clear evidence of pelvic disease can be discerned. *b*. Following aspiration of the fluid, endometriotic implants are revealed.

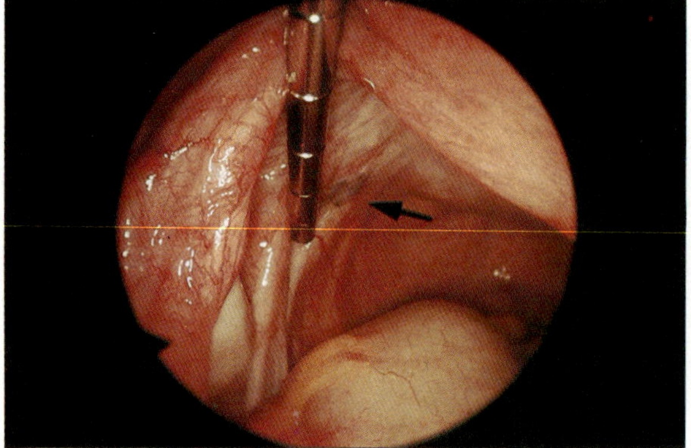

Figure 3.38 Endometriotic foci on the left uterosacral ligament. Their proximity to the left ureter interdicts any attempt to treat this condition translaparoscopically.

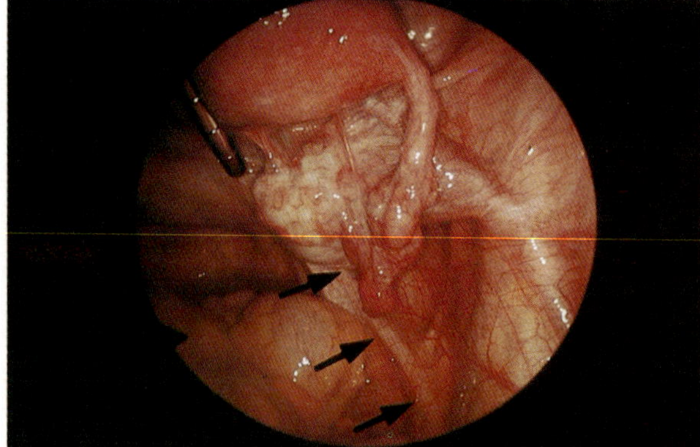

Figure 3.39 Follow-up diagnostic laparoscopy after extensive surgery for pelvic endometriosis. Persistent utero-ovarian and tubo-ovarian adhesions are seen. The course of the right ureter is seen (arrows). Laparoscopy proves helpful in planning future therapy for such cases.

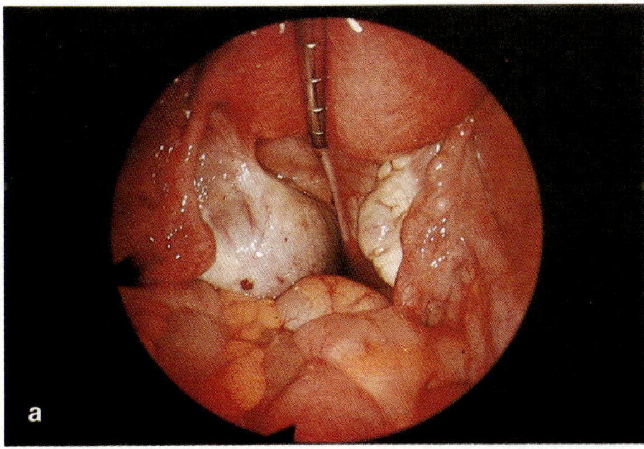

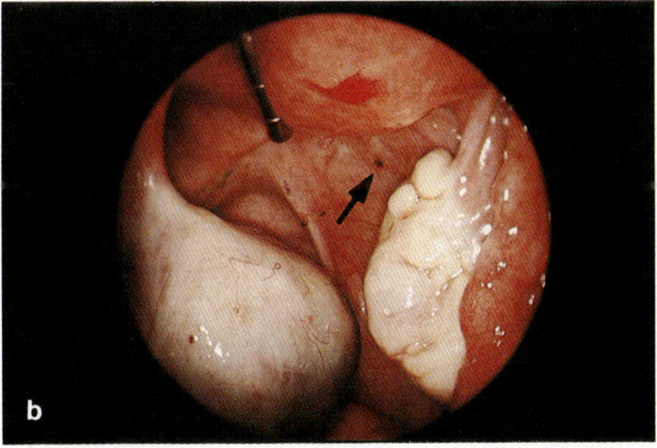

Figure 3.40 Aspiration of peritoneal fluid to disclose disease. *a*. Left ovarian cyst and bloody-tinged fluid obstruct the view of the posterior cul-de sac. *b*. Following aspiration of the peritoneal fluid and mobilization of the left ovarian cyst, multiple endometriotic implants can be seen seeding both uterosacral ligaments. One focus of endometriosis is located at the site where the right ureter crosses the uterine artery (arrow). This is not amenable to translaparoscopic destruction by fulguration.

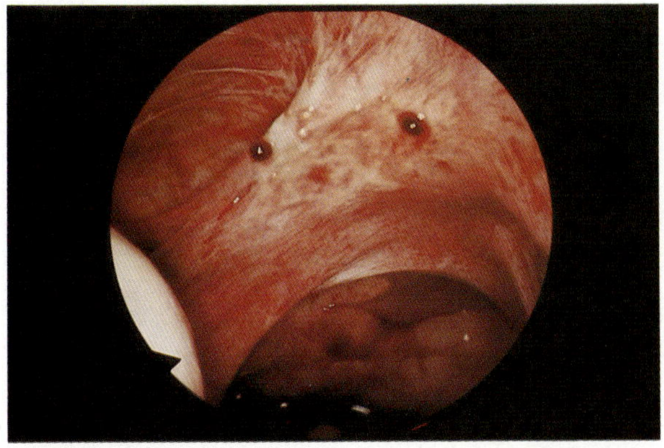

Figure 3.41 Endometriotic implants on the left utero-ovarian ligament and posterior uterine wall serosa. Translaparoscopic fulguration is feasible and appropriate for this type of lesion.

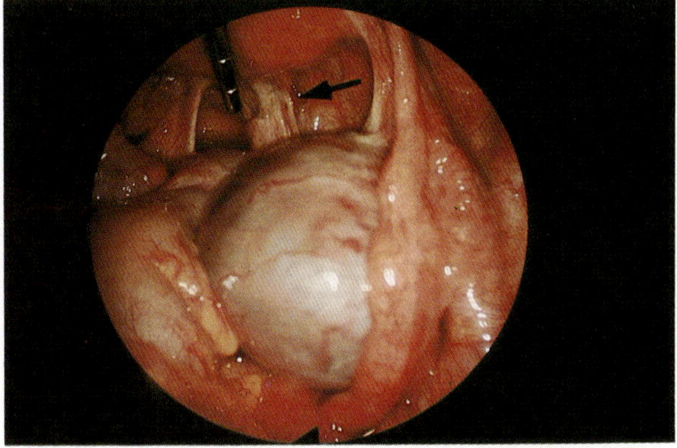

Figure 3.42 Endometrioma on the right ovary. Fibrotic right uterosacral ligament can also be seen (arrow) indicating long-standing pelvic endometriosis.

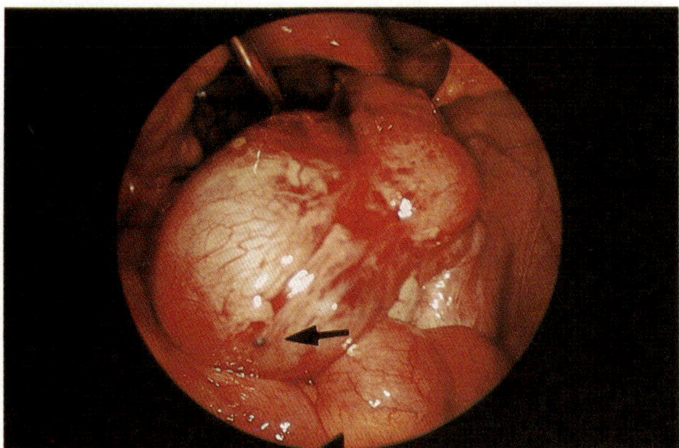

Figure 3.43 Endometriotic implant on the right ovary (arrow). This was an incidental finding during a diagnostic laparoscopy in a woman with known tubal disease. Right pyosalpinx is seen overlying the enlarged right ovary.

Endometriotic implants on the serosa of the bowel are usually incidental findings. While the entire length of the bowel cannot be visualized by laparoscopy, a panoramic view of the abdominal contents often reveals the obvious implants. The status of the appendix and mesoappendix should be evaluated since it is not unusual for endometriosis to involve this area.

Genital Tract Anomalies. Laparoscopy can be used for evaluation of congenital anomalies of the reproductive system to confirm a presumptive diagnosis. Normal tubes and ovaries may be seen accompanying an hypoplastic uterus in patients with Rokitansky-Küster-Hauser syndrome (congenital absence of vagina). Streak ovaries are identifiable in patients with Turner syndrome. Because urinary tract and genital anomalies often coexist, endoscopic evaluation of the female reproductive organs should be made whenever an anomaly of the urinary tract is found (such as double ureter or unilateral renal agenesis).

Laparoscopy is considered essential in patients who are suspected of having a congenital reproductive abnormality before a therapeutic plan is established. In cases in which a septate uterus is identified by hysterosalpingography, only laparoscopy can differentiate between a simple intrauterine septum and a bicornuate or didelphic uterus. The surgical method chosen for correction may vary accordingly.

Salpingitis. Infection or inflammation of the fallopian tubes with subsequent healing is a source of tubal obstruction, peritubal adhesions, and intraluminal anatomic distortion (Figures 3.44 to 3.49). The last is considered a major cause of reproductive wastage because it may cause ectopic pregnancy.

Salpingitis in its acute or chronic phases can be limited to the fallopian tubes, and gives rise to minimal overt manifestations. Rosenfeld et al reported that less than 25 percent of patients with laparoscopically confirmed hydrosalpinx had a prior history of acute pelvic inflammatory disease and/or pelvic pain.[15]

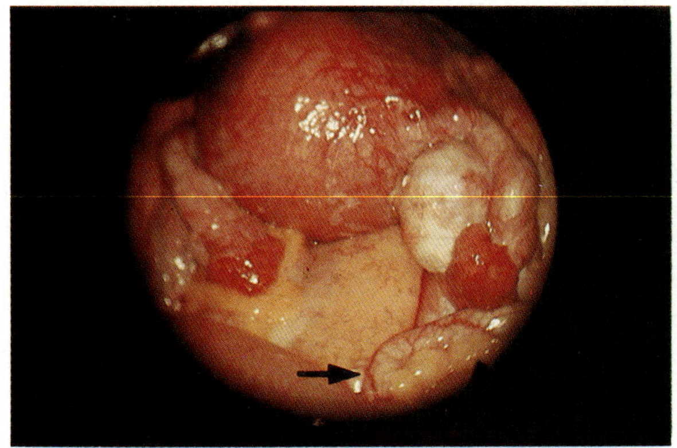

Figure 3.44 Acute salpingitis. Uterine hypervascularity and bilaterally inflamed fimbria confirm the diagnosis. Diagnostic laparoscopy was performed to rule out appendicitis. A normal appendix is seen overlying the pelvic brim (arrow).

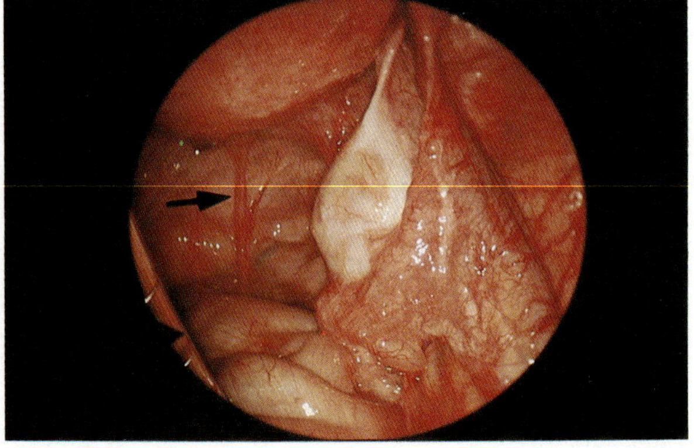

Figure 3.45 Tubo-ovarian adhesions distort the right fallopian tube. An adhesive band crosses the posterior cul-de-sac (arrow).

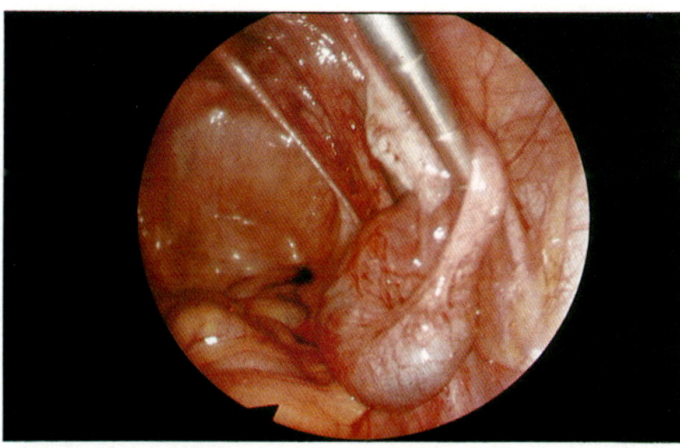

Figure 3.46 Right hydrosalpinx. Multiple tubo-ovarian adhesions further distort the anatomy of the fallopian tube.

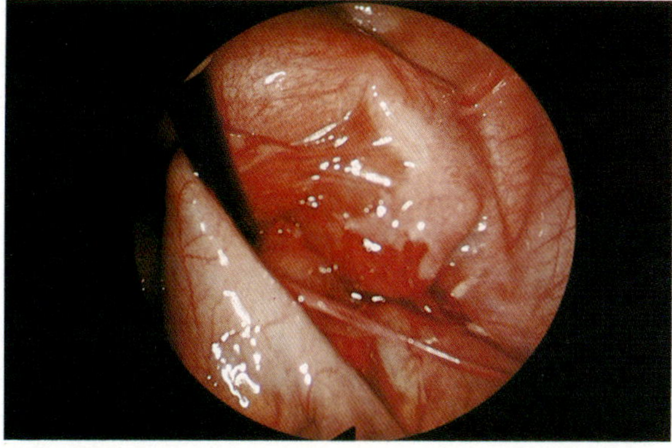

Figure 3.47 Acute pelvic inflammatory disease (same case as Figure 3.10). Right pyosalpinx and moderate amount of exudate confirm the diagnosis. The right ovary is not seen, suggesting that it could be part of a tubo-ovarian abscess.

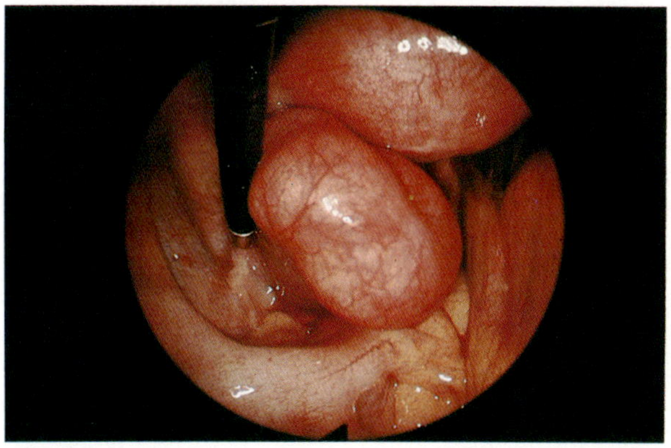

Figure 3.48 Dilated fallopian tube, left. Absence of peritubal adhesions suggest hydrosalpinx as the most likely diagnosis. However, sterile purulent material was obtained from the tube at laparotomy making the diagnosis of chronic sterile pyosalpinx.

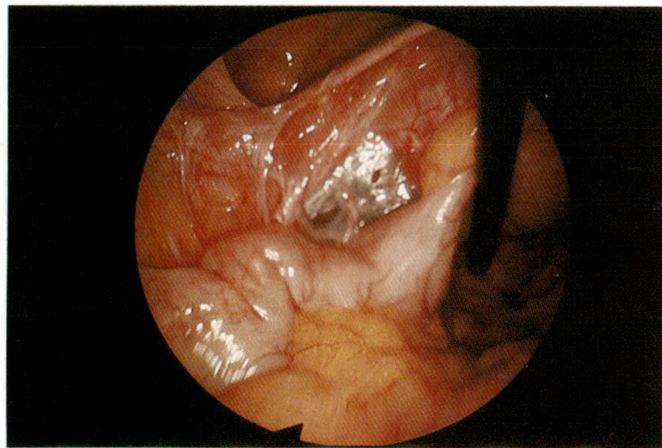

Figure 3.49 Multiple adhesions between uterus, bowel, and left adnexa in a patient with a history of recurrent pelvic inflammatory disease. Inability to visualize the left fallopian tube required laparotomy because tubal pregnancy was suspected; left ectopic pregnancy was found.

They recommended that endoscopic visualization of the female reproductive organs should be considered early in the course of an infertility investigation. Furthermore, in view of the minor symptoms and possible insidious nature of salpingitis, the diagnosis should be suspected in young sexually active patients with nonspecific gynecologic complaints. In such cases, early diagnosis would lead to early treatment and possibly avoid destructive sequelae.

Second-Look Laparoscopy. Second-look laparoscopy in infertile women is not limited to evaluation for further therapy after corrective surgery. The multifactorial aspects of infertility may require prolonged periods of medical therapy in patients in whom surgery was not clearly indicated at the outset. As in many other areas of medical practice, infertility need not be a static condition, but may vary with time. Repeated reevaluations of the patient, therefore, may yield new information on responsible etiologic factors.

Diagnostic laparoscopy should be repeated in patients who fail to conceive within 2 to 3 years of the original endoscopic evaluation if there is no other reason for their infertility. Pelvic adhesions, endometriosis, and fimbrial disease are sometimes found even though they were not present at the original laparoscopy. Testing tubal patency by transcervical pertubation with indigo carmine should be an integral part of this reevaluation. A more in-depth discussion of second-look laparoscopy is detailed in the last section of this chapter (see p. 85).

EVALUATION FOR POSSIBLE UTERINE PERFORATION

Uterine perforation occurring at the time of a diagnostic or therapeutic endometrial curettage is a potentially serious complication. Whenever it is suspected, the surgery should be stopped and careful evaluation undertaken. If the uterus is perforated during a diagnostic curettage with a blunt or sharp instrument, the event mandates discontinuation of the procedure and close observation. Postoperative complications, such as persistent pain and falling hematocrit, require additional investigation to assess for evidence of intraperitoneal damage.

Laparoscopy should be done expeditiously in cases with complicated postoperative recovery. The procedure is helpful for making a correct diagnosis. Sites of persistent slow bleeding are amenable to translaparoscopic hemostasis (see Chapter 17) (Figures 3.50 and 3.51). Perforation of the urinary bladder, if diagnosed promptly, is sometimes easily corrected by continuous bladder drainage (see Chapter 19). Injury to a segment of the gastrointestinal tract requires exploration and surgical repair or resection; such damage is much more readily correctable if diagnosed before disseminated peritonitis develops (see Chapter 18).

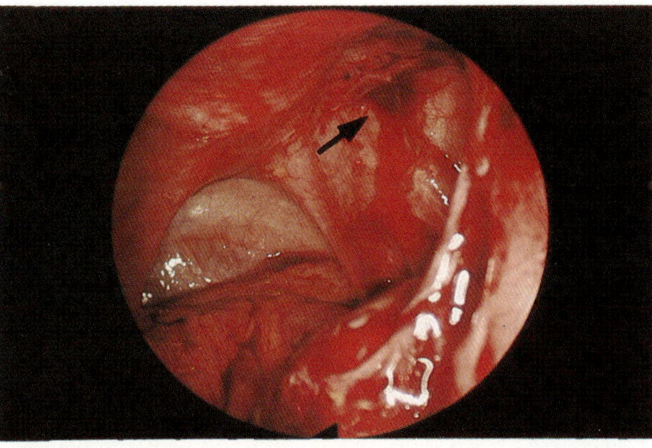

Figure 3.50 Uterine perforation, with an active bleeding site (arrow). Hematoma of the right broad ligament was confirmed at laparotomy. Laparoscopy was helpful in prompting early intervention.

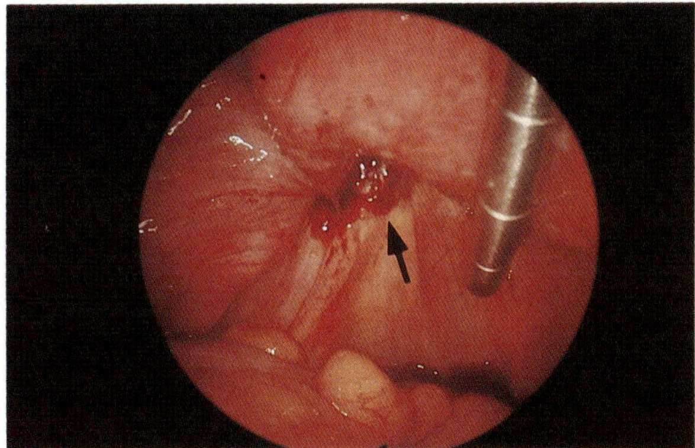

Figure 3.51 Uterine perforation following a diagnostic uterine curettage. Adequate hemostasis was achieved by the translaparoscopic application of microfibrillar collagen (Avitene).

When a uterine perforation is suspected at the time of a suction curettage, the procedure must be discontinued at once. Diagnostic laparoscopy enables the surgeon to evaluate whether any intraperitoneal organ has been damaged. If the perforation has occurred before the conclusion of the primary procedure, the curettage can be completed under laparoscopic guidance.

SECOND-LOOK LAPAROSCOPY

In the early developmental stages of endoscopy, a history of prior low abdominal surgical procedure was considered a contraindication to laparoscopy. As experience accumulated, selective screening of patients encouraged the increasingly liberal use of laparoscopy in lieu of laparotomy for exploratory purposes even in these cases. At the present time, with the exception of a few remaining absolute contraindications (see Chapter 6), endoscopy is being widely used in patients who have had previous abdominal surgery.

The value of laparoscopy for postsurgical reexamination is not limited to its diagnostic capabilities. Recently, it has been utilized for therapy and prognosis after major abdominal procedures. Second-look laparoscopy has been advocated for (1) follow-up of infertility surgery, (2) evaluation of therapy for ovarian neoplasm, and (3) assessment of fertility following treatment of acute salpingitis.

Infertility. This application has been alluded to earlier. Originally, second-look laparoscopy (SLL) was proposed as a method to evaluate the efficacy of new surgical techniques for infertility.[19] It has also been used for evaluating the effectiveness of drugs placed in the peritoneal cavity to prevent the formation of postoperative adhesions. The discovery that hydrocortisone forms plaques postoperatively prompted the discontinuation of intraperitoneal steroid use after infertility surgery.

The optimal time to perform a SLL for lysis of adhesions seems to be between 4 and 8 weeks from the original operation.[5] At that time, the newly formed adhesions have minimal tensile strength and are easily separated by blunt dissection with a probe. If more than 10 weeks transpire between the surgery for infertility and the SLL, the adhesions are dense and vascularized. They require electrocoagulation and sharp division to prevent bleeding. Another advantage of a short interval for the SLL is to permit one to dilate stenotic fimbria following fimbrioplastic procedures. In addition, electrocauterization of small areas of residual endometriosis can be carried out.

At the present time, the benefits of SLL are considered to be mostly theoretical. Improvement in the appearance of the pelvic anatomy following translaparoscopic lysis of adhesions may or may not have real therapeutic value. Systematic evaluation by Raj and Hulka of 60 patients following infertility surgery showed SLL to have little therapeutic or prognostic value after tubal reanastomosis or implantation because the incidence of postoperative adhesions was extremely low.[14] There are no data showing improved pregnancy rates. The incidence of adhesion reformation following lysis at the time of SLL is unknown; this cast doubts on the practical importance of this procedure. There is clear need for well controlled studies before SLL can be accepted as a routine follow-up procedure.

Gynecologic Oncology. Recent advances in adjunctive chemotherapy after extensive extirpative surgery have improved remission rates in patients with advanced ovarian carcinoma. Even small clusters of viable tumor cells, if left untreated, inevitably result in a relapse of the disease. Therefore, every effort should be made to verify a disease free state before therapy is discontinued. The usual means of reevaluation heretofore consisted of a secondary laparotomy to corroborate the clinical impression of complete remission. The impracticality of performing multiple laparotomies limited their use to a single operation at the conclusion of a planned course of therapy for purposes of excluding persistent disease.

Significant risk of developing acute nonlymphocytic leukemia after prolonged alkylating agent therapy prompted the use of shorter regimens and earlier second-look evaluations. Discontinuation, modification or reinstitution of chemotherapy is based on the operative and histologic findings at the time of reexploration. Laparoscopy has successfully filled the void by allowing repetitive exploratory evaluations with minimal morbidity and discomfort to the patient.

Piver et al reported the use of SLL in patients with ostensibly complete clinical remission after prolonged chemotherapy for advanced ovarian carcinoma.[13] Evidence of persistent ovarian cancer was documented in 36 percent of these cases, thus avoiding the need for a laparotomy. Moreover, in half of the patients, malignant cells in cytologic washings were the only laparoscopic evidence of persistent ovarian cancer. Berek et al evaluated SLL to follow clinically disease-free patients treated for ovarian cancer; they suggested that a negative laparoscopy confirmed by biopsy and cytology is associated with a significant prolongation in survival.[2]

Disadvantages associated with SLL in patients treated for ovarian cancer include the limited ability to examine the anterior abdominal wall and the entire pelvic cavity and the inability to evaluate the retroperitoneal lymph nodes. These limitations may justify exploratory laparotomy in patients who show no evidence of persistent malignancy at the time of the SLL before discontinuation of effective chemotherapy. Complications associated with the use of SLL in oncologic patients will be further described in Chapter 16.

Pelvic Inflammation. Wolner-Hanssen and Westrom, early supporters of laparoscopy as a means to confirm the primary diagnosis of pelvic infection, recently reported their experience with SLL in patients previously diagnosed with acute salpingitis.[21] In 13 patients, primary laparoscopy had revealed dense peritubal adhesions; eight of them had a normal pelvis at the time of the SLL 6 months later. The authors concluded that the acute-stage adnexal adhesions disappear after the primary disease subsides. These results are preliminary and should be interpreted cautiously since laparoscopy cannot evaluate the degree of intraluminal tubal damage. Long-term fertility follow-up is required to disclose the prognostic value of SLL in patients with acute salpingitis before it can be routinely recommended.

References

1. Anteby SO, Schenker JG, Polishuk WZ. The value of laparoscopy in acute pelvic pain. Ann Surg 1975; 181:484-486.
2. Berek JS, Griffiths TC, Leventhal JM. Laparoscopy for second-look evaluation in ovarian cancer. Obstet Gynecol 1981; 58:192-198.
3. Cassell GH, Younger JB, Brown MB, et al. Microbiologic study of infertile women at the time of diagnostic laparoscopy: Association of ureaplasma urealyticum with a defined subpopulation. N Engl J Med 1983; 308:502-505.
4. Cunanan RG, Courey NG, Lippes J. Laparoscopic findings in patients with pelvic pain. Am J Obstet Gynecol 1983; 146:589-591.

5. Daniell JF, Pittaway DE. Short-interval second-look laparoscopy after infertility surgery: A preliminary report. J Reprod Med 1983; 28:281-283.
6. El-Minawi MF, Hadi MA, Ibrahim AA, Wahby O. Comparative evaluation of laparoscopy and hysterosalpingography in infertile patients. Obstet Gynecol 1978; 51:29-32
7. Goldstein DP, Cholnosky C, Emans SJ, Leventhal JM. Laparoscopy in the diagnosis and management of pelvic pain in adolescents. J Reprod Med 1980; 24:251-256.
8. Jacobson L, Westrom L. Objectivized diagnosis of acute pelvic inflammatory disease: Diagnostic and prognostic value of routine laparoscopy. Am J Obstet Gynecol 1969; 105:1088-1098.
9. Jones GS, Maffezzoli RD, Strott CA, et al. Pathophysiology of reproductive failure after Clomiphene induced ovulation. Am J Obstet Gynecol 1970; 108:847-867.
10. Kleinhaus S, Hein K, Sheran M, Boley SJ. Laparoscopy for diagnosis and treatment of abdominal pain in adolescent girls. Arch Surg 1977; 112:1178-1179.
11. Lundberg WI, Wall JE, Mathers JE. Laparoscopy in evaluation of pelvic pain. Obstet Gynecol 1973; 42:872-876.
12. Musich JR, Behrman SJ. Infertility laparoscopy in perspective: Review of five hundred cases. 1982; 143:293-303.
13. Piver MS, Lele SB, Barlow JJ, Gamarra M. Second-look laparoscopy prior to proposed second-look laparotomy. Obstet Gynecol 1980; 55:571-573.
14. Raj SG, Hulka JF. Second-look laparoscopy in infertility surgery: Therapeutic and prognostic value. Fertil Steril 1982; 38:325-329.
15. Rosenfeld DL, Seidman SM, Bronson RA, Scholl GM. Unsuspected chronic pelvic inflammatory disease in the infertile female. Fertil Steril 1983; 39:44-48.
16. Semchyshyn S. Fitz-Hugh and Curtis syndrome. J Reprod Med 1979; 22:45-48.
17. Sweet RL, Mills J, Hadley KW, et al. Use of laparoscopy to determine the microbiologic etiology of acute salpingitis. Am J Obstet Gynecol 1979; 134:68-74.
18. Sweet RL, Draper DL, Schachter J, et al. Microbiology and pathogenesis of acute salpingitis as determined by laparoscopy: What is the appropriate site to sample? Am J Obstet Gynecol 1980; 138:985-989.
19. Swolin K. Laparoscopy as an operative tool in female sterility. Fertil Steril 1977; 19:167-170.
20. The American Fertility Society. Classification of endometriosis. Fertil Steril 1979; 32:633-634.
21. Wolner-Hanssen P, Westrom L. Second-look laparoscopy after acute salpingitis. Obstet Gynecol 1983; 61:299-303.

4 OPERATIVE LAPAROSCOPY

Infertility Surgery
Ectopic Pregnancy
Therapy for Endometriosis
Ovarian Cyst Aspiration
Ovarian Biopsy
Removal of Intraperitoneal Foreign Body
Uterine Suspension

In most instances, diagnostic laparoscopy is an integral component of the basic infertility work-up. Early attempts to combine diagnosis and therapeusis through the laparoscope were hampered by the lack of appropriate instrumentation and experience. The advent of microsurgical techniques further delayed the application of translaparoscopic surgery for the treatment of infertility. The success of operative laparoscopy for infertility reported by pioneers like Gomel, Semm and Swolin compared favorably with similar procedures done through a laparotomy incision.[10,21,26] Procedures that lend themselves to performance through the laparoscope include: lysis of peritubal and periovarian adhesions; lysis of adhesions to reconstruct the posterior cul-de-sac; fimbrioplasty, and salpingoneostomy.

INFERTILITY SURGERY

Lysis of Adhesions. Filmy adhesions between abdomino-pelvic structures may occur spontaneously or as a result of intraperitoneal surgery (Figures 4.1 to 4.3). Adhesion formation as a consequence of a pelvic inflammatory process is a common cause of infertility. Peritubal and periovarian adhesions produce sterility by interfering with the physiologic process of ovum capture from the ovary by the fimbriated end of the tube. It is also believed that the anatomic integrity of the pouch of Douglas contributes to the normality of the fertilization process. The laparotomy done for adhesiolysis may itself induce the formation of new adhesions. Electrocoagulation and division of those adhesions at the time of the initial diagnostic laparoscopy has proven effective in restoring the normal pelvic anatomic configuration.

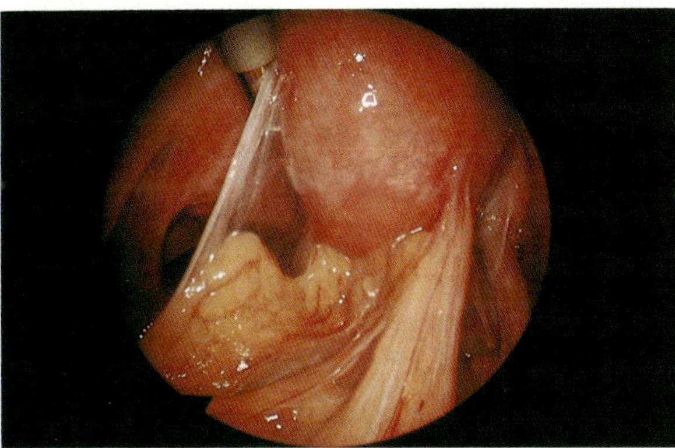

Figure 4.1 Filmy adhesions between uterus, omentum, and bowel in a patient who had had a posterior uterine wall myomectomy 2 years earlier. Lysis of adhesions through the laparoscope requires one or more auxiliary trocar punctures to provide access for probes to place the adhesions on stretch.

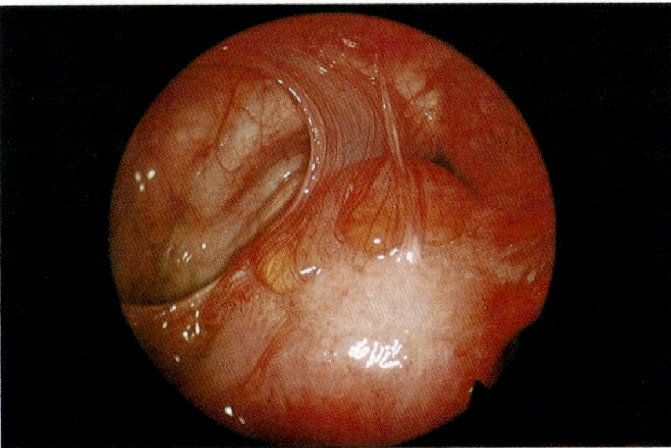

Figure 4.2 Adhesion between anterior pelvic wall and uterine fundus. A fundal myomectomy had been performed 5 years earlier. The number of vessels traversing this adhesion requires it to be electrocoagulated prior to division. This type of adhesion on the anterior uterine wall needs to be divided only if the patient is symptomatic from it. Otherwise, it merely acts to suspend the uterus.

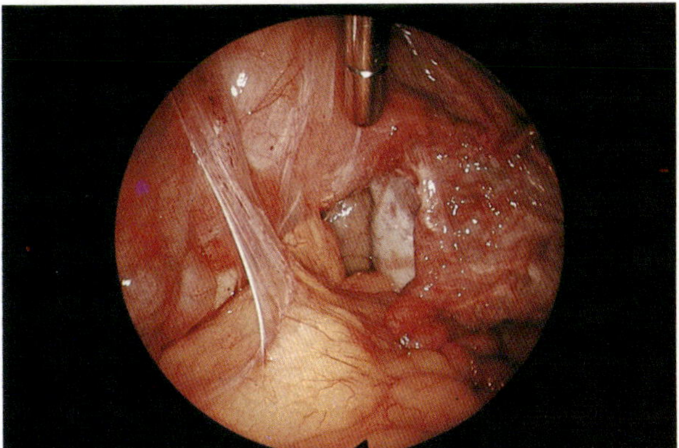

Figure 4.3 Adhesion between omentum and posterior uterine wall. A prior left salpingo-oophorectomy was carried out 3 years before. Translaparoscopic division of the adhesion facilitated visualization of the pouch of Douglas.

Periovarian Adhesions. Fibrinous filmy adhesions encasing the ovary are not unusual. They act as a barrier between the fimbrial end and the ovarian follicle impeding ovum pick up into the tubal lumen (Figures 4.4 to 4.6). Incising this type of adhesions is not sufficient; division and removal is the procedure of choice. In order for this to be performed translaparoscopically, it may require two or more accessory trocar punctures. The ovary and periovarian structures must be held firmly by means of an atraumatic forceps or a solid metal probe before such surgery is attempted (Figure 4.7).

Thin avascular filmy adhesions can be incised with sharp scissor-forceps without the need of electrical current.[10] Division of dense and vascularized adhesions necessitates electrocoagulation before they are sharply cut. Caution should be exercised to recognize that an adhesion put on stretch may mistakenly appear to be avascular. Whenever vascularization of an adhesion is uncertain, electrocoagulation must always precede cutting it (Figure 4.8). Placing the adhesion on stretch facilitates its division; this may require the use of insulated probes through the accessory laparoscope channel or by way of additional trocar punctures.

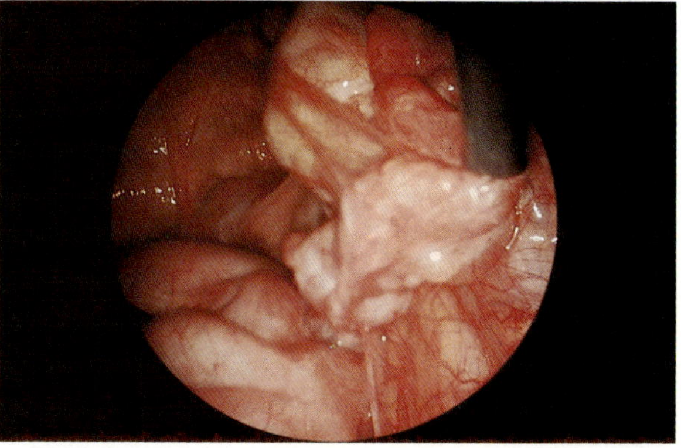

Figure 4.4 Tubo-ovarian adhesion. The ovary is fixed to the lateral pelvic wall and the tubal fimbria are kept away from the ovary by the filmy adhesive band. There had been no prior surgery in this patient.

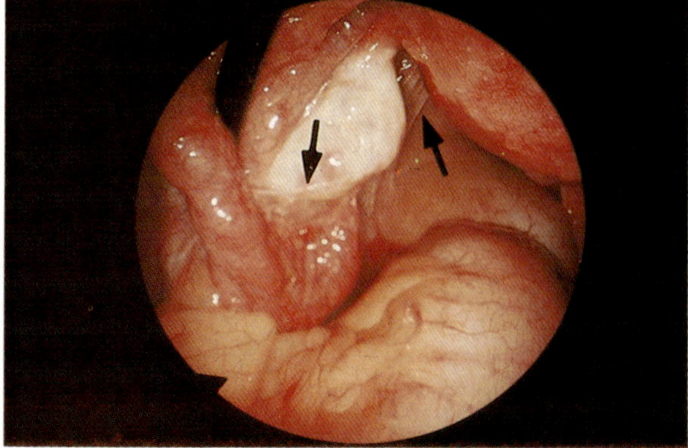

Figure 4.5 Tubo-ovarian adhesion (left arrow) disturbs the normal spatial relationship between those organs. The avascularity of this adhesion permits it to be cut with scissors without the need for prior electrocoagulation. There is also a fimbrial adhesion to the posterior leaf of the left broad ligament (right arrow).

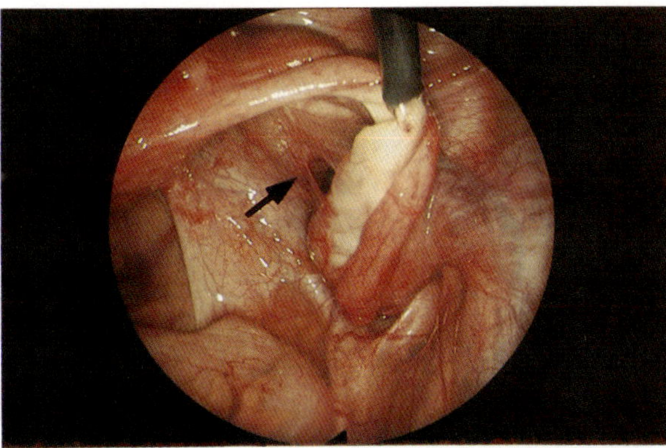

Figure 4.6 Adhesion between ovary and posterior leaf of the right broad ligament. This filmy adhesion encases the ovary entirely. It acts as a barrier to the normal ovum pickup by the fallopian tube. Lysis of this adhesion is required in order to evaluate the condition of the right tubal fimbria.

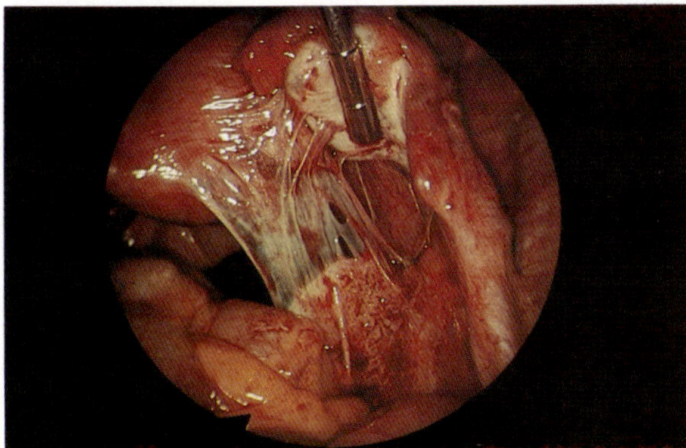

Figure 4.7 Adhesions between right adnexa and uterus are placed on stretch by the auxiliary probe. Scissors introduced through a third auxiliary puncture are used to divide them after bipolar electrocoagulation.

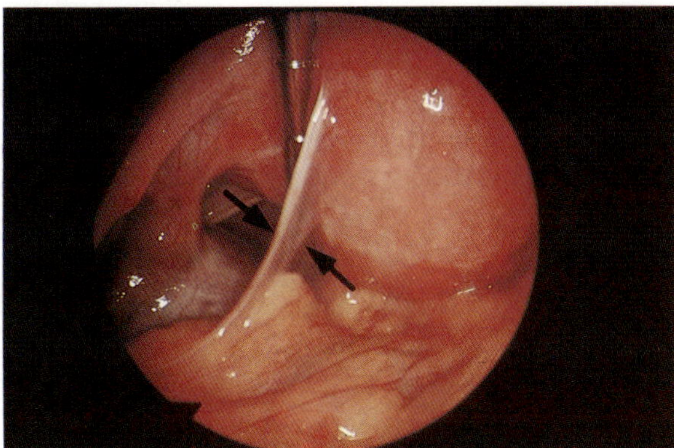

Figure 4.8 Fibrotic adhesion between sigmoid and posterior uterine wall. The thickness of the adhesive band makes identification of vessels within it uncertain. Possible areas of vascularity are identified (arrows). When in doubt, it is prudent to use electrocoagulation before sharply dividing the adhesion.

Peritubal Adhesions. Adhesions involving the tubal serosa may vary from the single, thin, avascular type which impedes the free apposition of fimbria and ovary to the densely vascular kind which significantly distorts tubal morphology (Figures 4.9 to 4.11). Similar to the procedure for lysis of periovarian adhesions, adhesions involving the fallopian tube should be placed on stretch before they are divided. Care must be taken to avoid applying unipolar electrocoagulating current to peritubal adhesions, because they are capable of conducting current and may therefore damage the tube itself. Electrocoagulation with a bipolar forceps followed by sharp division with scissor-forceps is the safest approach.

A complete evaluation of the pelvic anatomy should be carried out before attempts to lyse adhesions through the laparoscope are made. Tubal patency ought to be determined (Figure 4.12). If correction of the tubal distortion re-

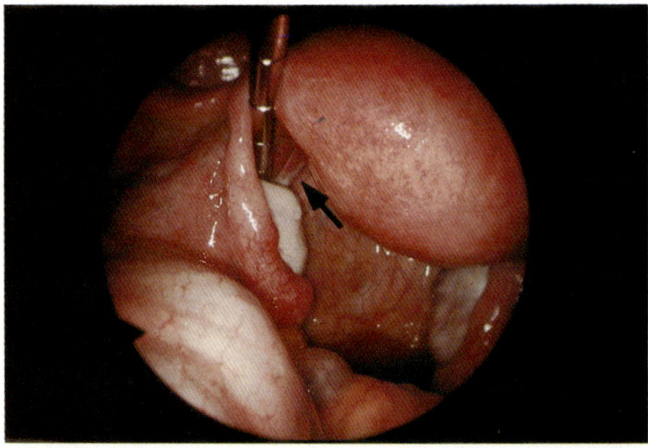

Figure 4.9 Single fibrotic band holding the left ovary and fimbria firmly against the posterior leaf of the left broad ligament. Division of this adhesion freed the entire left adnexa and averted additional surgery.

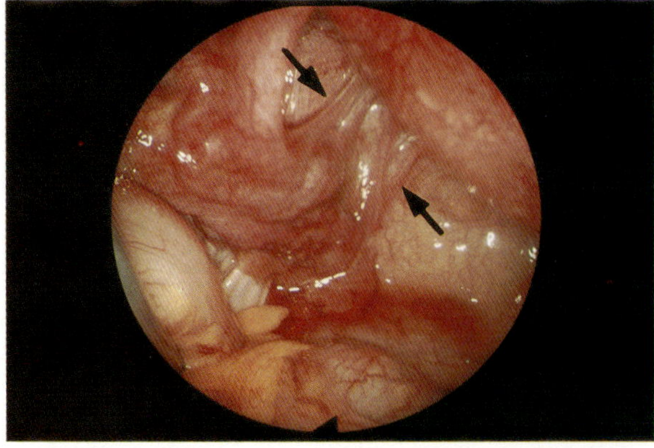

Figure 4.10 Broad filmy adhesion between ampullary segment of the left tube and the base of the left broad ligament. Blood vessels traverse the adhesion (arrows), making preliminary electrocoagulation mandatory in order to avoid bleeding from the cut edges.

quires a major surgical procedure, it is superfluous (and therefore inappropriate) to attempt translaparoscopic surgery. The risk outweighs the benefit since further corrective surgery will have to be performed subsequently.

Fayez reported restoration of normal tubo-ovarian relationships in 60 patients undergoing translaparoscopic lysis of adhesions (salpingolysis, ovariolysis and salpingo-ovariolysis).[7] Tubal patency was confirmed in 100 percent of these patients with a 60 percent conception rate in the first 12 months following the procedure. Benefits of operative laparoscopy for adhesiolysis include: a single anesthetic for diagnosis and treatment of patients harboring pelvic adhesions, reduced hospitalization and costs, and shortened postoperative recovery time. Furthermore, the ability to carry out repetitive corrective attempts without subjecting the patient to additional major surgery should not be underestimated.

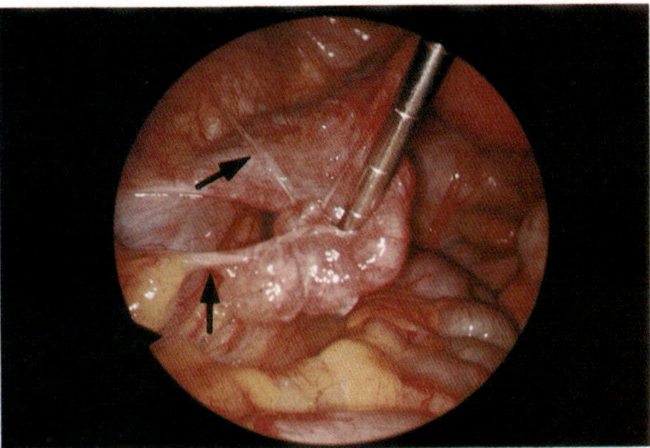

Figure 4.11 Tubal configuration distorted by multiple peritubal adhesions. Fibrotic bands (arrows) stretch the left fallopian tube so that the fimbrial end of the tube is held away from the ovary (not seen here).

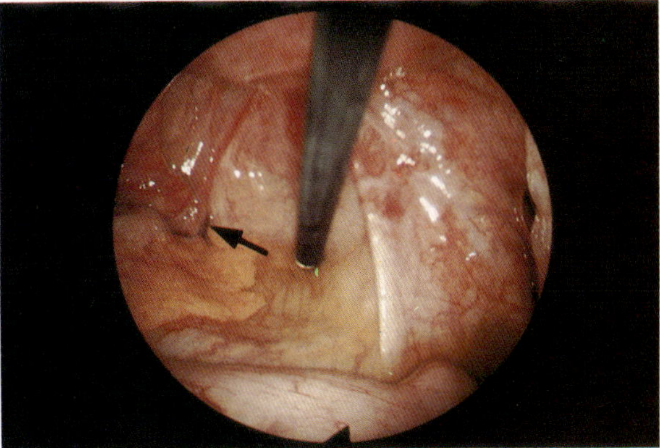

Figure 4.12 Confirmation of tubal patency by free flow of indigo carmine (arrow). This suggests that the disease process is limited to the adhesions exterior to the fallopian tube. This patient, who had two years of primary infertility, conceived within two months after the adhesions were lysed.

Salpingostomy. Fimbrial obstruction with hydrosalpinx formation is not an unusual finding in the infertile female population (Figure 4.13). Salpingostomy performed in these patients has been accompanied by limited success. Persistent tubal patency is low and the conception rate is even lower following this type of corrective surgery. Reoperation on patients whose tubes become occluded once again is unwarranted. Salpingostomy through the laparoscope has emerged as a procedure of last resort in such women. Gomel reported an 80 percent rate of tubal patency in patients in whom prior reconstructive surgery had failed.[9] Furthermore, he found an encouraging 50 percent pregnancy rate in patients with confirmed tubal patency following laparoscopic salpingostomy.

The technique of translaparoscopic salpingostomy requires several accessory puncture channels. These are usually placed in the lateral lower abdominal quadrants. The tube must be immobilized with atraumatic grasping forceps, and traction is applied by means of lateral uterine displacement. Doing so facilitates the operative procedure. Indigo carmine is injected transcervically to distend the terminal end of the tube for identification of the fimbrial dimple. Scissors are used to cut through the thin tubal wall and hemostasis is achieved by pressure or pinpoint electrocoagulation. Bleeding areas should be irrigated, thus permitting precise identification of the bleeding vessel. Coagulation of tissue is kept to a minimum to reduce cellular destruction and potential adhesion formation. At the conclusion of the procedure, the pelvis should be lavaged with copious amounts of physiologic solution.

Subsequent studies in larger groups of patients yielded somewhat lower success rate than the aforementioned report. Mettler et al reported less than 70 percent tubal patency in patients undergoing a laparoscopic salpingostomy as the primary corrective surgical procedure.[19] Pregnancy following such a procedure occurred in only 26 percent. Fayez reported even more disappointing results following translaparoscopic salpingoneostomy.[7] Tubal patency was confirmed in 31 percent of patients during follow-up hydrotubation; the overall pregnancy rate was just 10 percent.

The disappointingly low success rate for laparoscopic salpingostomy does not support its use as a primary operation for hydrosalpinx. However, in women in whom a previous salpingostomy by the laparotomy route has failed, it offers a realistic (although not optimistic) alternative. Newer translaparoscopic microsurgical suture techniques may permit performance of the same surgical procedure usually done in the course of a laparotomy.

Fimbrioplasty. Fimbrial phimosis may coexist with periadnexal adhesions. Agglutination of the fimbria by fibrinous material or a filmy serosal adhesion covering the tubal fimbria is the usual appearance. Blunt enlargement of the fimbrial opening can be accomplished by placing a closed alligator forceps into the tubal lumen and withdrawing it with its open jaws, as described by Gomel.[9] Sharp incision of tenacious adhesive bands is carried out with laparoscopic scissors.

The incidence of ectopic gestation following translaparoscopic fimbrioplasty has ranged from 5 to 40 percent. Reagglutination with partial or complete tubal obstruction is not infrequent. It has been suggested that patients who have had a fimbrioplasty performed through the laparoscope may benefit from a repeat follow-up laparoscopy 3 months following the original procedure, just as those may benefit who have had other types of translaparoscopic tubal surgery. This allows for evaluation of the results of the primary surgery as well as an opportunity for relysing any freshly formed adhesions.

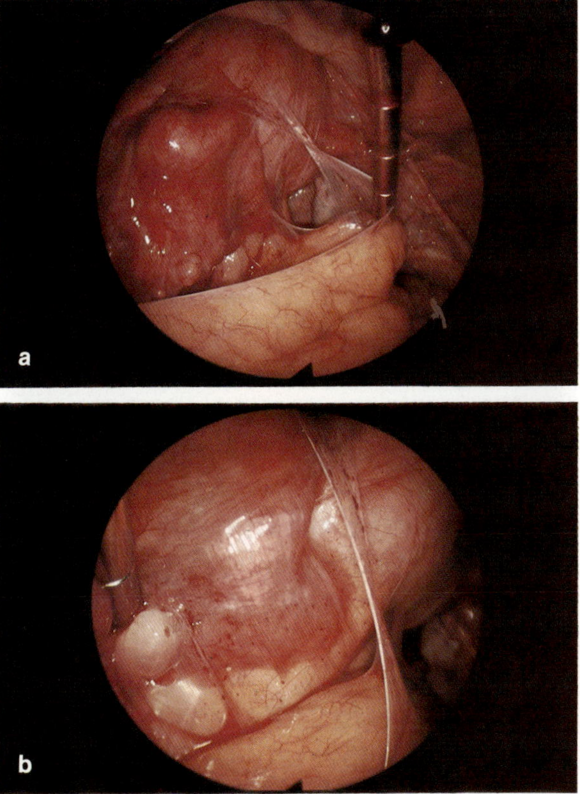

Figure 4.13 Multiple adhesions in a patient with a confirmed history of pelvic inflammatory disease. *a*. Left tube is dilated in the form of a hydrosalpinx and is curled over itself. The entire tube is adherent to the posterior wall of the uterus. The posterior cul-de-sac appears to be intact because there are no adhesions obstructing it. *b*. Close up view of the left tubal fimbria, showing filmy adhesions encasing it. Sharp division of these adhesions disclosed normal fimbria. A follow-up laparoscopy will be required to verify the resolution of the left hydrosalpinx.

ECTOPIC PREGNANCY

The incidence of ectopic pregnancy has been steadily increasing. The use of radioimmunoassay measurement of human chorionic gonadotropin (beta-subunit) and pelvic sonography has enhanced the early diagnosis of pregnancy overall. As to extrauterine (tubal) gestation, laparoscopy has facilitated identification prior to rupture in a great number. Standard therapy for ectopic pregnancy, until recently, consisted of partial or total salpingectomy. The diagnosis of an unruptured tubal gestation in women desiring to preserve their fertility has encouraged the development of more conservative surgical techniques. Salpingotomy with removal of the eccyesis at the time of laparotomy may allow preservation of the affected tube. Normal intrauterine pregnancies have been reported following this type of surgery.

Application of laparoscopy has remained limited principally to confirmation of the ectopic location of the pregnancy. In 1973, Shapiro and Adler reported the first translaparoscopic partial salpingectomy for removal of an early isthmic tubal pregnancy.[22] They recommended this procedure only for patients in whom the preservation of tubal function was not required. I have performed translaparoscopic partial salpingectomy in cases of failed tubal sterilization. Distal segment ectopic pregnancies are more preponderant in sterilization failures. (Figure 4.14). Absent the need to preserve normal tubal physiology makes them more susceptible to translaparoscopic extirpation. Partial salpingectomy through the laparoscope requires close attention to the vascularization of the tube. Hemostasis is achieved by extensive coagulation of the mesosalpingeal vessels beyond the resection margins.

In those patients in whom retention of normal tubal function is desired to preserve fertility, a linear salpingotomy is the procedure of choice. Bruhat et al reported 60 cases of ectopic pregnancy treated by tubal aspiration or salpingotomy at the time of the initial diagnostic laparoscopy.[2] Tubal aspiration was used when the conceptus was located in the distal part of the ampulla or fimbrial portion of the tube. Linear salpingotomy was used when the gestation was located in the isthmic or proximal portion of the tubal ampulla.

Bruhat et al reported a 72 percent pregnancy rate in those women desiring to become pregnant following the translaparoscopic treatment of an ectopic gestation.[2] They also reported a 12 percent rate of repeat ectopic gestation. This compares favorably with other more radical treatment for this condition. DeCherney et al reported a 50 percent conception rate in women undergoing translaparoscopic salpingotomy with expression of the tubal gestation.[4] Furthermore, tubal patency was confirmed by hysterosalpingography in those women who did not attempt to conceive following this type of treatment.

When salpingotomy is performed through the laparoscope, the tube is incised on its antimesenteric border (Figures 4.15 and 4.16). Utilizing electrical

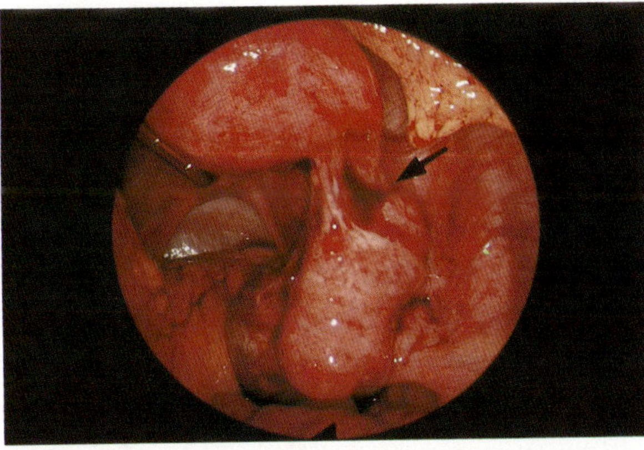

Figure 4.14 Ampullary ectopic pregnancy in the distal segment of the right tube in a previously sterilized patient. The area of tubal occlusion can be readily seen (arrow). Distally, the advanced eccyesis is close to rupturing the tube. Electrocoagulation of the mesosalpinx devascularized the distal segment of tube. Division and extraction of the ectopic pregnancy was easily accomplished thereafter.

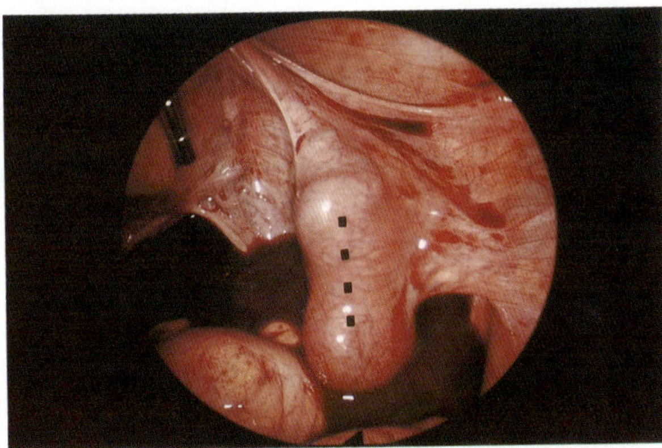

Figure 4.15 Early isthmic ectopic pregnancy (5 to 6 weeks from last menstrual period) with hemoperitoneum (same case as Figure 3.15). At this stage, translaparoscopic salpingotomy is feasible. The incision site for the extraction of the eccyesis is delineated (broken line).

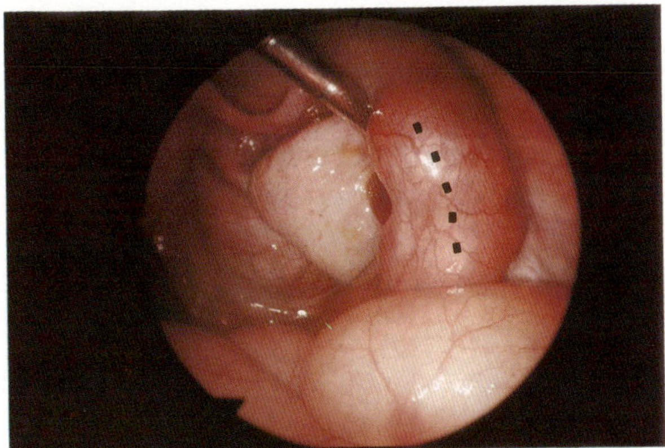

Figure 4.16 A more advanced gestation in the tubal isthmus (7 weeks), but still amenable to translaparoscopic salpingotomy. The anticipated tubal incision is shown (broken line).

scissors, one opens the tube over the area of tubal distention, and the conceptus is extruded by gentle compression with atraumatic forceps. Bleeding points on the tubal edge are controlled with pinpoint unipolar cautery. To avoid excessive tissue damage, Bruhat et al recommend atraumatic forceps compression of the bleeding vessels for hemostasis. In the future, the use of laser through the laparoscope for the initial incision on the tube may permit one to carry out the entire procedure with minimal bleeding.

Prevention of postoperative adhesions following translaparoscopic removal of an ectopic pregnancy is of importance. Rinsing the peritoneal cavity with normal saline at the conclusion of the procedure is recommended. Injection of 200 cc of high molecular dextran before removing the auxiliary laparoscopic trocar has also been suggested.[12]

Advantages associated with the conservative treatment of ectopic pregnancy through the laparoscope include shorter duration of surgery, reduced postoperative patient discomfort, and shortened hospitalization. Patient selection is of obvious importance. Only the earliest gestational duration cases are acceptable, and the patient's cardiovascular system must be stable. The contralateral tube should appear grossly normal and no coexistent pelvic pathology (such as pelvic adhesions) should be present. Experience with laparoscopic surgery is indispensable before this therapeutic approach can be considered.

THERAPY FOR ENDOMETRIOSIS

The mechanism by which endometriosis reduces fertility is unknown. The rate of conception has been shown to improve following therapy of the endometriotic implants. Surgical excision or destruction by electrocoagulation as the primary form of therapy is advocated by some. Others support a more conservative approach by medically suppressing gonadotropic stimulation of endometriosis with consequent atrophy as a result of hypostimulation of the endometrial stroma. While the primary mode of therapy for endometriosis remains controversial, little doubt exists about the need to confirm such a diagnosis prior to initiating any form of treatment. Direct visualization of the endometriotic foci is required for staging of the disease in accordance with the classification of the American Fertility Society. Laparoscopy has emerged as the most accurate diagnostic technique to verify the existence of intraperitoneal endometriosis.

Experience has shown that no relationship exists between the extent of endometriosis and the degree of infertility. Thus, Stage I endometriosis, which is usually represented by small numbers of scattered endometriotic sites, was deemed amenable to attempts to translaparoscopic ablation. Sulewsky et al reported a 40 percent pregnancy rate in 100 consecutive women undergoing treatment of endometriosis at initial laparoscopy for infertility.[24] All their patients had mild to moderate endometriosis with or without pelvic adhesions. Unipolar cautery was used to fulgurate the endometriotic implants and lyse any adhesion present at the time of laparoscopy. Additionally, they reported that 77 percent of the women who had preoperative dysmenorrhea were relieved of pain following the translaparoscopic ablation of endometriotic implants.

The wide variation in size and location of the ectopic endometrium made early attempts of translaparoscopic fulguration less than safe. The use of electrocautery in areas too close to vital structures (bowel, ureter) made them unsuitable for routine use (see Chapter 2). Furthermore, extensive thermal injury to large areas of peritoneum predisposed to formation of postoperative adhesions.

Daniell and Brown first reported treatment of endometriosis by means of carbon dioxide laser through the laparoscope.[3] Translaparoscopic laser beam surgery offers several advantages. It allows precise destruction of the endometriotic focus with control of depth and minimal damage to adjacent tissues. This coupled with its hemostatic effect makes it suitable for the ablation of lesions in close proximity of essential structures such as ureter or infundibulopelvic vessels.

One of the shortcomings of the carbon dioxide laser is that it loses power when it passes through the intraperitoneal carbon dioxide.[27] This requires one to increase the output power to compensate. Also, because carbon dioxide laser vaporizes tissue, it produces some smoke, known as ''smoke plume,'' which may obstruct clear vision in the closed abdominal cavity.

Development of the argon laser, which is capable of being used through the laparoscope, has overcome many of these difficulties.[14] The argon laser beam photocoagulates instead of vaporizing the tissues with which it comes into contact. Selective absorption of the argon energy by the hemoglobin containing endometriosis permits its use for the destruction of endometriotic implants on bowel, bladder or ureter.

The ability to treat endometriosis through the laparoscope in a safe fashion has many advantages. First, it allows therapy to be carried out at the time of the original diagnostic procedure. Second, it averts the discomfort associated with a laparotomy incision. Third, it avoids the delay in attempting conception in those patients who would have to undergo prolonged hormonal suppression therapy. Finally, the ability to perform the surgery on an outpatient basis reduces hospitalization with its attendant increased cost.

OVARIAN CYST ASPIRATION

Identification of an ovarian cyst at the time of laparoscopy is not unusual. Whether the finding is incidental or occurs during the evaluation for pelvic pathology, the operator is confronted with a diagnostic dilemma when an ovarian cyst is encountered. There is acknowledged difficulty in correctly diagnosing a cystic growth on the ovary merely by its external appearance. This shortcoming compounds the problem.

Although some European laparoscopists have advocated routine aspiration of simple ovarian cysts through the laparoscope, gynecologists in the United States have been less enthusiastic about routinely endorsing this approach. Alleged benefits of translaparoscopic ovarian cyst aspiration include: reduction in size and weight, thus decreasing the likelihood of adnexal torsion; restitution of the normal tubo-ovarian spatial relationship, and avoidance of a laparotomy procedure for the treatment of a functional cyst.

Shortcomings associated with this technique are not just theoretical in nature. Adequate experience in endoscopic surgery is required. Some patients undergoing laparoscopy for diagnostic purposes may require immediate laparotomy when it becomes clear that what was thought to be a benign functional cyst turns out to be an endometrioma or benign cystic teratoma. Of even greater importance is the delay it may cause in correctly diagnosing a malignant ovarian process when a random biopsy of its wall is reported as benign. To prevent such occurrence, some endoscopic surgeons have recommended that the cyst wall should be fenestrated to permit the direct visualization of the cystic cavity to rule out the presence of papillary excrescences.[15]

Certain criteria have to be fulfilled before one can proceed with the aspiration of an ovarian cyst through the laparoscope. As to its external appearance, the capsule must be smooth and thin walled. It should be translucent and transilluminate with ease. No adhesion should restrict its free movement. Its size ought not to exceed 8 cm in largest diameter (Figure 4.17 to 4.19). Biopsy of the cyst wall and fenestration should be performed in conjunction with aspira-

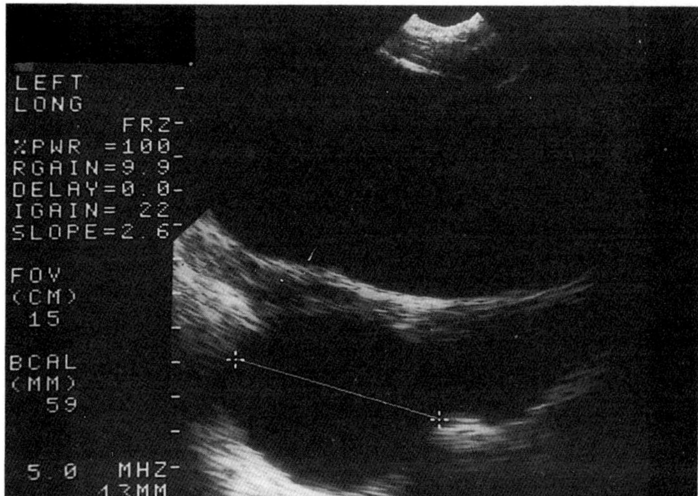

Figure 4.17 Pelvic ultrasonogram in a woman with a palpable pelvic mass, showing a cyst measuring 59 mm in diameter apparently located in the left ovary. The absence of intracavitary echoes suggests that the cyst has but a single cavity.

tion of the ovarian cyst fluid. Pathologic confirmation of the benign nature of the cyst wall is essential.

The presence of multiloculation on a preoperative pelvic sonogram contraindicates translaparoscopic aspiration of an ovarian cyst. Even though intraperitoneal spillage of fluid from a malignant ovarian lesion does not appear to alter the prognosis for survival, adequate staging and therapy mandate laparotomy. Immediate laparotomy must follow the identification of a benign cystic teratoma; spillage of its contents can give rise to a severe and potentially fatal reactive peritonitis.

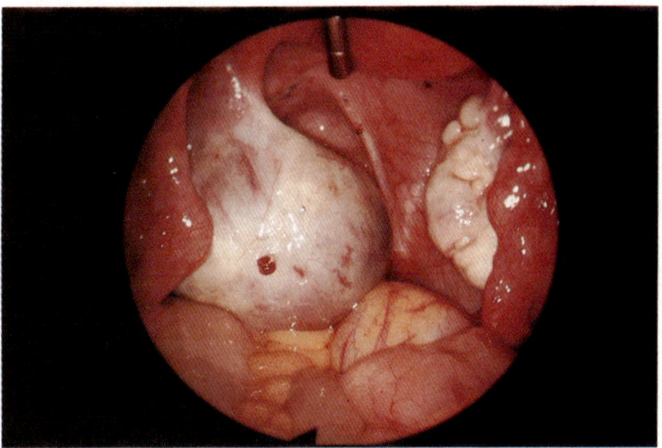

Figure 4.18 Ovarian cyst, left, encountered at laparoscopy in the patient whose ultrasonogram is presented in Figure 4.17. The cyst has a smooth capsule with no adhesions to any adjacent structure. Evaluation and aspiration of this cyst are shown in the ensuing Figures 4.19 to 4.22.

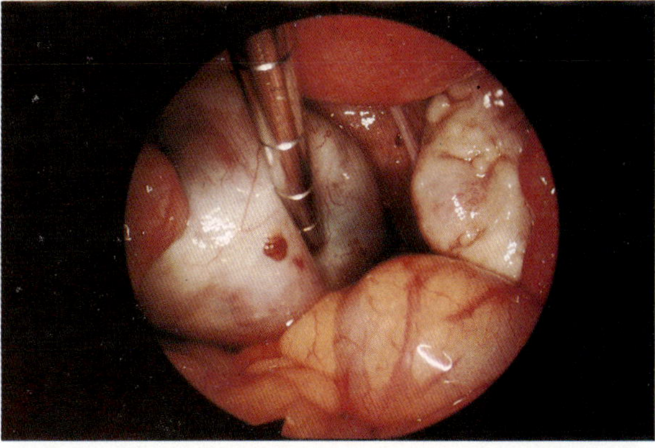

Figure 4.19 Ovarian cyst being palpated with a solid probe to confirm its soft consistency and demonstrate that it is fluid filled. This observation in combination with the ultrasonographic description makes it amenable to translaparoscopic aspiration.

Aspiration of an ovarian cyst may require the use of additional auxiliary punctures. The solid probe inserted through the midline suprapubic secondary puncture is utilized to immobilize the cyst (Figure 4.20). This facilitates its perforation by the aspirating needle because it offers a firm, fixed surface to be pierced.

The aspirating needle is usually inserted directly through the anterior abdominal wall. A long 16-gauge needle is recommended. The bevelled tip should be sharp to facilitate perforation of the cyst wall. The tip of the needle should be inserted deep into the cystic cavity to an imaginary point located at the center of the cyst (Figure 4.21). This prevents the needle from pulling out of the cyst as it deflates during aspiration of its fluid contents (Figure 4.22).

The operator should try to aspirate the entire content of the cystic cavity with a single puncture. Repeated puncture of the cyst becomes more difficult once deflation of the cavity has begun. The wall of the cyst is easily indented as the internal tension diminishes. Multiple punctures of the cyst wall predisposes to leakage of the cyst contents into the peritoneal cavity. Whenever possible, this ought to be avoided.

Ovum Collection. Oocyte harvest for in vitro fertilization under laparoscopic guidance is a very common indication for ovarian cyst aspiration. Its use is limited to individuals and centers involved in on going in vitro fertilization programs. It differs from the aspiration of an ovarian cyst found incidentally at laparoscopy (already noted) in that it is done under controlled conditions. Patients are known to be free of ovarian pathology based on previous laparoscopic investigation. The growth and development of the follicular cyst(s) are continuously monitored by pelvic sonography and hormone evaluation. Obtaining an oocyte confirms the functional nature of the cyst. These patients are subjected to intense, close follow-up after the procedure.

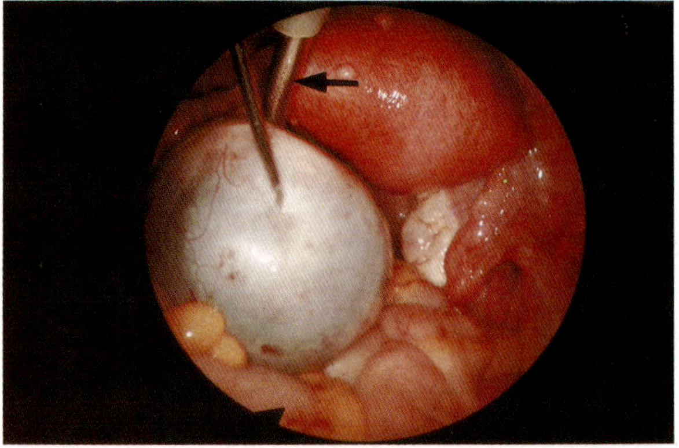

Figure 4.20 Long 16-gauge needle is inserted transabdominally. Solid metal probe (arrow) is used to immobilize the ovary. The needle should be inserted with a single firm thrust to avoid lacerating the cystic wall.

The technique of oocyte aspiration requires experience and precision in its execution. Perforation of the follicular cyst wall is done with a fine needle. This is to avoid the extrusion of the ovum through the puncture site if the oocyte is not obtained at the first try. Following aspiration of the follicular fluid, microscopic identification of the oocyte is done immediately. Irrigation of the follicular cavity and reaspiration enhances the rate of ovum collection. Because patients undergoing this procedure usually receive ovulation inducing agents, multiple follicles are often found at the time of laparoscopy. Care should be exercised to puncture each follicle individually under direct visualization. It is important to avoid intraovarian bleeding which may disrupt the hormonal production following oocyte aspiration.

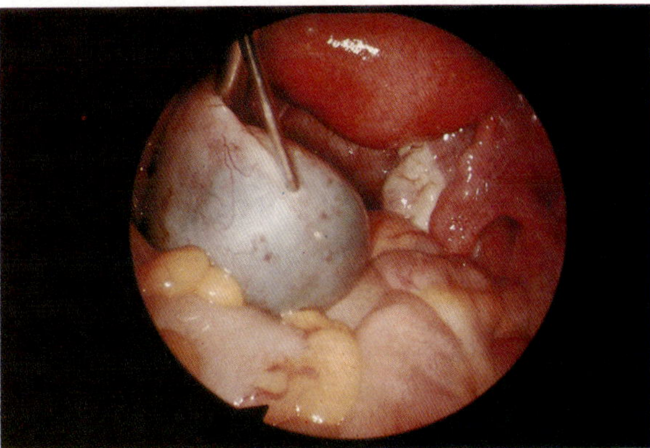

Figure 4.21 Aspiration needle is inserted aiming at the center of the cystic cavity. As the cystic fluid is being aspirated, the cavity decreases in volume and its walls tend to slide down the needle toward the tip. If the needle is inserted too superficially, one risks the tip becoming dislocated out of the cavity as the cyst deflates. Reinsertion of the needle is more difficult because the cyst walls are increasingly more elastic.

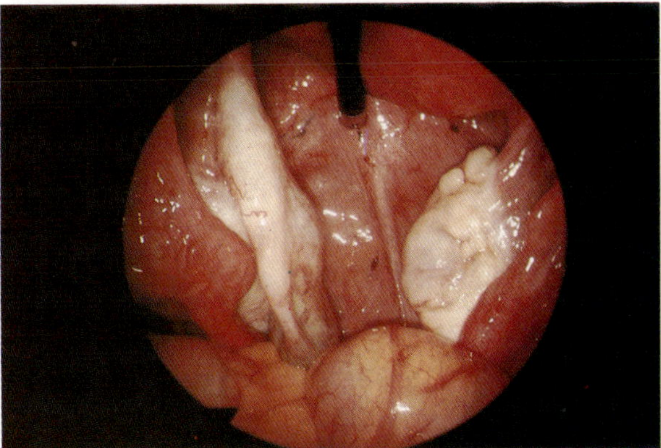

Figure 4.22 Ovarian cyst deflated following fluid aspiration. Extraction of straw-colored fluid suggested this was a corpus luteum cyst. Fenestration of the cyst wall was not performed in this case.

OVARIAN BIOPSY

Translaparoscopic ovarian biopsy has been suggested as a tool to assess gonadal function.[6,28] A critical evaluation of the recommended indications reveals that this procedure is not hazard free and is occasionally associated with serious morbidity. Sutton reported the division of a ureter in the course of attempts to biopsy a streak ovary; the injury necessitated a ureteral neocystostomy at a subsequent date.[25] Similarly, Duignan et al described the development of a ureterovaginal fistula as a result of the biopsy of a streak ovary.[5] Hemorrhagic complications requiring a laparotomy are not uncommon following a laparoscopic ovarian biopsy.

Advances in reproductive endocrinology have further diminished the need for direct sampling of ovarian tissue. Nevertheless, some of the original indications for this procedure have not yet found an alternative diagnostic modality. Thus, direct sampling of ovarian tissue may sometimes be indispensable for the diagnosis, prognosis and choice of therapy. The demonstration of the absence of germinal cells can directly influence the management of patients with Turner syndrome or with a 46XX karyotype and dysgenetic gonads. Confirmatory evidence of premature ovarian failure can only be obtained histologically. A confirmed pathologic diagnosis relieves the patient and physician from prolonged investigations and unnecessary stimulation tests while concomitantly providing early substitutional therapy.

When indicated, laparoscopic ovarian biopsy requires a double puncture technique; technically a Palmer forceps yields the best results. Electrocoagulation can be used to stop bleeding from biopsy sites. Also described is the translaparoscopic application of microfibrillar collagen which could avert the need for a major procedure to achieve hemostasis.[1]

Wedge resection of the ovary is the accepted modality of treatment for Stein-Leventhal syndrome following failure of a trial of hormonal therapy to reinstitute normal ovulatory cycles. However, extensive postoperative adhesions arising as a consequence of such surgery may themselves become the cause of postoperative sterility. There have, therefore, been other, less aggressive methods proposed, but they must still be considered as unproved. Swolin reported normal ovulatory cycles following translaparoscopic cuneiform incision of the ovaries in these types of patients.[26] Gjonnaess utilizing unipolar electrocautery of the ovarian capsule (4 to 8 cauterized holes) restored ovulation in 92 percent of women with hormonally confirmed polycystic ovaries within 3 months following the procedure.[8] A pregnancy rate of 69 percent within the first year after the corrective surgery compares favorably with other more invasive techniques. Reduced postoperative adhesions on repeat laparoscopy and reduced cost and length of hospitalization are some of the advantages associated with these modes of therapy.

REMOVAL OF INTRAPERITONEAL FOREIGN BODY

Intraperitoneal migration of an intrauterine contraceptive device (IUD) is not an infrequent complication. When it occurs at the time of insertion, removal is facilitated by traction on the tail string. Most often, the extrauterine location of an IUD is diagnosed after the patient or her physician fails to identify the transcervical tail or after an unwanted pregnancy has occurred.

Use of the laparoscope to remove an intra-abdominal IUD has been advocated in the past. The type of IUD, the material it is made of, and the length of time it has been translocated are important pieces of information for planning the therapeutic approach. IUDs made of purely inert plastic material are generally amenable to translaparoscopic removal. At times, the procedure requires the use of one or more accessory trocar punctures.

Removal of a copper-containing IUD by laparoscopy is only feasible if attempted shortly after the transuterine migration has taken place, specifically if perforation was recognized at the time of insertion. The inflammatory response, which occurs in tissues coming into contact with metallic copper in the peritoneal cavity, produces multiple adhesions.[20] Adherence or encasement by omental or bowel adhesions makes their translaparoscopic removal difficult if not altogether impossible. Patients wearing a copper-containing device must be counseled about the probable need for a laparotomy to remove the IUD from the abdominal cavity if laparoscopy should fail to accomplish the task.[18]

The use of laparoscopy to retrieve a foreign body from the abdominal cavity is not limited to the extraction of IUDs. Manganiello and Lee reported the translaparoscopic removal of a sewing needle from the posterior cul-de-sac in one patient.[16] Small surgical sponges left behind in an intra-abdominal procedure have also been removed under laparoscopic guidance through an accessory trocar puncture. Plastic catheter tips from ventriculoperitoneal shunts are similarly amenable to removal transendoscopically.[11]

A rare condition associated with the use of intraperitoneal drains is their breakage or migration into the abdominal cavity. At one time, removal of such displaced drains usually required a second laparotomy with its associated morbidity and inconveniences. Herbsman et al reported the translaparoscopic removal of a Penrose drain lost in the peritoneal cavity following drainage of a cholecystectomy site.[13] A similar technique was used to remove a peritoneal lavage catheter which also migrated into the abdominal cavity.

UTERINE SUSPENSION

Currently, uterine suspension is rarely performed as a primary operation. Controversy still exists over the valid indications for this type of surgery. Nevertheless, it is acceptable to perform a ventrosuspension of the uterus as part of the conservative surgical therapy for infertility in patients with endometriosis. The removal of the uterine corpus from direct contact with the posterior cul-de-sac following the lysis of peritoneal adhesions is helpful in preventing them from forming again, thereby avoiding a subsequent fixed uterine retroversion. With an increase in translaparoscopic surgery done for the correction of infertility, hysteropexy under laparoscopic visualization should be considered as a potential adjunctive therapeutic measure. Originally described by Steptoe, the first step is a routine diagnostic laparoscopy for pelvic inspection. By transillumination, an avascular area 5 cm from the midline and 3 cm above the inguinal ligament is chosen in each lower abdominal quadrant.[23] The skin is incised and a secondary trocar inserted under direct visualization. The round ligament is grasped with forceps approximately 5 cm from its uterine implantation. The round ligament is then extraperitonealized and pulled through the rectus fascia by withdrawing the forceps and investing cannula sheath together. The round ligament loop is grasped with an atraumatic forceps and the procedure repeated on the contralateral side. The tension is adjusted under laparoscopic visualization, and concomitantly, while the uterus is pulled upward, the pneumoperitoneum is partially evacuated to relax the anterior abdominal wall. The round ligament loop is then stitched to the anterior rectus fascia or the external oblique aponeurosis with nonabsorbable suture material.

Avulsion of the round ligament is the most common complication accompanying this procedure.[17] It is usually the result of excessive traction placed on the round ligament loop at the time it is being advanced anteriorly or when it is being sutured into position. Reduction of the pneumoperitoneum aids in preventing undue tension on the ligaments while at the same time ensuring that the suspension will not be too lax. Additionally, one should be cautious to locate the auxiliary lower abdominal entrance site far enough laterally so as to avoid forming a gap between the shortened round ligament and the anterolateral pelvic wall. Such an opening could potentially become the ring through which a loop of intestine may herniate. This procedure has also been performed in patients with severe uterine retroversion and dyspareunia, but with inconsistent success.

References

1. Borten M, Friedman EA. Translaparoscopic hemostasis with microfibrillar collagen. J Reprod Med 1983; 28:804-806.
2. Bruhat MA, Manhes H, Mage G, Pouly JL. Treatment of ectopic pregnancy by means of laparoscopy. Fertil Steril 1980; 33:411-414.
3. Daniell JF, Brown DH. Carbon dioxide laser laparoscopy: Initial experience in experimental animals and humans. Obstet Gynecol 1982; 59:761-764.
4. DeCherney AH, Romero R, Naftolin F. Surgical management of unruptured ectopic pregnancy. Fertil Steril 1981; 35:21-24.
5. Duignan NM, Jordan JA, Coughlan BM, Logan-Edwards R. One thousand consecutive cases of diagnostic laparoscopy. J Obstet Gynaecol Br Commonw 1972; 79:1016-1024.

6. Fayez JA, Jonas HS. Assessment of the role of laparoscopic ovarian biopsy. Obstet Gynecol 1976; 48:397-402.
7. Fayez JA. As assessment of the role of operative laparoscopy in tuboplasty. Fertil Steril 1983; 39:476-479.
8. Gjonnaess H. Polycystic ovarian syndrome treated by ovarian electrocautery through the laparoscope. Fertil Steril 1984; 41:20-25.
9. Gomel V. Salpingostomy by laparoscopy. J Reprod Med 1977; 18:265-268.
10. Gomel V. Salpingo-ovariolysis by laparoscopy in infertility. Fertil Steril 1983; 40:607-611.
11. Guzinski GM, Meyer WJ, Loeser JD. Laparoscopic retrieval of disconnected ventricular-peritoneal shunt catheters. J Neurosurg 1982; 56:587-589.
12. Holtz G, Baker ER, Tsai C. Effect of thirty-two percent Dextran 70 on peritoneal adhesion formation and reformation after lysis. Fertil Steril 1980; 33:660-662.
13. Herbsman H, Gardner B, Alfonso A. The value of laparoscopy in general surgery. J Reprod Med 1977; 18:235-240.
14. Keye WR, Dixon J. Photocoagulation of endometriosis by the argon laser through the laparoscope. Obstet Gynecol 1983; 62:383-386.
15. Kleppinger, RK. Ovarian cyst penetration via laparoscopy. J Reprod Med 1978; 21:16.
16. Manganiello PD, Lee JH. Removing a sewing needle from the pelvic cul-de-sac with an operative laparoscope. J Reprod Med 1978; 20:30-32.
17. Mann WJ, Stenger VG. Uterine suspension through the laparoscope. Obstet Gynecol 1978; 51:563-566.
18. McKenna PJ, Mylotte MJ. Laparoscopic removal of translocated intrauterine contraceptive devices. Br J Obstet Gynaecol 1982; 89:163-165.
19. Mettler L, Giesel H, Semm K. Treatment of female infertility due to tubal obstruction by operative laparoscopy. Fertil Steril 1979; 32:384-388.
20. Osborne JL, Bennett MJ. Removal of intra-abdominal intrauterine contraceptive devices. Br J Obstet Gynaecol 1978; 85:868-871.
21. Semm K. Modern endoscopy in gynecology and obstetrics. Clin Excerpts 1972; 34:1094-1103.
22. Shapiro HI, Adler DH. Excision of an ectopic pregnancy through the laparoscope. Am J Obstet Gynecol 1973; 117:290-291.
23. Steptoe PC. Laparoscopy in Gynaecology. Edinburgh-London: E&S Livingstone, 1967:78-80.
24. Sulewski JM, Curcio FD, Bronitsky C, Stenger VG. The treatment of endometriosis at laparoscopy for infertility. Am J Obstet Gynecol 1980; 138:128-132.
25. Sutton C. The limitations of laparoscopic ovarian biopsy. J Obstet Gynaecol Br Commonw 1974; 81:317-330.
26. Swolin K. Laparoscopy as an operative tool in female sterility. J Reprod Med 1977; 19:167-170.
27. Tadir Y, Kaplan I, Zuckerman Z, Edelstein T, Ovadia J. New instrumentation and technique for laparoscopic carbon dioxide laser operations: A preliminary report. Obstet Gynecol 1984; 63:582-585.
28. Yuzpe AA, Rioux JE. The value of laparoscopic ovarian biopsy. J Reprod Med 1975; 15:57-59.

5 STERILIZATION

Counseling for Sterilization
Unipolar Electrocoagulation
Bipolar Electrocoagulation
Tubal Occlusion with Silastic Bands
Tubal Occlusion using Clips
Thermal Cautery
Sterilization Reversal

In the 1970s, acceptance of tubal occlusion as a method for fertility control encouraged the development of safe and effective techniques. Traditionally, female sterilization required a laparotomy or colpotomy for transection of the fallopian tubes. Frequently, hysterectomy was the procedure elected.

The use of laparoscopy as an alternative technique for tubal occlusion was an important development. In addition to its standard diagnostic use, it offered the opportunity to use the laparoscope as an operative tool. Undoubtedly, the ability to perform sterilization procedures translaparoscopically ought to be credited with the rebirth and popularization of laparoscopy in this country.

For the beginner, knowledge of the various modalities enables the operator to select the most appropriate method for a particular patient. Furthermore, the skill to carry out the proposed procedure in a variety of different ways proves useful if complications arise with the primary method selected. A description of the most common complications associated with laparoscopic sterilization appears in Chapter 22.

Once it became generally available, translaparoscopic tubal occlusion soon became the most popular and widely used method to accomplish sterilization in women. Its appeal was multifactorial. From the patient's point of view, it offered the same effectiveness as previously used procedures without the need for a cosmetically less-than-desirable surgical scar. Furthermore, avoidance of a major transabdominal or transvaginal procedure reduced the discomfort and duration of the postoperative period. From the physician's point of view, the procedure was short and simple and when properly performed free of complications. Additionally, it allows the operator to explore the surrounding abdominopelvic structures visually; thus the procedure offers him or her the opportunity to diagnose the presence of any concomitant abnormal condition. Finally, the socioeconomic aspects derived from the application of laparoscopic sterilization procedures was not without significance. Reduced hospitalization resulted in an overall decrease in costs for the procedure and reduced the period of time the patient was away from her regular daily activities.

Several methods to accomplish occlusion of the fallopian tubes under laparoscopic visualization have been developed. Some techniques were designed to overcome shortcomings of other methods, whereas some were aimed at facilitating the surgical procedure as a whole. Translaparoscopic tubal occlusive methods can be divided into those electrical and nonelectrical in nature. Techniques classified as electrical are those in which electric current of variable frequency and voltage is used to accomplish the localized destruction of a segment of fallopian tube. They include the monopolar and bipolar types of electrocauterization. Nonelectrical techniques achieve tubal obstruction by mechanical occlusion of the tubal lumen by utilization of a variety of clips, rings or sutures. Interruption of tubal continuity without the use of electrical current traversing the patient's tissues can also be accomplished utilizing heat generated by a portable battery in the form of thermal cautery.

COUNSELING FOR STERILIZATION

No description of sterilization procedures would be complete without a discussion concerning counseling. Proper information and in-depth analysis of the reasons and concerns surrounding the decision to undergo sterilization must precede the surgical procedure.

Studies evaluating emotional responses to sterilization suggest that some patterns are recurrent.[3] Few of the problems encountered relate to the technical aspects of the procedure. The advent of translaparoscopic sterilization—with its low risk minimal scarring, relatively minor discomfort, and short hospitalization—has encouraged many women to undergo the procedure who would not otherwise have accepted major surgery for this purpose.

Regrets about having undergone the sterilization procedure appear to be present in a small proportion of most populations studied. Early remorse is reported within the first 12 months postoperatively in 2 to 5 percent. The frequency increases somewhat thereafter and subsequently decreases by 2 years. Further investigation into patient characteristics reveals that the younger the patient or the more she lacks complete understanding of the irreversibility of the procedure, the greater the risk of future emotional problems. A particular group of patients has been identified in most follow-up studies as being at high risk, namely those undergoing sterilization at the time of cesarean section or immediately post partum. Compared to other women, these patients expressed misgivings about their decision to accept sterilization ten times more often. Complaints with regard to libido and sexual satisfaction tended to correlate with poor knowledge of the procedure and especially with lack of full understanding and acceptance of its irreversibility.

These findings suggest that great discretion should be used in recommending sterilization to women in the following groups or situations:

Young women of low parity
Women in unstable relationships
Women with a history of failed alternative contraception
At the time of cesarean section or during the puerperium
In combination with abortion
In combination with other procedures for convenience

A history of psychiatric illness is by itself not a contraindication for sterilization but a more in-depth evaluation is in order. Patients with severe personality disorders are more likely to be dissatisfied at a later date. Similar results are seen in women requesting sterilization because of sexual dysfunction; this should never be attempted as treatment for this condition.

The informed consent process concerning sterilization procedures works two ways. Even though a woman requests sterilization, physicians can and should refuse to perform the operation when they judge her to be incompletely counseled or lacking complete understanding of the nature and implications of such a procedure. A sterilizing operation should not be treated as a routine technical procedure. Doubts and fears should be discussed and evaluated on their own merits because different social and religious backgrounds shape attitudes towards the procedure. The physician must detach his own feelings concerning birth control, sexual activity, and social morals while counseling a patient for sterilization. Although a woman as an individual has the right to choose sterlization, experience has shown that a better decision is made by the couple as a unit.

It cannot be sufficiently emphasized that a woman should never be accepted as a candidate for a sterilization procedure until she has a full understanding of the concept of the "definitive and irreversible" nature of the operation. An ill-advised or less than completely counseled patient is the most likely candidate to regret her decision in the future. Despite the advances in microsurgical reanastomosis of the fallopian tubes and its widespread advertisement we should not confuse tubal patency with success—success meaning a full term pregnancy.

UNIPOLAR ELECTROCOAGULATION

Unipolar or monopolar electrocoagulation of the fallopian tubes was originally the most widely used method for laparoscopic sterilization.[14] The technique was facilitated by the existence of the required electrogenerators in most surgical operating suites. A detailed description of the generator has already been given in Chapter 1. The instrument will be described here.

Palmer Forceps. The Palmer forceps is made up of a double-barrelled metal cylinder with a central pair of forceps tongs capable of conducting electrical current (Figure 5.1). The grasping forceps is in the open position when completely extruded from the inner cylinder. When the forceps is retracted, the tongs close up grasping the tissue between them. The outer cylinder has a sharp edge and is moved up and down the inner cylinder by turning it in a circular motion over the main stem of the instrument. The forceps is connected to the electrogenerator by a high frequency cord.

The essence of unipolar electrocoagulation for tubal sterilization consists of passage of electrical current between a forceps applied to the fallopian tube and a dispersive plate attached to the patient's skin at a location nearby. Passage of current produces dessication of the grasped tissue by driving water out and coagulating the cellular components. Since the current seeks out the dispersive electrode (plate), the dessication of the tissue spreads radially away from the area grasped by the forceps. This process continues as long as current is being transmitted through the primary electrode (forceps) thus accomplishing the desired amount of tissue destruction with a single application of the forceps to the fallopian tube.

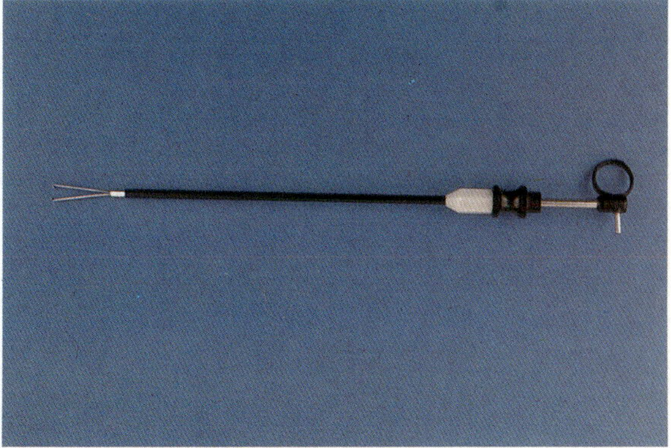

Figure 5.1 Palmer unipolar forceps. Grasping forceps are shown in the open extruded position.

During unipolar electrocoagulation, the tissue being dessicated first turns light brown and as the coagulation process continues it becomes white (Figure 5.2). This results from the denaturation of the cellular proteins and concomitant devascularization of the affected tissues. Tissue subjected to dessication becomes necrotic and subsequently is reabsorbed by phagocytosis.

During the early stages of unipolar tubal sterilization, several variations of the technique were used in attempts to ensure complete tubal occlusion: burn only; burn and divide the cauterized segment; and burn and resect a portion of burned tube.

Burn Only. The burn only technique consisted of applying unipolar high frequency coagulation to a segment of tube and mesosalpinx measuring approximately 3 to 5 cm in length. The tube is grasped with a Palmer coagulation forceps at the isthmic portion about 4 to 5 cm from the uterine cornu. Use of the fulguration (coagulation) current produces tissue dessication while minimizing the amount of concentrated heat delivered to the tissue. This in turn reduces the amount of water transformed into steam without obliterating the view through the laparoscope. This procedure is repeated on the contralateral tube.

Burn and Divide. Concern about the possibility of leaving a patent tubal lumen after the coagulation was completed led some laparoscopists to recommend surgical division of the fallopian tube. This was accomplished by passing a cutting current for electrosurgical division or by means of translaparoscopic scissors for sharp transection. Additional coagulation was applied if the tubal lumen still appeared to be incompletely cauterized.

Burn and Resect. The desire to obtain pathologic confirmation of the operated tissue prompted the development of special instruments that were capable of performing the dual task of cauterization and division. To accomplish this following the coagulation of an adequate portion of fallopian tube and mesosalpinx, the outer cannula of the unipolar forceps is screwed downward by rotating it clockwise while simultaneously applying intermittent cutting current (Figure 5.3). By this means division of the fallopian tube and mesosalpinx allows one to remove the portion of salpinx that was being held by the forceps (Figure 5.4). This dessicated portion of tissue is then submitted for pathologic evaluation.

Originally widely used, unipolar tubal electrocoagulation has fallen into disfavor at the present time.[2] Limitations and complications associated with these methods of sterilization are responsible for their abandonment in favor of safer techniques. Complications are described in Chapter 22.

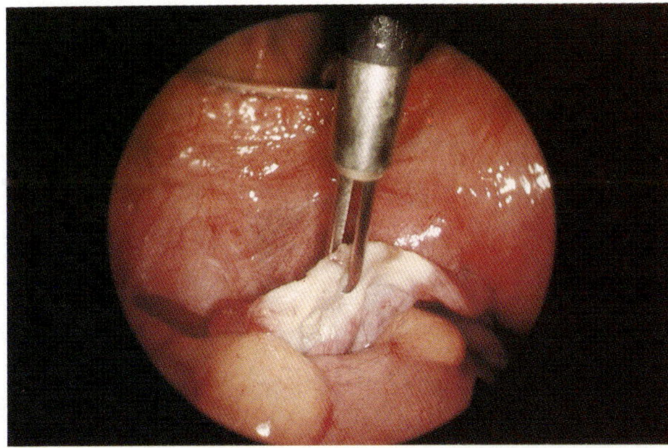

Figure 5.2 End-stage of unipolar electrocoagulation of the left fallopian tube. Approximately 3 cm of tube are visibly damaged. Injury to the endosalpinx extends even further in both directions (proximally and distally) from the burned area.

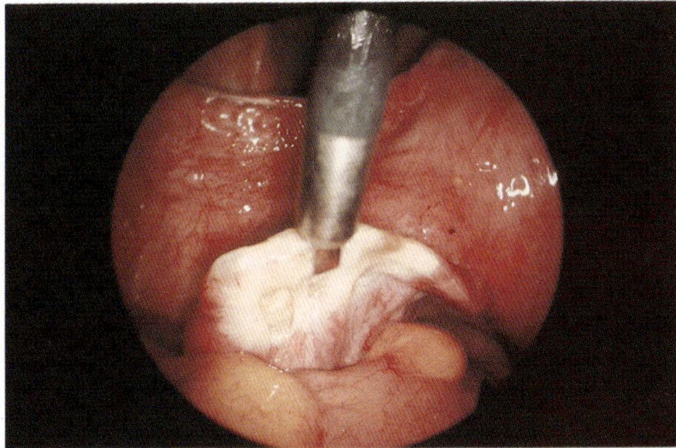

Figure 5.3 Outer sleeve of the unipolar forceps is screwed down over the grasping forceps. Simultaneous application of cutting current allows the removal of the tissue within the grasping forceps.

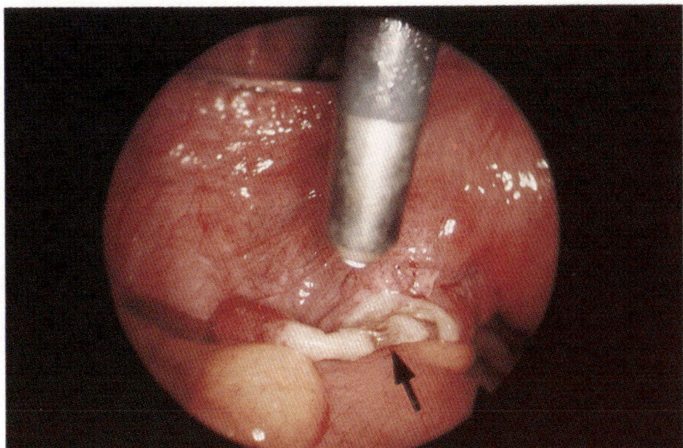

Figure 5.4 Segment of tube is removed for pathologic evaluation. The gap in continuity of the fallopian tube is apparent (arrow).

BIPOLAR ELECTROCOAGULATION

Complications related to the pathway of dispersion of the electrical current used with unipolar electrocoagulation led to the development of bipolar electrocoagulating forceps. This instrument incorporates the return electrode into one of the forceps tongs. The circuit thus created (bipolar circuit) limits the passage of electricity and electrical dessication to the tissue grasped between the jaws of the forceps. Additional advantages associated with the bipolar electrocoagulation technique are as follows: coagulation of the tissue treated is circumscribed to the area in contact with the forceps tongs; the rest of the patient is never part of the electrical circuit; lower voltage and wattage are required to achieve tissue coagulation; free sparks do not occur within the abdominal cavity; and the ground plate is not needed as a dispersing electrode.

The most commonly used bipolar electrocoagulating forceps for tubal sterilization is the one designed by Kleppinger (Figure 5.5). This device has features which are specifically designed for tubal surgery.[8] The upper loop is insulated to avoid contact between the forceps jaws and the outer sleeve of the forceps. The lower ovoid loop encloses the fallopian tube within its perimeter. The flat, serrated tong-tips are designed to appose each other when the mesosalpinx is grasped. Dessication of the mesosalpinx is recommended to ensure that both proximal and distal occluded ends fall away from each other following reabsorption of the electrocoagulated segment of tube.

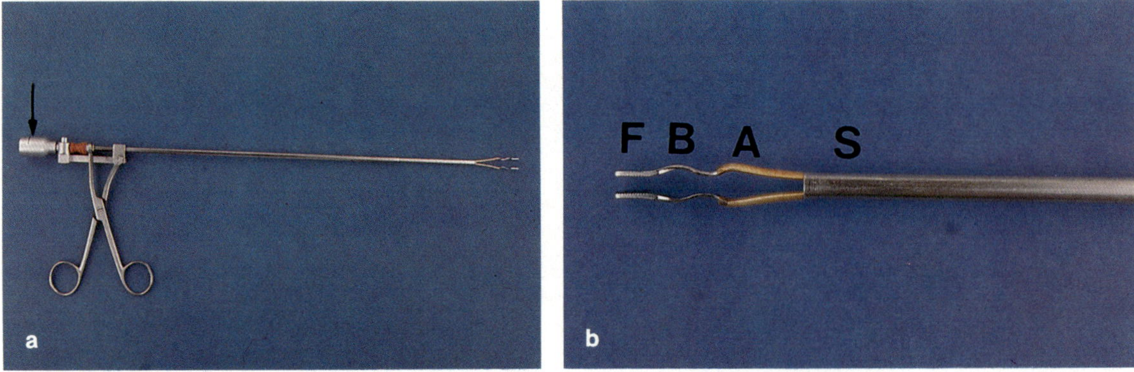

Figure 5.5 Kleppinger bipolar forceps. *a.* Bayonet receptacle above the scissors-grip handle is where the bipolar grounded cord is connected (arrow). *b.* Close-up of the distal tip. Upper loop (A) is insulated preventing contact between the active electrode and the outer sleeve (S). Lower ovoid loop (B) encloses the fallopian tube. Flat serrated tong-tips (F) are designed to cauterize the mesosalpinx beneath the segment of burned tube.

The operative procedure involves the electrofulguration of a segment of tube approximately 2 to 3 cm in length. Because the bipolar forceps confines the tissue destruction to the segment of tube included between the forceps tongs, it requires two or three adjacent applications to achieve the desired extent of tubal destruction. The fallopian tube is grasped at its isthmic segment starting from the distal end of the desired segment to be burned (that is, the portion closest to the fimbria). The additional burn or burns should be more proximal to the initial cauterization. The purpose of placing the second and third burns closer to the cornu is to enhance the safety of the procedure. This practice eliminates the possibility of electrons overflowing centrifugally to any adjacent organs, such as bowel. Instead, any excess of electrons will travel in the direction of the uterine cornua.

As the electrical current travels between the forceps tongs, the tissue being held undergoes dessication (Figures 5.6 to 5.14). The outflow of water and electrolytes decreases the ability of the tissue to conduct electrical current, a phenomenon known as resistance to the flow of electrons. The greater the resistance offered by dessicated tissue, the less the flow of electrons between the forceps tongs. A total lack of electrical flow between the electrodes marks the end point of the fulguration process. The steps are repeated until the desired amount of tube is fulgurated.

Proper execution of a tubal sterilization with bipolar forceps requires a bipolar generator. This electrogenerator must produce low voltage and constant wattage power output. As previously stated, the flow of electrons is inversely proportional to the resistance offered by the tissue between the forceps jaws.

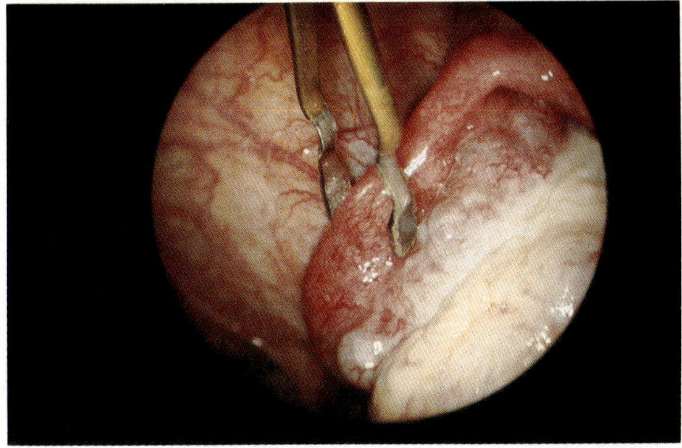

Figure 5.6 Selecting the optimal site on the tubal isthmus to apply the bipolar forceps. The forceps tongs are atraumatic and can be used to mobilize the delicate tubal tissues for proper application.

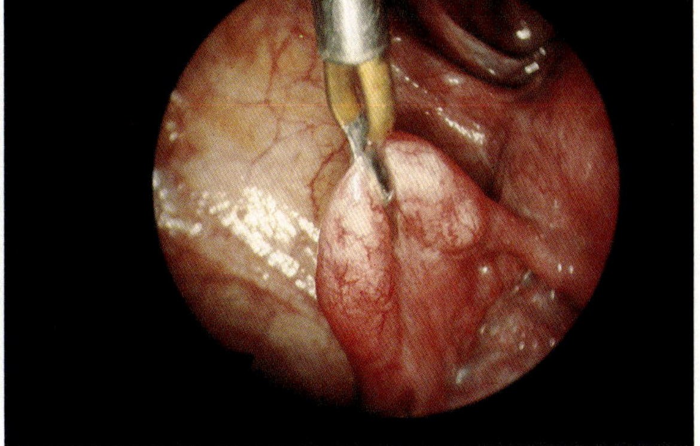

Figure 5.7 Correct application of the Kleppinger bipolar forceps. Noninsulated loop encircles the portion of the tube to be cauterized. Flat serrated tong tips appose each other on the underlying mesosalpinx.

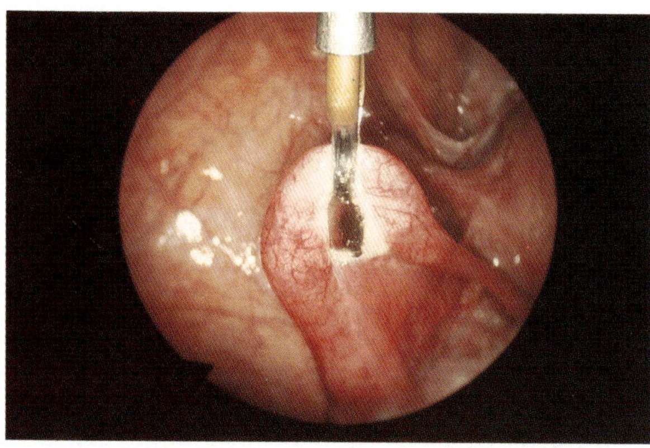

Figure 5.8 Application of bipolar electrocoagulation. Instrument and segment of tube being held are under direct vision and are verified not to be in contact with any adjacent structure. Electric current is applied to the bipolar forceps.

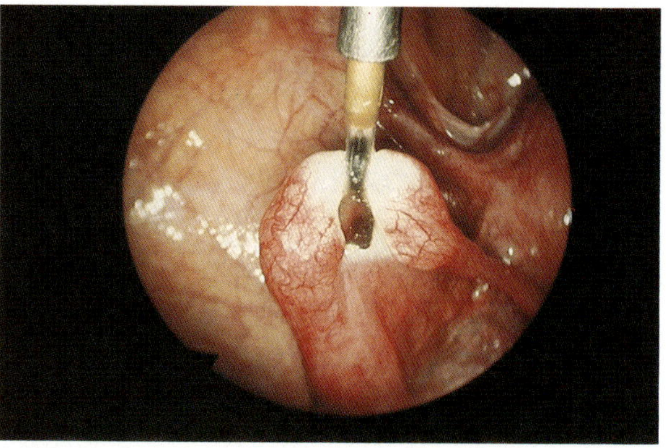

Figure 5.9 Application of bipolar electrocoagulation. Blanching of the tubal peritoneum occurs immediately. Flow of electrons continues until the tissue grasped between the forceps tongs is completely cauterized. Total resistance to the flow of electrons confirms complete cauterization of the operated segment.

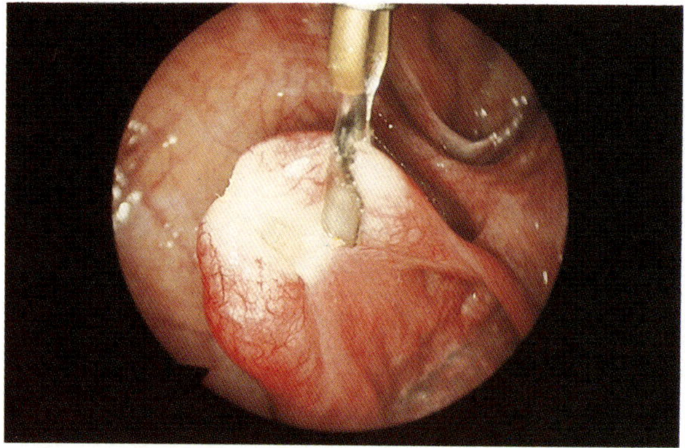

Figure 5.10 Application of bipolar electrocoagulation. The procedure is repeated for the second time at a site just proximal to the first and closer to the uterine cornu.

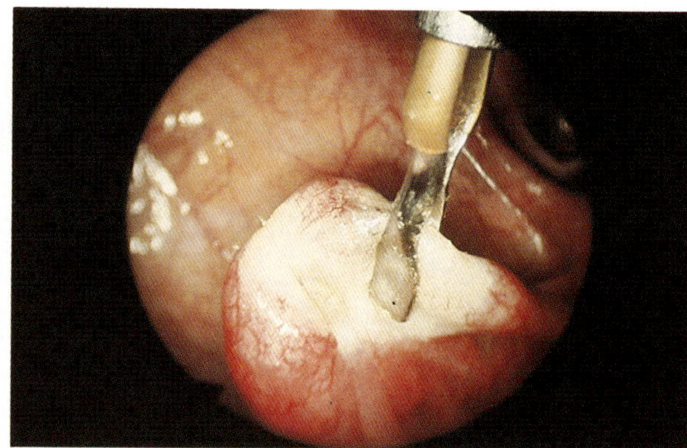

Figure 5.11 Application of bipolar electrocoagulation. The second burn is continued until all electron flow ceases.

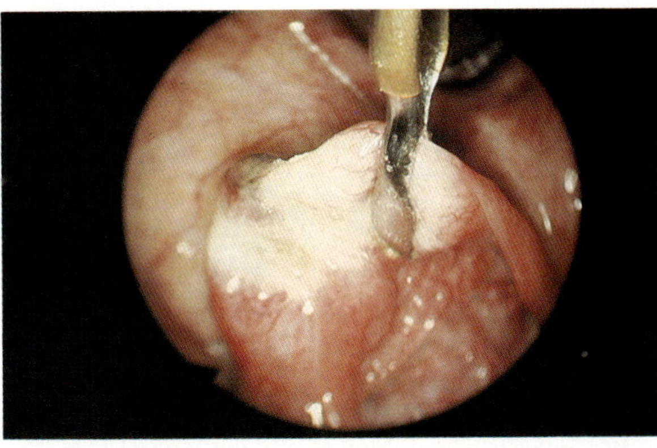

Figure 5.12 Application of bipolar electrocoagulation. The second and third additional cauterizations are placed proximal to the first. This prevents overflowing electrons from travelling distally to any adjacent organ, such as bowel. Instead any excess of electrons will travel in the direction of the uterine cornu.

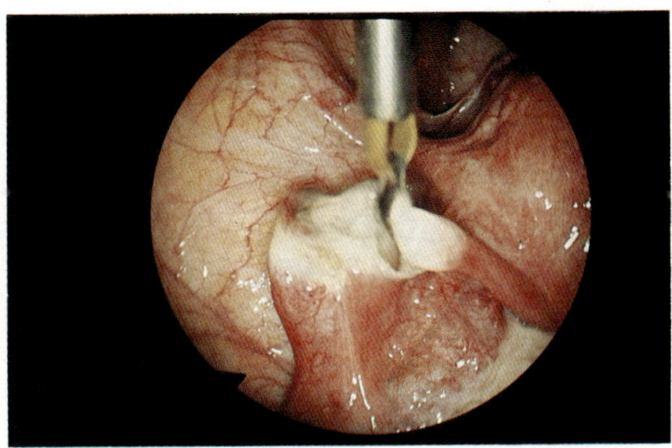

Figure 5.13 Application of bipolar electrocoagulation. The procedure is completed on one side and then repeated on the opposite side.

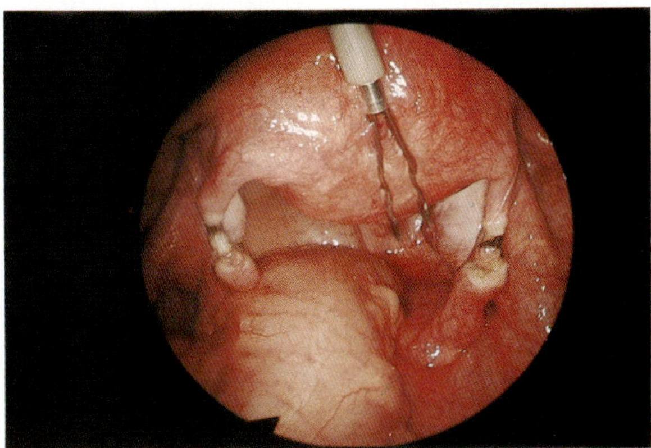

Figure 5.14 Panoramic view of the completed procedure. Areas of adequate tubal cauterization can be seen bilaterally.

Some units come equipped with an electron flow measuring device (ammeter) (Figure 5.15). This gauge is an important safety feature since it measures the amount of current flowing between the forceps tongs. Gradual diminution of electron flow to zero demonstrates maximal resistance and complete coagulation of the tissue grasped by the forceps. This electron flow indicator can also be used prior to the initiation of the procedure to check the integrity of the bipolar circuit. Personally, I prefer to set the bipolar current power to provide a medium flow of electrons (for example, the No. 3 setting on the Wolf generator).

It is recommended that a dispersive electrode be attached to the patient even though it is not required for a procedure with bipolar instruments. This suggestion is a safety precaution in case the bipolar circuit malfunctions. Breakdown of the integrity of the bipolar circuit results in the instrument acting as a unipolar electrocoagulator; thus, it requires a dispersive electrode to retrieve the electrical current applied to the tissues. Complications connected with this sterilization method are detailed in Chapter 22.

The infrequent, but serious complications of translaparoscopic electrocauterization of the fallopian tubes (see Chapter 22) led to the development of nonelectrical methods. Among the nonelectrical techniques designed, the silastic band introduced by Yoon et al in 1974 has gained widespread acceptance.[18] Spring-loaded clips have also been used around the world.[7]

Every one of the aforementioned methods has been promoted by its developers as the safest and simplest to apply. However, experience with each has shown that none of them is completely free of undesirable side effects and complications (see Chapter 22). Knowledge of the indications and limitations of all methods is essential if complications are to be averted.

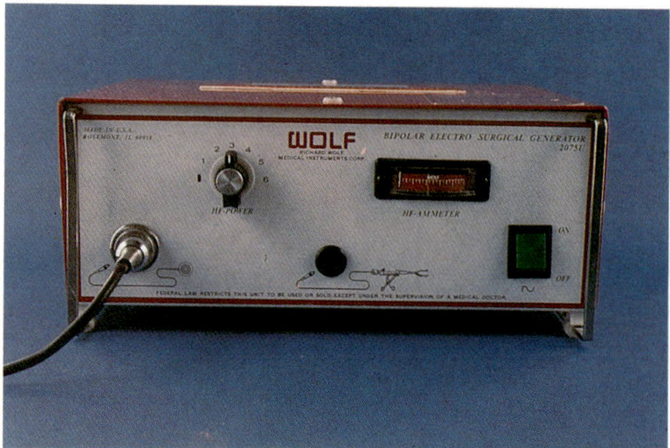

Figure 5.15 Bipolar generator. Visual display of the flow of electrons is depicted by the ammeter at the right upper front face of the instrument. Bipolar current power switch is set at a position that delivers moderate flow (setting No. 3 on this instrument).

TUBAL OCCLUSION WITH SILASTIC BANDS

Since their introduction by Yoon et al in 1974, the silastic band method for tubal occlusion has been adopted worldwide.[18] The method consists of applying an elastic, siliconized ring over a knuckle of the fallopian tube at its midportion. Obstruction of the vascular supply to that segment of the tube results in atrophic fibrosis with interruption of the continuity of tubal lumen.

The method has enjoyed a rapid spread in popularity that is due principally to its simplicity.[9] This was augmented by the concomitant appearance of reports of serious complications associated with the use of unipolar electrocauterization of the tubes. The initial enthusiasm for the use of silicone bands for sterilization was further enhanced by the appreciation of several additional advantages. Decreased operating time, smaller amount of pneumoperitoneum needed, and the feasibility of applying the ring by various routes (transvaginally, via minilaparotomy, and so forth) all contributed to their acceptance. Similar to any other surgical procedure, knowledge of the instruments and the materials required for the procedure facilitates understanding their advantages and limitations.

Silastic Band. The silastic bands are composed of dimethylopolysiloxane impregnated with 5 percent barium sulfate. Roentgenographically, the silicone rings can be identified at the site of application in most cases. The tubal ring has an outer diameter of 3.6 mm and an inner opening of 1 mm. It is 2.2 mm thick and possesses a good elastic memory (Figure 5.16); the ring regains its predistention measurements if not stretched beyond 6 mm or for a prolonged period of time (more than 5 minutes).

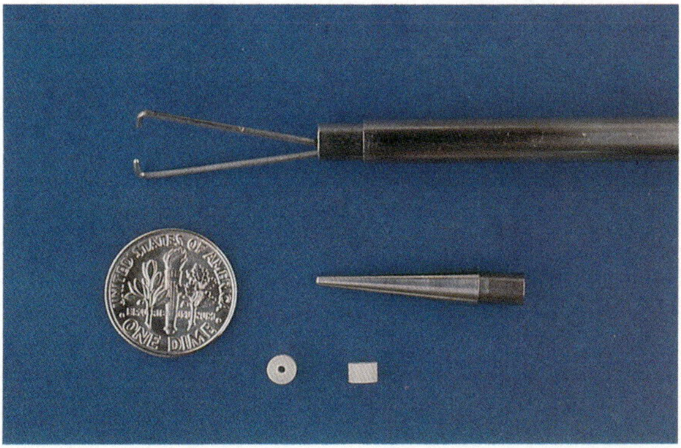

Figure 5.16 Silastic band (lowermost), frontal and lateral views. Intra-abdominal end of the band applicator is also shown with its extended open grasping forceps (uppermost). The conical ring loader appears in the middle with a dime (14 mm) for size comparison.

Ring Applicator. The silastic ring applicator consists of a double-barrelled metal cylinder with central atraumatic grasping forceps. The inner cylinder protrudes approximately 7 mm beyond the end of the outer cylinder. It is over this protrusion that the stretched silastic ring is loaded. The outer cylinder has a spring-like movement that allows it to be displaced down over the inner cylinder; thus it dislodges the stretched ring. The central grasping forceps is in the open position when extruded from the inner cylinder (Figure 5.16). It closes when retracted into the lumen of the cylinder. The grasping tongs withdraw 1 cm into the inner cylinder when completely recessed.

The ring applicator has a special ring loader. This is a conical device with a base diameter of 6 mm, which is equal to the outer diameter of the inner hollow cylinder (Figure 5.16). Its only function is for the gradual stretching of the silastic ring to be loaded onto the applicator. It must be removed before the instrument is inserted into the abdomen.

The Falope ring applicator has a maximal diameter of 7 mm at its stem (Figure 5.17). Because its width is unusual (all other laparoscopic instruments are 5 mm, 8 mm, or 10 mm in diameter), it has its own trocar and sleeve. Caution must be exercised not to interchange trocar sleeves because one that is smaller than 7 mm does not allow the ring applicator to be inserted; a larger sleeve will predispose to gas leakage and loss of pneumoperitoneum.

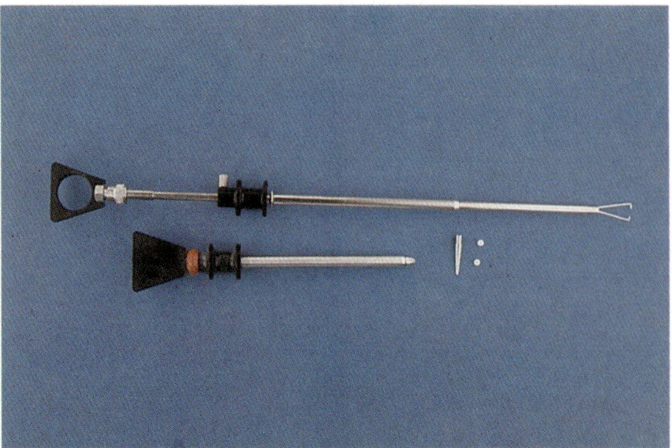

Figure 5.17 Falope ring applicator and special 7 mm accessory puncture trocar. Conical ring loader and a set of silastic bands (lower right) complete the required instrumentation for silastic ring sterilization.

Application of Silastic Ring

Once the laparoscope is in place, the ring applicator sleeve with its corresponding sharp trocar in place is inserted in the midline suprapubically. This midline introduction site allows movement toward either side of the uterus. The unloaded ring applicator, with the forceps tongs withdrawn in a closed position, is introduced into the abdomen. In this manner it can be used as a probe to move the intra-abdominal organs (bowel, omentum) away from the fallopian tubes.

The tubal thickness and any involvement with peritubal adhesions are then evaluated by the operator. If the tube is too thick or immobilized by adhesions, the procedure should not be undertaken. The central forceps of the applicator is extruded and the relative width of the tube measured against the distance between the tong tips. Experienced operators are able to assess the suitability of the tubes for this method by visual inspection of the pelvis.

The ring applicator is then removed from the abdomen for loading of the silastic ring. Following the aforementioned steps reduces the length of time the silastic ring remains in a stretched position. Prolonged stretching may impair the elastic memory of the silastic ring and thereby compromise its occlusive properties.

The tube is grasped at its isthmic portion not less than 3 cm from the cornual insertion. To minimize the width of the tubal loop or knuckle to be formed, only the tube itself should be included between the forceps tongs; the mesosalpinx should be avoided. If only the tube has been grasped, slight tenting of the tube by lifting the applicator upward will reveal an area of blanching. This elevation of the tube also verifies its mobility and lack of restriction by peritubal adhesions (Figures 5.18 to 5.22).

Following verification of the prior step, retraction of the tube into the inner sheath of the ring applicator is undertaken. It should be done slowly and with a steady motion. Elevating the tube into the inner cylinder of the band applicator forms the tubal loop or knuckle. It is essential to perform this maneuver under direct vision. The operator must see the tube advancing up into the instrument's compartment at the same speed as the forceps tongs are being retracted. If doubt exists about the proper formation of the tubal loop, the forceps tongs should be extruded and the prior step repeated as often as required. Indentation at the base of the retracted loop (Figure 5.23) verifies the size of the retracted tubal knuckle.

The entire applicator with the tubal loop in place should be advanced caudally before the silastic band is applied. Application of the Falope ring is done in a single steady motion under direct vision (Figure 5.24). The operator ought to be able to see the silastic band shrinking to its prestretched dimension as the band is extruded past the end of the applicator. This serves to ensure that the band is completely off the inner applicator cylinder (Figure 5.25).

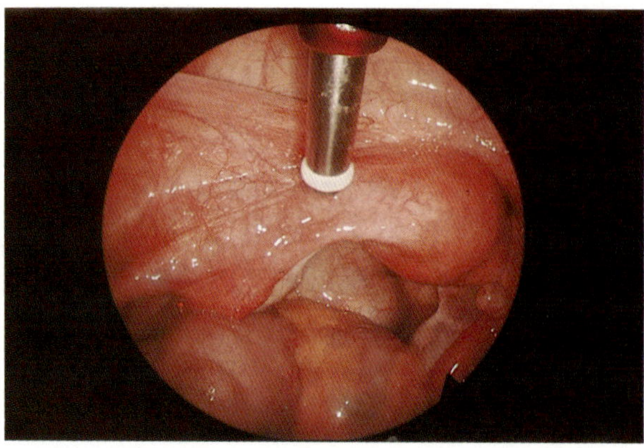

Figure 5.18 Silastic ring sterilization. The auxiliary trocar is in place. Insertion of the trocar in the midline allows movement toward either side of the uterus. A silastic band is in its loaded position. The relative size of the tubes in relation to the distended Falope ring can be appreciated here.

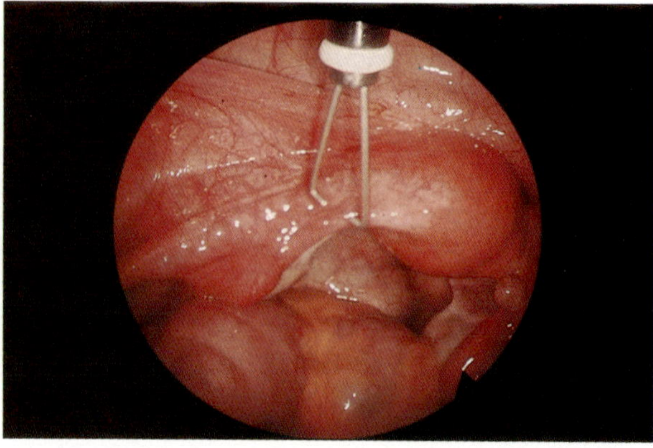

Figure 5.19 With the Falope ring loaded on the outer cylinder, the inner forceps tongs are extended into their open position under direct vision. The tube is grasped at its isthmic portion, no less than 3 cm from the cornual insertion. Relative thickness of the tube can be measured against the distance between the forceps tongs in its open position.

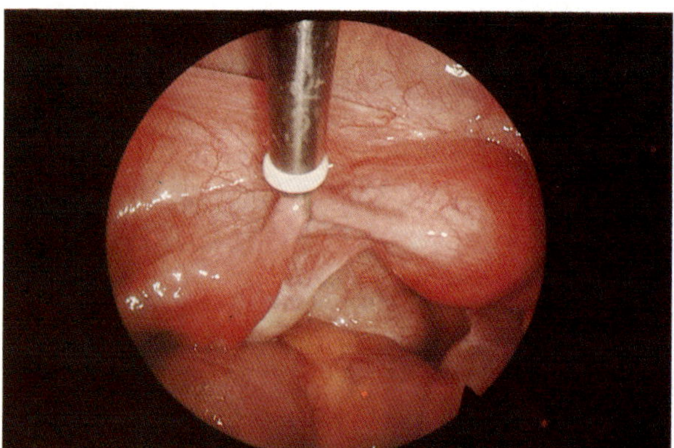

Figure 5.20 To minimize the width of the tubal loop or knuckle that is formed, only the tube should be included between the forceps tongs. Slight tenting of the tube by lifting it upward reveals an area of blanching if only the tube has been grasped.

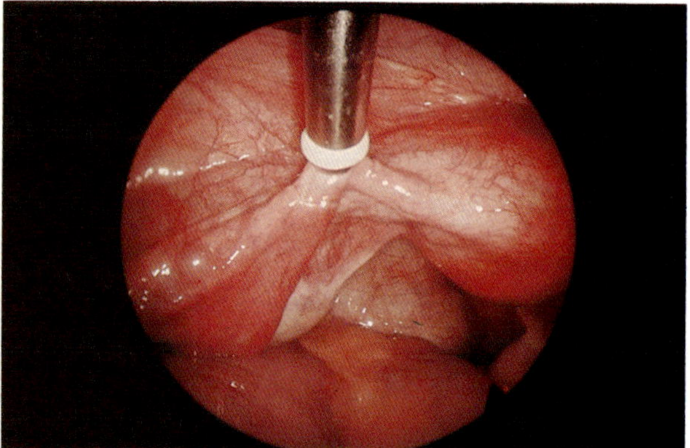

Figure 5.21 Forceps tongs are slowly retracted to elevate the tube. This assures that there are no peritubal adhesions that can limit the normal motility of the tube.

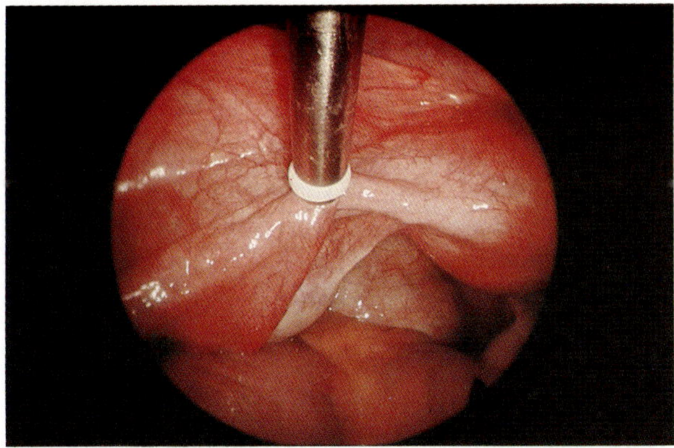

Figure 5.22 Retraction of the tube into the inner sheath of the ring applicator should be done slowly and in a steady motion. The tube is elevated so that it feeds into the inner cylinder of the band applicator under direct vision. The surgeon must see the tube ascending into the instrument's compartment at the same speed as the forceps tongs are being retracted.

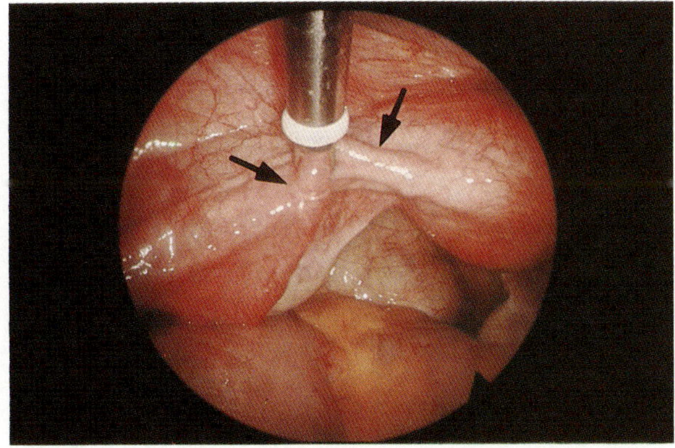

Figure 5.23 The operator must be sure that the entire tubal loop or knuckle is within the inner cylinder. This should be verified prior to the application of the Falope ring to the tube. The prior step may be repeated as often as required if doubt exists about the proper formation of the tubal loop. The indentations left on the tube by the elevation and formation of the tubal loop are important landmarks (arrows).

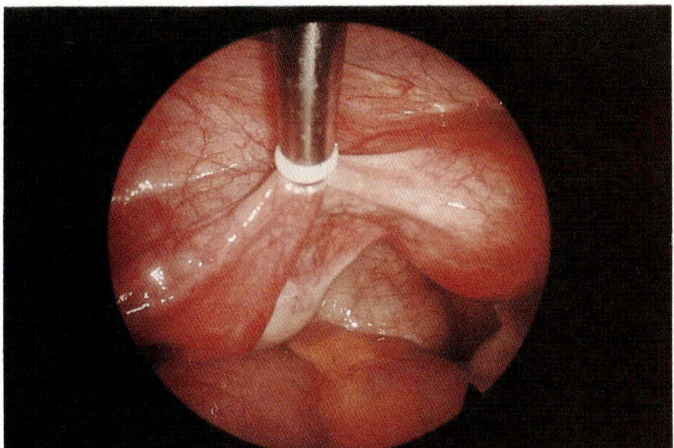

Figure 5.24 The entire applicator with the tubal loop in place should be advanced caudally before the silastic band is applied. Application of the Falope ring is done in a single steady motion under direct vision. The operator should be able to see the silastic band shrinking back to its prestretched dimension.

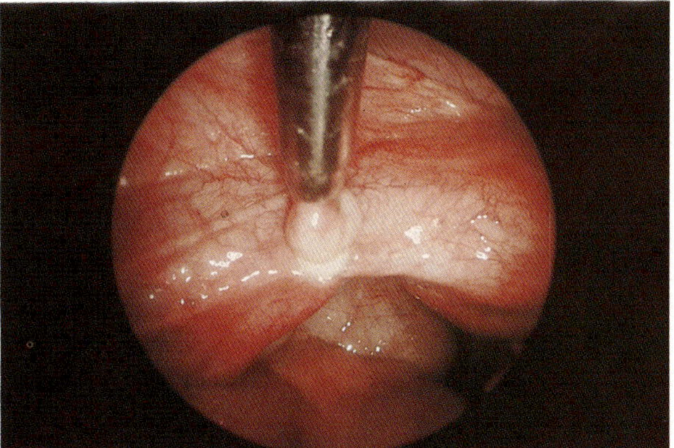

Figure 5.25 Release of the recently formed tubal knuckle should be accomplished in a slow and uniformly steady fashion. Integrity of the tubal knuckle can be appreciated immediately upon extrusion of the tubal loop from the inner cylinder of the applicator.

Release of the recently formed tubal knuckle should be accomplished in a slow and uniformly steady fashion. Integrity of the tubal knuckle can be appreciated immediately upon extrusion of the tubal loop from the inner sheath of the applicator. Release of the forceps tongs is accomplished by a lateral motion freeing up one tong at a time (Figures 5.26 and 5.27). The procedure is then repeated on the contralateral tube (Figure 5.28).

The silastic ring produces vascular obstruction at the base of the tubal knuckle. Evidence of blanching of the tubal loop is progressive and becomes more pronounced within the next few minutes after the application of the silastic band. This blanching confirms that the ring has been properly placed (Figure 5.29). Blanching of both tubal knuckles should be observed before the procedure is terminated. Complete devascularization of the tubal loop is shown by the fact that surgical incision of the tubal loop can be done without evidence of bleeding from the cut edges.

The ischemic tubal knuckles, which result from the application of silastic rings, undergo fibrinoid degeneration. Anatomic and histologic damage to the fallopian tube is limited to the portion of salpinx included in the original devascularized loop. Laparoscopic evaluation at 1 month has shown the occluded ends of the tube separated by a fibrotic band (Figure 5.30). The silastic ring is usually covered by a layer of fibrin (Figure 5.31). Occasionally, it is possible to see that, although the occluded tubal ends are separated by the aforementioned fibrotic band, the tubal knuckle remains intact. This is believed to result as a consequence of neovascularization developed from the adjacent tissues (Figure 5.32).

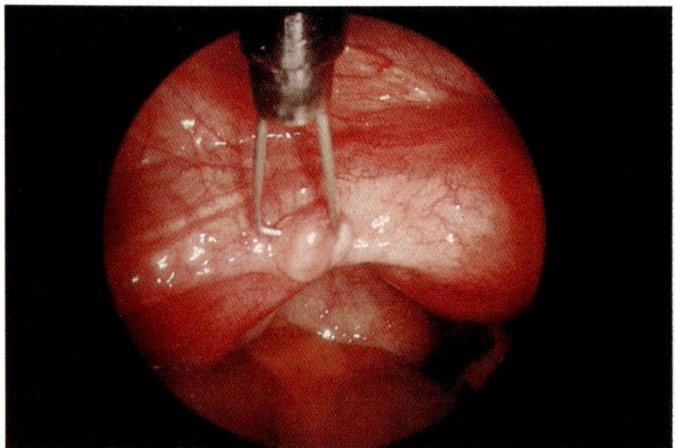

Figure 5.26 The forceps tongs are completely extended. Formation of a tubal loop may have enlarged the tubal dimension, preventing spontaneous release of the forceps tongs. Release of the forceps tongs is accomplished by a lateral motion.

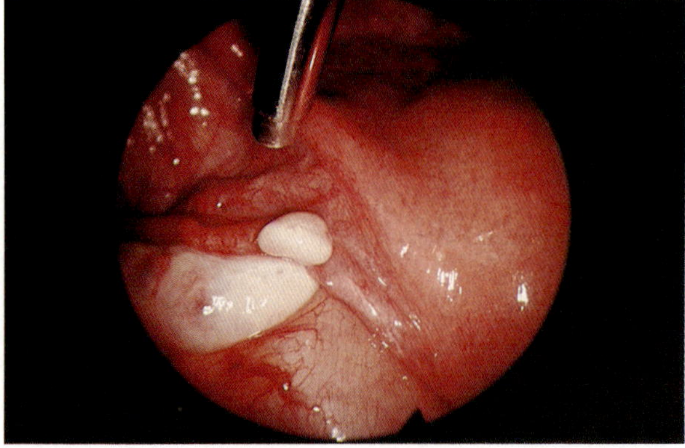

Figure 5.27 The Falope ring applicator can be used as a probe to mobilize pelvic structures. This facilitates exploration to confirm the proper location of the silicone band. To avoid accidental damage to any abdominopelvic structure, the forceps tongs should always be withdrawn into the inner cylinder of the ring applicator in the closed position.

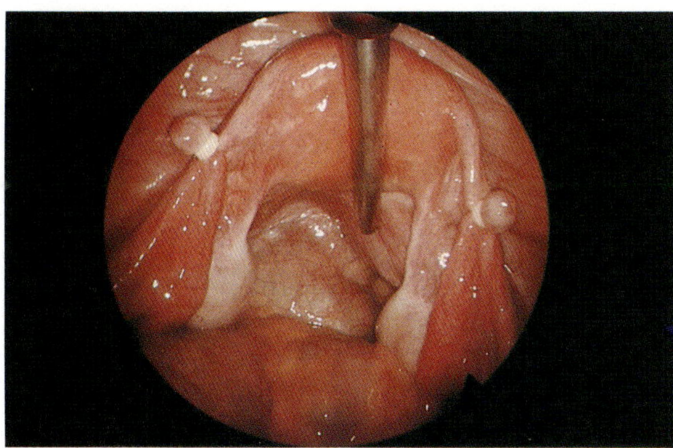

Figure 5.28 Panoramic view of the pelvis after the procedure has been completed and both Falope rings have been applied.

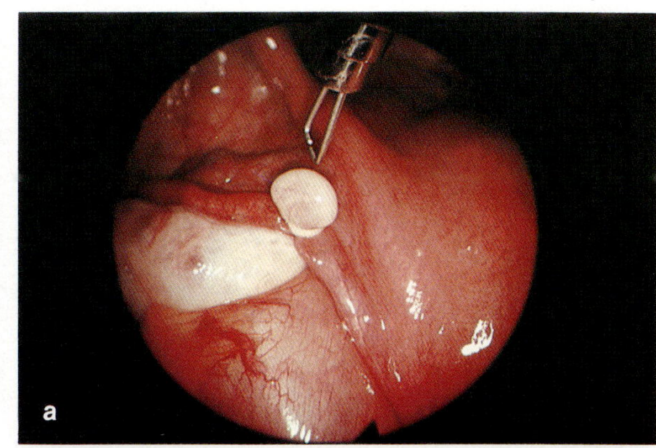

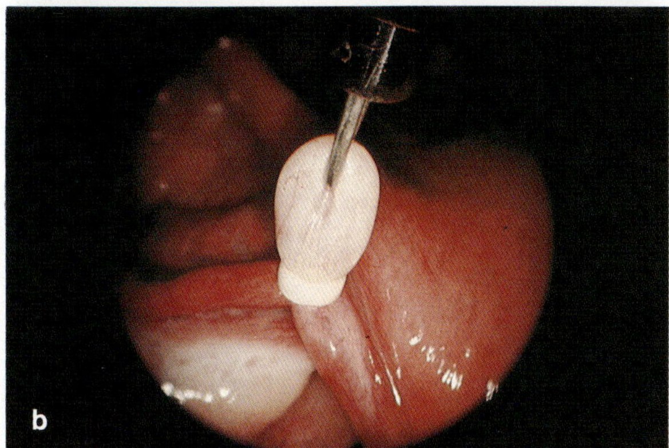

Figure 5.29 Evidence of blanching of the tubal knuckle can be seen one minute after the application of the silastic band. *a*. This blanching confirms that the Falope ring has been properly placed. It reflects complete vascular occlusion to that portion of the fallopian tube. *b*. The ring applicator can be used to help confirm both the proper location of the silastic band and the blanching of the tubal loop.

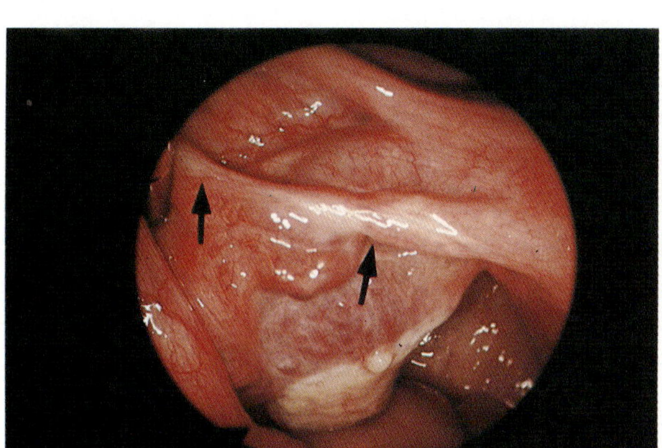

Figure 5.30 Laparoscopic evaluation of a patient who previously underwent a laparoscopic silastic ring sterilization. Anatomic and histologic damage is limited to the portion of tube included in the original loop. The proximal (right) and distal (left) obstructed ends of the remaining portions of the tube have separated (arrows).

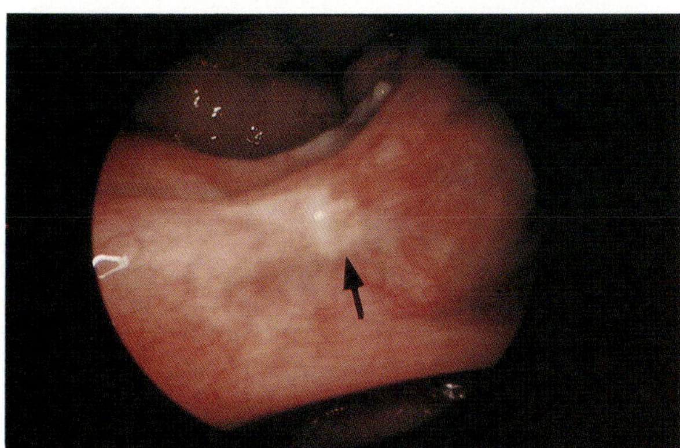

Figure 5.31 The silastic ring is usually found between the separated tubal segments covered by filmy adhesions (arrow). These filmy adhesions are composed of celomic serosal epithelium and may also reveal some muscularis.

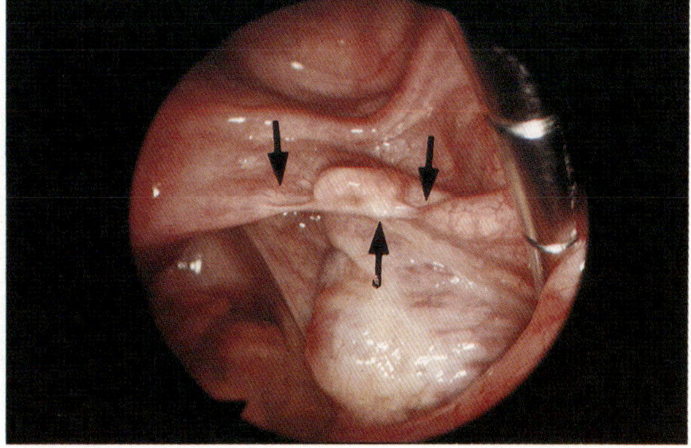

Figure 5.32 Tubal knuckle can occasionally be found intact. The occluded ends of the tubal segments (lateral arrows) are attached to the loop by fibrotic bands. Serosa covers the silastic ring (center arrow).

In patients undergoing this operation under local anesthesia, pain associated with silastic band sterilization has been reported to occur at the time of surgery. This pain is the result of manipulation of the sensitive peritoneum covering the fallopian tube. Any sudden motion of the tube while it is being held by the forceps tongs increases the discomfort. Peritubal adhesions that limit the free movement of the tube are also associated with more pain than ordinarily expected at the time of silastic band application.

Diminution of intraoperative pain during Falope ring sterilization can be accomplished by topically applying a local anesthetic agent to the portion of tube to be operated.[13] Direct injection into the tubal wall is contraindicated because swelling of the tube will make it impossible to form a suitable knuckle over which the band can be applied. More often, the so-called dry technique is used; in this procedure 4 percent lidocaine is dripped over the segment of tube to be grasped by the forceps tongs. A similar anesthetic effect has been reported to be obtained by submerging the operative end of the applicator in 2 percent lidocaine jelly. Whichever method of local tubal anesthesia is used, pain can be minimized by applying the silastic rings in a slow and uniformly steady fashion.

Postoperative pain lasting for 24 to 48 hours is common in patients sterilized with Falope rings irrespective of the type of anesthesia used for the procedure itself.[1] Levinson reported that 35 percent of patients operated by this method experienced marked to severe postoperative pain requiring strong narcotics for relief.[10] Because pain related to this surgical procedure is considered a complication of the technique, the reader is referred to Chapter 22 for a more in-depth discussion of the subject.

TUBAL OCCLUSION USING CLIPS

Attempts to simplify female sterilization gave rise to the use of clips for tubal occlusion. Rigid tantalum clips, similar to those employed to control bleeding during surgical procedures, were first employed.[5] Failure to completely obliterate the tubal lumen resulted in a high rate of poststerilization pregnancies.

In 1973, Hulka et al first reported the use of a spring-loaded clip for human sterilization.[6] Prior studies in pigs verified the adequacy of tubal occlusion achieved with this type of clip. Additionally, the limited destruction produced by the application of this device suggested that reanastomosis with reestablishment of tubal patency was likely to be feasible.

Technical difficulties with the application of the original design of spring-loaded clips led to subsequent modifications of both applicator and clip. A description of the applicator and clips in current use facilitates understanding of their advantages and limitations. A step-by-step description of the technique follows.

Spring-loaded Clip. The spring-loaded clip consists of two plastic jaws united by a metal pin on one end. The inner surface of the jaws contains opposing lined teeth; when apposed the teeth anchor into the grasped tube preventing displacement of the clip. A gold-plated, stainless steel spring holds the clip jaws in an open position. This metal spring when pushed over the plastic jaws closely approximates them over the tissue being held. The plastic jaws cannot be opened after the gold-plated spring has closed them (Figure 5.33). Spring-loaded clips come packaged in pairs in the open position.

In its closed position, the spring-loaded clip measures 1.1 cm in length and 3 × 4 mm in cross-sectional diameter. The inner surface of the plastic jaws measures 7 mm. This restricts its application to fallopian tubes of less than 7 mm in width.

Clip Applicator. The original applicator, designed by Hulka and Clemens, was a single puncture applicator with fixed optics. Its large size (12 mm) and restricted movement were its main disadvantages.

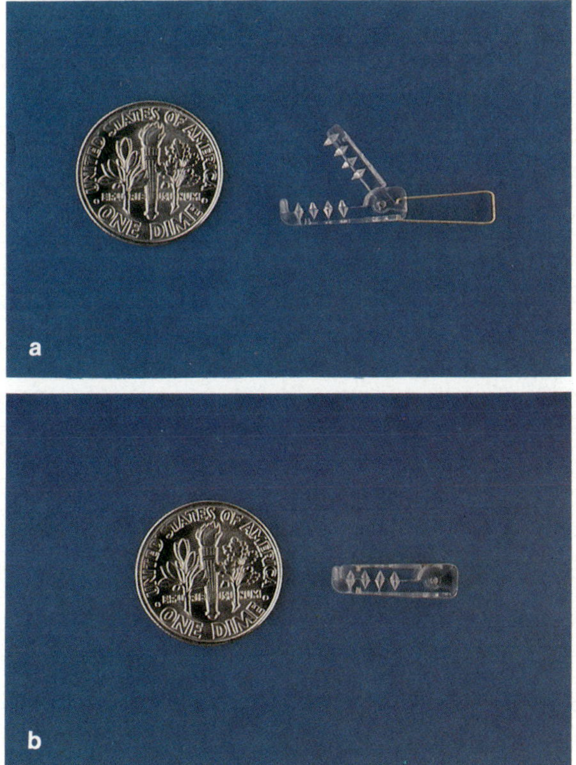

Figure 5.33 Spring-loaded clips. *a*. Clip in the open position. *b*. Closed clip with gold-plated spring holding its jaws together. Dime (14 mm) is shown for size comparison.

The two-puncture applicator (Figure 5.34) is favored at the present time. It contains interlocking springs designed to accomplish loading, application, and dislodgement of the clip with a single set of manipulations. Mastering the complex sequence of movements ought to be accomplished in the laboratory prior to using this technique in the operating room.

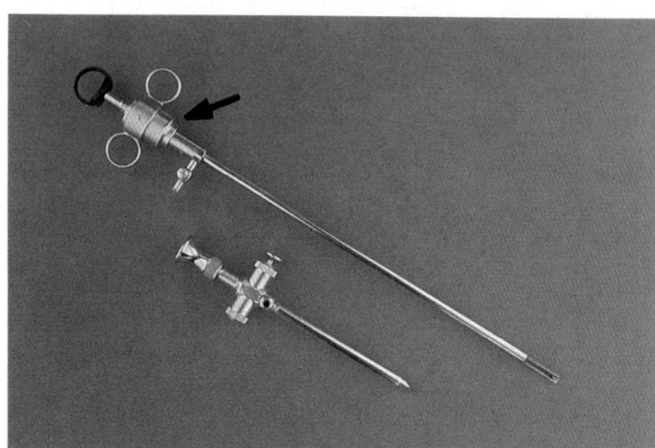

Figure 5.34 Two-puncture spring-loaded clip applicator. Instrument has a chamber (arrow) containing the interlocking springs designed to accomplish loading, application, and dislodgement of the clip in a single set of manipulations.

Spring-Loaded Clip Application

Under direct laparoscopic visualization, the applicator sleeve and trocar are inserted (Figure 5.35). The spring-loaded clip, which is placed onto the applicator in its open position, must have its plastic jaws approximated to traverse the applicator sleeve. Caution should be exercised not to push the gold-plated spring over the jaws (Figure 5.36). The plastic jaws are opened once the applicator is beyond the lower edge of the applicator sleeve. This step must be carried out under direct vision to prevent accidental release of the spring-loaded clip. The relative size of the tubes should be compared with the size of the clip's open jaws (Figure 5.37).

The tube is hooked at its isthmic segment onto the posterior jaw of the clip. Tenting of the mesosalpinx pushed up by the inferior end of the applicator confirms that the tube is well within the occlusive portion of the plastic jaws (Figure 5.38). The plastic jaws can be gently closed to assess tubal occlusion (Figure 5.39). This step may be repeated as often as required if doubt exists about proper placement of the clip.

Only after proper placement of the spring-loaded clip has been verified may the gold-plated spring be pushed down over the plastic jaws (Figure 5.40). This step should be accomplished in a slow and uniformly steady motion. The applicator must remain stable. Movements are triggered by pressing and releasing the thumb rod located at the operator's end of the applicator.

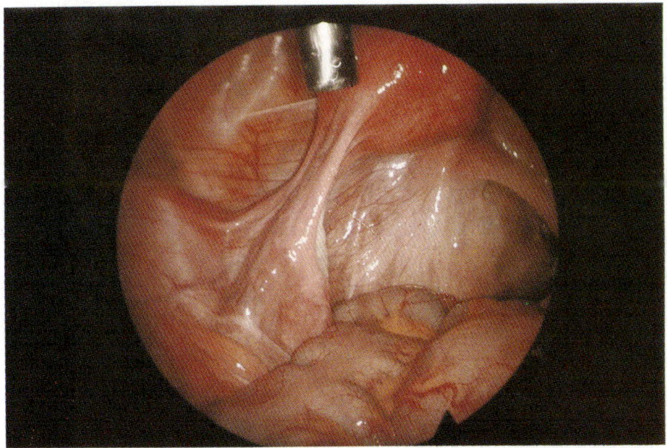

Figure 5.35 Spring-loaded clip applicator entering the abdominal cavity. The plastic jaws of the clip are apposed (but not locked) in order to traverse the applicator sleeve.

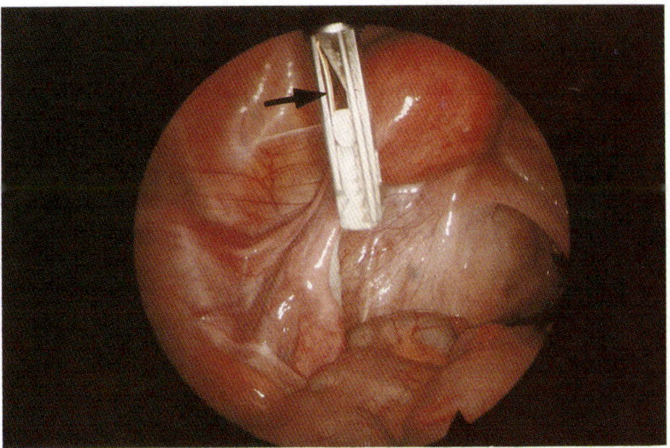

Figure 5.36 When closing the plastic clip for introduction into the abdominal cavity or to test its applicability to a particular tube, caution should be exercised not to push the gold-plated spring over the jaws. This would lock the clip permanently. The extended (open) gold-plated spring is shown (arrow).

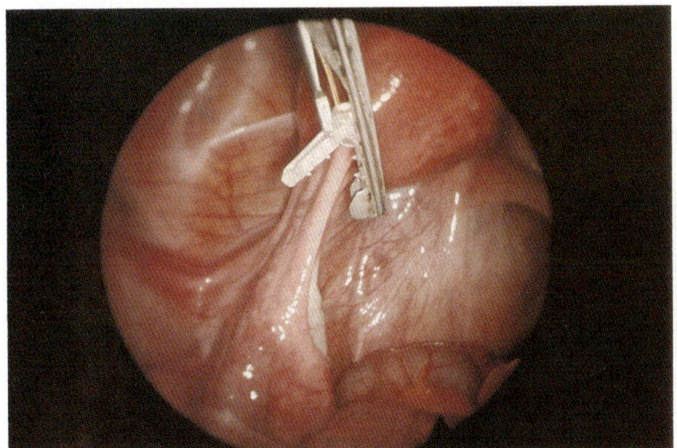

Figure 5.37 Once in the abdomen, the plastic jaws are opened in order to assess their suitability for that particular tube. The tube must be completely covered by the plastic jaws when in their closed position. Selection of the appropriate site of application of the clip to the tube is carried out.

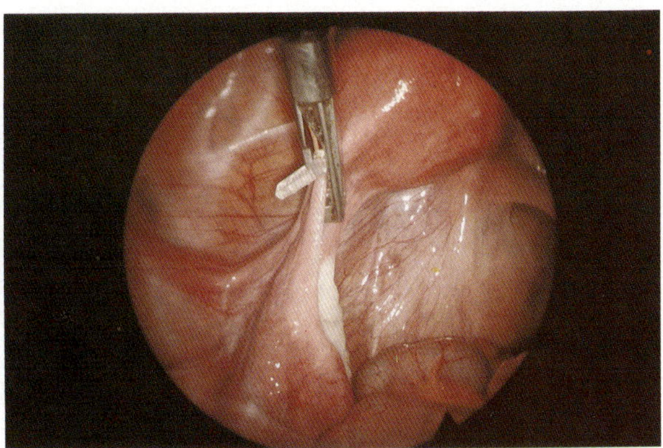

Figure 5.38 The fallopian tube is hooked at its isthmic portion onto the posterior jaw of the clip. Tenting of the mesosalpinx pushed up by the inferior end of the applicator confirms the proper positioning of the instrument.

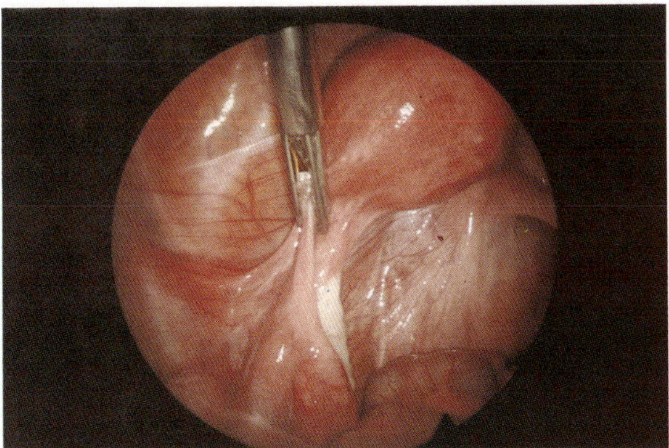

Figure 5.39 The plastic jaws are gently approximated to assess the degree of tubal occlusion. Before proceeding, the operator must be sure that the entire thickness of the fallopian tube will be covered by the clip. The prior step may be repeated as often as required if there is any doubt about the proper occlusion of the tube.

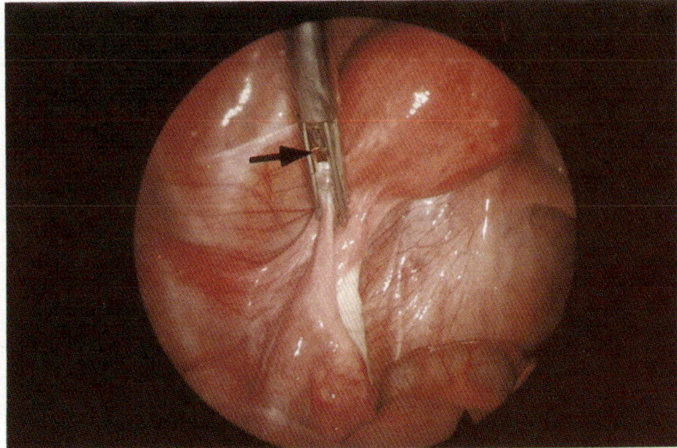

Figure 5.40 Only after correct placement of the clip has been clearly verified may the spring be pushed down over the plastic jaws to lock them in place. The center rod of the applicator (arrow) pushes the gold-plated spring down.

With the clip locked into place, the central thumb rod is slowly withdrawn under direct vision. Only when the anterior rod is entirely withdrawn into the applicator stem is the clip unrestricted (Figure 5.41). Complete release of the applied clip is achieved by pivoting the applicator tip posteriorly (Figure 5.42). Release of the clip must take place gently to prevent dislodging the clip from the tube. Complete obliteration of the fallopian tube must then be visually verified (Figure 5.43). If one is not satisfied with the clip application, a second clip may be placed adjacent to the first one. A similar procedure is repeated on the contralateral tube (Figure 5.44).

Spring-loaded clip sterilization lends itself to translaparoscopic technique under local anesthesia. Analogous to the silastic band procedure, the woman experiences pain when the clip is closed on the tube. Lidocaine 4 percent sprayed on the tubes or lidocaine gel placed topically on their surface reduces the intraoperative discomfort considerably. The incidence of postoperative pain following clip application is also the same as in patients sterilized by Falope rings.

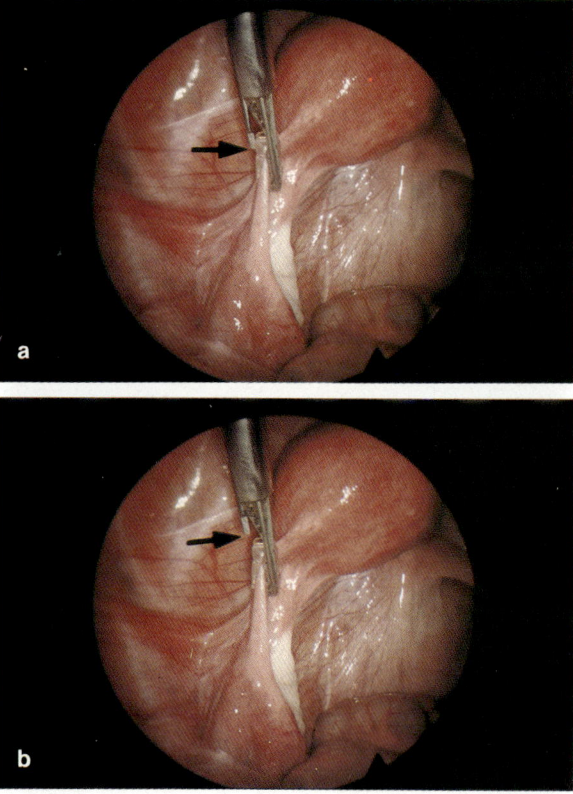

Figure 5.41 Withdrawing applicator. The spring completely covers the clip's plastic jaws. The clip is locked in place. *a*. The anterior rod of the applicator which was holding the clip loaded in place is retracted (arrow). *b*. The anterior rod is completely withdrawn. This frees the clip. The final position of the anterior rod is shown (arrow) before release of the clip is attempted.

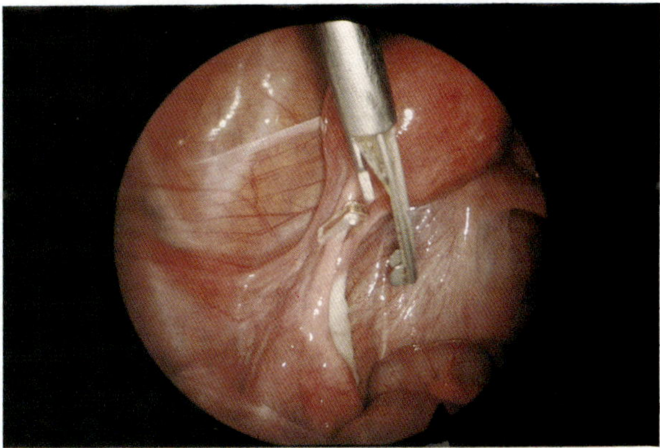

Figure 5.42 Release of the locked clip is achieved by pivoting the front end of the applicator posteriorly.

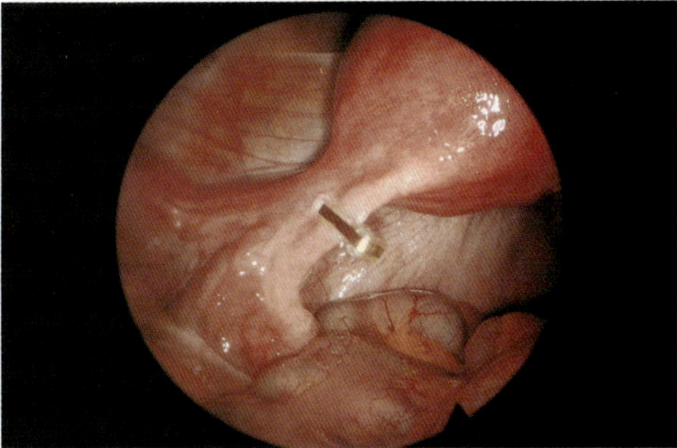

Figure 5.43 Spring-loaded clip locked in place. The entire width of the fallopian tube is seen collapsed between the plastic jaws of the clip.

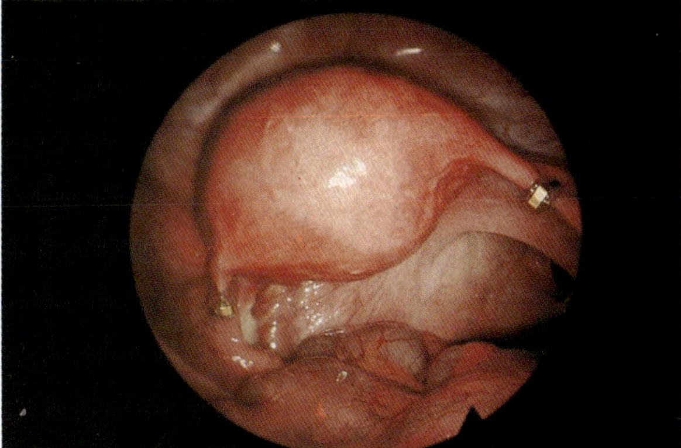

Figure 5.44 Panoramic view of the pelvis after the procedure has been completed with both spring-loaded clips seen in place. If the operator is not satisfied with either clip application, a second clip may be placed adjacent to the first one. No attempt should be made to remove a clip already locked into place translaparoscopically.

THERMAL CAUTERY

Translaparoscopic thermal cauterization of the fallopian tubes was developed as an alternative to tubal electrocoagulation. This method utilized a low voltage rechargeable battery to produce heat. The heat is transmitted through a Teflon coated wire to a disposable metal hook inserted into the abdomen through a secondary puncture. The tube is grasped 3 to 4 cm from its cornual implantation. The hook is heated to 300 ° to 400 °F which cauterizes the tube.

Gunning et al performed thermal sterilization in 393 women.[4] They reported no major complications in their series. In 10 patients without tubal pathology undergoing hysterectomy, they compared thermal coagulation of one tube with unipolar electrocoagulation of the contralateral side. Pathologic evaluation of the specimen revealed the mean total gross burn produced by the two methods was not significantly different.

To the present time, thermal cauterization of the fallopian tubes has not gained widespread acceptance. The low rate of reported complications is encouraging. Further evaluation is required to establish its potential.

STERILIZATION REVERSAL

Improvements in safety and availability of sterilization coupled with sociologic changes (increase in divorce and remarriage rates) underlie the increased demand for procedures to reverse tubal sterilization. A detailed discussion of the work-up and techniques used to accomplish this goal is beyond the intent or scope of this book. Nevertheless, because there seems to be a direct relationship between the method and the quality of the sterilization performed and the successful outcome of tubal occlusion reversals, it deserves some consideration.[15,16] Among the factors determining the success or failure of sterilization reversal procedures, the type of tubal sterilization and available length of viable tube left appear to be most important.

Type of Sterilization. As they were introduced, methods of laparoscopic sterilization were judged by their rate of efficacy in preventing conception. Success rates for tubal occlusion with electrical instruments (unipolar, bipolar) were found to be in direct proportion to the degree of tubal destruction. Thus, the greater the damage to the tubes, the better the procedure was deemed to be. A similar principle applied to the silastic bands.

Requests to restore fertility coupled with new microsurgical techniques encouraged consideration of tubal reanastomosis operations. It soon became evident that the results with some types of sterilization were more amenable to tubal reconstruction than those with other procedures. The reanastomosis success rate proved to be inversely proportional to the degree of tubal damage.

Destruction of tubal architecture was greater with electrical sterilization methods than with mechanical ones.

Lesions encountered as a result of tubal damage include flattening of the mucosal folds, deciliation of the endosalpinx, and formation of mucosal polyps.[17] Some of these changes are not evident until 3 years or more after the sterilization procedure. Tubes extirpated immediately following tubal electrocauterization showed endosalpingeal destruction greater than can be appreciated translaparoscopically by the unaided eye.[12]

By contrast, tubal damage as a result of mechanical tubal occlusion is usually limited to the site of tubal obliteration. Silastic bands tend to obliterate 3.0 to 3.5 cm of salpinx. The smallest extent of tubal destruction is seen with the spring-loaded clips. Injury to the tube as a consequence of clip occlusion is no greater than 5 to 6 mm. An additional advantage offered by clip sterilization is the minimal damage it produces in the mesosalpinx and the blood supply to the remaining portions of the tube. Preservation of the mesosalpingeal vasculature increases the probability of healing of the reanastomosis.

Although sterilization procedures must still be considered a permanent method of contraception, their potential reversibility ought to play an important role when counseling a woman for this procedure. Of special importance in this regard are young and low parity women (vide supra). The choice of mechanical versus electrical methods of sterilization has to be considered in these cases.[11]

References

1. Cognat MA, Audebert A, Larue-Charlus S, Barakat S. Poststerilization pain: A comparison of band versus clip. J Reprod Med 1980; 25:29-30.
2. Engle T. Laparoscopic sterilization: Electrosurgery or clip application? J Reprod Med 1978; 21:107-110.
3. Gonzales BL. Counseling for sterilization. J Reprod Med 1981; 26:538-540.
4. Gunning JE, Tomasulo JP, Garite T. Laparoscopic tubal sterilization using thermal coagulation. Obstet Gynecol 1979; 54:505-509.
5. Haskins AL. Oviductal sterilization with tantalum clips. Am J Obstet Gynecol 1972; 114:370-377.
6. Hulka JF, Fishburne JI, Mercer JP, Omran K. Laparoscopic sterilization with a spring clip: A report of the first fifty cases. Am J Obstet Gynecol 1973; 116:715-718.
7. Hulka JF, Omran K, Lieberman BA, Gordon AG. Laparoscopic sterilization with the spring clip: Instrumentation development and current clinical experience. Am J Obstet Gynecol 1979; 135:1016-1020.
8. Kleppinger RK. Ancillary uses of bipolar forceps. J Reprod Med 1977; 18:254-256.
9. Kumarasamy T, Hurt WG. Laparoscopic sterilization with silicone rubber bands. Obstet Gynecol 1977; 50:351-358.
10. Levinson DJ, Daily HI, Marko MW, Richardson DC. Nonelectric laparoscopic sterilization: Experience with a silastic band. Obstet Gynecol 1975; 48:494-496.
11. Lindenmayer JP, Steinberg MD, Bjork DA, Pardes H. Psychiatric aspects of voluntary sterilization in young, childless women. J Reprod Med 1977; 19:87-91.
12. Malhotra RP, Cera PJ, Bates JS. Evaluation of the fallopian tube section obtained at laparoscopic fulguration. J Reprod Med 1977; 18:38-40.
13. Pelland PC. The application of lidocaine to the fallopian tubes during tubal fulguration by laparoscopy. Obstet Gynecol 1976; 47:501-502.
14. Phillips JM, Hunka JF, Hunka B, Corson SL. 1979 AAGL membership survey. J Reprod Med 1981; 26:529-533.
15. Rock JA, Bergquist CA, Zacur HA, et al. Tubal anastomosis following unipolar cautery. Fertil Steril 1982; 37:613-618.

16. Seiler JC. Factors influencing the outcome of microsurgical tubal ligation reversals. Am J Obstet Gynecol 1983; 146:292-298.
17. Vasquez G, Winston RML, Boeckx W, Brosens I. Tubal lesions subsequent to sterilization and their relation to fertility after attempts at reversal. Am J Obstet Gynecol 1980; 138:86-92.
18. Yoon IB, Wheeless CR, King TM. A preliminary report on a new laparoscopic sterilization approach: The silicone rubber band technique. Am J Obstet Gynecol 1974; 120:132-136.

6 CONTRAINDICATIONS

Just as with any other elective surgical procedure, there are a number of contraindications to laparoscopy. These can be classified as either absolute or relative. Over the years, as extensive experience has been accumulated, some of the earlier absolute proscriptions against performing a laparoscopic procedure have become less constraining and are now being left up to the discretion of the operating surgeon. Furthermore, the development of the open technique for laparoscopy allows us to take advantage of the endoscopic aspects of this method while averting contraindications based on hazards attributed to the blind insertion of the Verres needle or the sharp laparoscopic trocar.

Analogous to principles applicable to other fields of clinical medicine, a relative contraindication in one patient may be an absolute one in another. Thus, each patient must be evaluated on an individual basis. When feasible, modifications in the routine laparoscopic operative technique may be introduced to suit a particular patient. For example, one can consider creating less abdominal distention by reducing gas insufflation in a patient with compromised respiratory function or utilizing a smaller degree of Trendelenburg tilt; sometimes one may have to resort to local anesthesia when general anesthesia is not suitable. These are some of the many variations that could permit one to perform a laparoscopy in a patient who might otherwise have been denied the benefits of the procedure.

ABSOLUTE CONTRAINDICATIONS

As the term implies, absolute contraindications are those circumstances in which a laparoscopic procedure is so likely to expose the patient to a serious complication that it should never be undertaken. Just as with any other diagnostic or therapeutic procedure, when the anticipated risks are greater than the benefits that can be expected to be derived from its use, it should not be utilized. Laparoscopy is not an exception to this valuable rule.

Contraindications to laparoscopy relate either to the patient's inability to tolerate the procedure or to the inherent technical risk of the method vis-à-vis some local intra-abdominal condition. An example of the former is the patient who suffers from hypovolemic shock in whom laparoscopy is likely to magnify the cardiovascular instability and thereby constitute a life-threatening hazard. Abdominal enlargement due to intestinal distention is the type of condition that seriously increases technical risks.

Patient Condition. An essential component of the laparoscopic technique is the need to create a pneumoperitoneum. As will be described in detail in Chapters 9 and 10, insufflation of gas into the abdominal cavity results in marked circulatory and respiratory changes. Such disturbances of the homeostatic mechanism, albeit well tolerated by the young, healthy, and stable subject, may cause cardiovascular decompensation in a patient with a preexisting circulatory or respiratory deficit.

Technical Difficulties. Abdominal distention resulting from paralytic ileus poses a technical problem. One is generally unable to distend the abdomen further to achieve a pneumoperitoneum. This may prove an insoluble dilemma. The situation is quite different from that of the patient with ascites in whom paracentesis for evacuation of the ascitic fluid makes room for the insufflating gas. Distended bowel from a paralytic ileus cannot be decompressed to provide space for the pneumoperitoneum. Hence, the overdistended loops of bowel may be injured; moreover, they obstruct the endoscopist's view, a constraint which is not easily overcome.

Hypovolemic Shock

The need to confirm the presence of a hemoperitoneum by laparoscopy prior to exploratory laparotomy is still controversial. Some gynecologists maintain that finding free, noncoagulable intraperitoneal blood by means of paracentesis or culdocentesis is sufficient information to permit one to proceed with an exploratory laparotomy for the purposes of identifying and treating the source of hemorrhage. To the contrary, those who advocate performing a diagnostic laparoscopy prior to laparotomy claim that the bleeding site can sometimes be identified (e.g., a hemorrhagic corpus luteum) and treated translaparoscopically for effective hemostasis. They feel they can thereby avoid laparotomy.

Cardiovascular changes occurring as a consequence of a laparoscopy (as will be described in detail in Chapter 9) are not without clinical significance. Altered venous return, cardiac output, heart rate, and blood pressure are easily compensated for in the young, healthy patient and thus go unnoticed most of the time. Such is not the case in a subject in whom there is a preexistent underlying circulatory derangement that results from an intra-abdominal hemorrhagic diathesis.

Pelvic laparoscopy requires the patient to be placed in the Trendelenburg position to facilitate visualization of the pelvic organs. This head-down position, previously thought to aid perfusion of vital organs (heart, brain) is now known to have adverse effects when used for treating patients in shock.[10] The initial increase in blood pressure, mainly due to the autoinfusion of blood from the lower extremities, rapidly drops, further compounding the peripheral circulatory failure. Rather than lowering the patient's head, adequate fluid repletion of the intravascular compartment is preferred.

The pneumoperitoneum required for a laparoscopic procedure raises the intra-abominal pressure. The increase in intraperitoneal pressure is paralleled by a proportional elevation in venous resistance secondary to compression of the inferior vena cava. This in turn may be reflected by a decrease in central venous return. The already compromised circulatory system of a patient with intra-abdominal bleeding will thus be aggravated.

The changes in cardiac output that occur during laparoscopy have been studied mainly in young healthy subjects (see Chapter 9). Cardiac output can fall to 60 percent of its baseline value due to the increase in intra-abdominal pressure and still be compensated for by the patient's own homeostatic mechanism. Adequate compensatory effects are reflected in the absence of any dramatic alteration in blood pressure, pulse rate, or peripheral circulation. This is not the case when hypovolemia is present. Using dogs rendered hypovolemic and anesthetized with halothane, Ivankovich et al showed that gradual increments in intra-abdominal pressure accentuated the hemodynamic disequilibrium, further predisposing to shock.[6]

During a laparoscopic procedure, the heart rate increases concomitantly with the insufflation of gas. Increased peripheral resistance results in elevation of blood pressure. This additional stimulus increases the heart rate.[9] In the hypovolemic patient, who is already tachycardic (because she is attempting to compensate for the circulatory deficit), any further increase in heart rate may trigger a still more serious circulatory imbalance as a consequence of cardiac arrhythmia.

Cardiac arrhythmias in patients undergoing laparoscopy are generally benign in nature and consist usually of ventricular extrasystoles.[8] There is an increased susceptibility to develop arrhythmias among hypovolemic-hypotensive patients with a central circulatory deficit, and this may be further aggravated by superimposing the burden of a laparoscopic procedure.

Young patients have great capacity to effect peripheral vasoconstriction. This permits them to sustain a normal or near normal blood pressure and pulse in the face of substantial intra-abdominal bleeding. Therefore, it is not possible to correlate the amount of blood loss with the clinical condition in these patients. Furthermore, when systemic responses such as hypotension or tachycardia are finally elicited, it should be clear that the compensatory mechanisms have been exhausted, thereby indicating a marked degree of hemodynamic disruption. These patients require stabilization of their hemodynamic status before laparoscopy can be attempted. Failure of the patient to respond to such stabilizing therapy absolutely contraindicates the use of laparoscopy.

Septic Peritonitis

Until recently, the performance of a laparoscopy in a patient with peritonitis was discouraged. It was thought teleologically that the inflammatory reaction was the peritoneum's attempt to circumscribe and combat the noxious agent. Abdominal distention produced by the pneumoperitoneum was believed to break down the protective peritoneal barrier, thereby facilitating intra-abdominal and systemic dissemination of the infectious process. A more thorough understanding of the pathophysiology of the peritoneal reaction to infection has modified our thinking in this regard. We now know that inflammation of the peritoneal layer can be localized or diffuse.

A localized peritonitis is usually limited to the peritoneum in close proximity to an inflamed organ (e.g., appendix or gallbladder) or circumscribed to a well defined area (such as lower lateral abdominal quadrant or pelvis). As described in Chapter 3, laparoscopy plays a very important role in the evaluation and diagnosis of patients with localized peritoneal reaction. In these patients, a timely laparoscopic evaluation may demonstrate that a major surgical operation is not needed. Therefore it may serve as a guide to the selection of more conservative therapy.

Diffuse or generalized peritonitis indicates a more serious insult to the defense mechanism offered by the peritoneum. The characteristic signs and symptoms of diffuse peritonitis that result (pain, rebound tenderness, guarding) yield the typical pattern of an acute surgical abdomen. The peritoneal space becomes a virtual abscess cavity. Because expeditious management is so critical in the patient with an acute surgical abdomen, the operative procedure must be both diagnostic and therapeutic at the same time. It is imperative to determine the cause and its source and to control further spread of the infection by treating the primary pathologic process as well as profusely irrigating and draining the area. These procedures can only be accomplished through an adequate abdominal incision and are thus not amenable to laparoscopy.

Intestinal Obstruction

One-fifth of general surgical emergency hospital admissions concern the treatment of intestinal obstruction. The most common causes of intestinal obstruction are adhesions, tumor, hernia, and diverticulitis. In patients who have had a previous abdominal operation, 90 percent of mechanical bowel obstruction is secondary to intra-abdominal adhesions.

Bowel distention occurs proximal to the point of obstruction as a result of gas and fluid accumulation. This third-space intraluminal distention is mainly responsible for the abdominal enlargement. The resulting increased intraluminal pressure may reach levels as high as 15 to 20 mm Hg, thereby raising the level of the diaphragm and impairing abdominal respiratory movements (see Chapter 10).

Similar abdominal distention can be seen as a result of a paralytic ileus. Common causes of paralytic ileus include intra-abdominal infection or inflammation (from appendicitis or pancreatitis, for example), generalized peritonitis (due to perforation of a viscus), pyelonephritis, and primary or metastatic malignancy. Gas and fluid accumulation in the bowel lumen occurs as a consequence of ineffective or nonpropulsive bowel motility. The small bowel and/or colon may be involved. Abdominal distention usually develops over a period of 2 or 3 days. The abdomen becomes tense and tympanitic, but the intraluminal bowel pressure does not increase to the high levels seen with mechanical obstruction.

Although some of the conditions that may give origin to bowel obstruction (adhesions) or paralytic ileus (appendicitis or neoplasia) are themselves indications for diagnostic laparoscopy, the concomitant appearance of bowel distention serves to contraindicate the method. This contraindication is absolute. Injury to a distended loop of bowel is most likely to occur as a consequence of the insertion of the Verres needle and/or sharp laparoscopic trocar, a procedure which is done blindly (see Chapter 18).

The open laparoscopic technique suggested by some is also contraindicated. This is based on the inability to achieve a suitable pneumoperitoneum. Poor visualization of the abdomino-pelvic structures is the result. Furthermore, the elevation of the diaphragm as a result of the distended bowel may already have compromised effective pulmonary ventilation. This adverse effect is aggravated by the creation of a pneumoperitoneum.

Large Abdomino-Pelvic Mass

The presence of an abdomino-pelvic mass, which can be palpated abdominally in the periumbilical area, is a contraindication to a laparoscopic procedure. Laparoscopy is contraindicated for several reasons: First, a mass that achieves large size requires excision even if it is benign in origin. Second, the sheer size of the mass limits its range of mobilization, thus precluding complete visualization of important areas such as the posterior cul-de-sac. Third, the risk of lacerating the mass in the process of inserting the laparoscopic instruments is much greater than at laparotomy.[5]

The use of laparoscopy for diagnostic purposes during the second trimester of pregnancy remains controversial. Serious complications may arise if the uterus, which is a very vascular organ at this stage of gestation, is inadvertently injured. Furthermore, to subject the circulatory system to the changes that normally occur during laparoscopy at the time of maximal hemodynamic stress in pregnancy is not only inadvisable but potentially hazardous.

RELATIVE CONTRAINDICATIONS

Relative contraindications distinguish themselves from absolute ones by the range of risk/benefit ratios that pertain to different patients presenting with a similar condition. Each individual case has to be evaluated on its own merits. A relative contraindication may become absolute in a particular patient. One factor that must be included in the decision making process is the experience of the surgeon with the technique of laparoscopy. Under certain conditions, the laparoscopist's limited experience tips the balance against endoscopy even though the patient's condition may warrant it. Before a laparoscopy is undertaken in a patient with a relative contraindication, it is essential to ensure that the surgeon is able to deal appropriately with any complication that may arise as a consequence of the patient's status.

Conditions considered to be relative contraindications to the performance of a laparoscopic procedure include multiple prior abdominal surgical procedures, antecedent peritonitis associated with an abdominal or pelvic operation, diaphragmatic hernia, severe cardiac disease, chronic obstructive lung disease, and intolerance to the Trendelenburg position.

Multiple Abdominal Surgical Procedures

A history of repeated abdomino-pelvic surgical operations, considered in the past to be an absolute contraindication to laparoscopy, is now believed to be a relative one.[3] Individual consideration should be given to the type of incision, the extent of the surgical procedure, and the primary indications for those operations.[1] These are important because they appear to correlate better with the risk of encountering intraperitoneal adhesions at laparoscopy. It is also useful to know if any complications occurred as a consequence of prior surgery. Postoperative infection, hemorrhage, dehiscence, and reexploration are all commonly associated with adhesion formation.

Type of Incision. Low transverse (Pfannenstiel) incisions appear to be less likely to produce parietal intraperitoneal adhesions postoperatively than do the standard subumbilical midline incisions. No clear explanation for this phenomenon exists since the peritoneum is incised in a similar fashion in both procedures. It has been suggested that the increased frequency of adhesions to the abdominal wall seen after midline incisions is related to the fact that this is the incision usually chosen in emergency cases with an acute surgical abdomen. Low transverse type incisions are utilized more often in elective surgical procedures. Thus, the condition which precipitates the surgery can explain the adhesions rather than the type of incision.

Type of Procedure. It is well recognized that some abdomino-pelvic surgical procedures are more likely than others to give rise to postoperative adhesions. Intraperitoneal drains left postoperatively increase the likelihood that one will later encounter adhesions at their site of exit from the abdominal cavity. Patients who have had a colostomy are also known to develop multiple intraperitoneal adhesions between loops of bowel and between bowel and abominal parietal peritoneum.

Closed laparoscopy in these cases carries an increased risk of injury to the abdominal contents. This untoward complication may result from damage produced by the Verres needle or by the laparoscopic trocar. The use of the open laparoscopy technique diminishes these risks considerably, but it does not eliminate them completely.

Indications for Previous Surgery. The peritoneum is an active protective barrier against infection and foreign matter. It has the capacity to become inflamed and to produce transudate and fibrinous exudate. Protection is also manifested by mechanisms that act to isolate and circumscribe an injurious process. On resolution of the infectious process, reabsorption of the exudated material takes place. This process may result in the formation of intra-abdominal adhesions.

It is not uncommon to find intra-abominal adhesions in patients previously operated on for ruptured appendix with disseminated peritonitis, diverticulitis, ruptured tubo-ovarian abscess, or any other inflammatory or infectious condition that produces a generalized peritonitic reaction. A patient who has had any of the aforementioned conditions is not a good candidate for a closed laparoscopic procedure. Nevertheless, one can minimize the risks associated with the blind steps of the method by use of the open laparoscopy technique. Thus, these patients can be offered the benefits of endoscopic evaluation with negligible risks of iatrogenic injury.

Postoperative Complications. No less important than the indications for the previous surgery is the need to know the nature of the postoperative course during the recovery from that surgery. Intraperitoneal infectious complications occurring during the postoperative period (even in the case of elective surgery) may also cause intra-abdominal adhesions to form. The unpredictable pattern of peritoneal adhesion formation under these circumstances mandates extreme caution. Direct visualization of the peritoneum at the entry site is necessary before introducing any instrument for purposes of creating a pneumoperitoneum. This is accomplished by using the open laparoscopy technique whenever intra-abdominal adhesions are suspected.

Laparoscopy is just as valuable for patients with previous abdomino-pelvic surgery as it is for those who have had no prior surgery. It is logical to postulate that patients who have already proved their propensity to form intraperitoneal adhesions are at great risk of developing more. Therefore, they should be subjected to the least possible amount of surgery required to obtain the necessary information or to carry out a needed procedure. This conservative approach should minimize the formation of new adhesions.

In patients in whom bowel adhesions are suspected, a diagnostic laparoscopy with a small diameter laparoscope (1.7 mm) has been suggested.[4] This miniaturized laparoscope can be used as the sole instrument for carrying out the endoscopic procedure. Conversely, it can be utilized to identify an area of abdominal wall free of adhesions through which a regular size laparoscope can be safely introduced. Inadvertent bowel puncture with this needle-sized laparoscope is reported to be relatively innocuous.[2]

Previous Peritonitis

Acute diffuse peritonitis in the past constitutes an absolute contraindication to the performance of a laparoscopy, as previously discussed. Similarly, closed laparoscopy is contraindicated in a patient who has had a bout of peritonitis that required surgical intervention. This is due to the fact that multiple intraperitoneal adhesions are frequently found at the time of subsequent laparotomy in these patients.

The risk of injuring an intra-abdominal structure while blindly inserting the Verres needle and/or laparoscopic trocar can be avoided by performing an open laparoscopy. Secondary and tertiary accessory punctures are recommended, using puncture trocars of the same dimension as the laparoscopic trocar. This permits one to interchange the entry site of the laparoscope if multiple adhesions prevent visualization of the entire pelvis.

Diaphragmatic Hernia

Diaphragmatic hernia may cause considerable respiratory difficulty and disability, but it may also go unnoticed until the adult years. Hernias through the posterolateral aspect of the diaphragm (foramen of Bochdalek) are most commonly seen in infants. Anterior retrosternal or parasternal hernias (through the foramen of Morgagni) are usually first detected in adults. Notwithstanding their different temporal appearance, they are both considered to be congenital defects of diaphragmatic fusion.

Hernias of the foramen of Bochdalek are usually symptomatic and diagnosed during infancy. Because they give rise to acute symptoms (including cyanosis, tachypnea, and increased respiratory effort), they usually require surgical correction before puberty. On the contrary, only 20 percent of foramen of Morgagni hernias are symptomatic, the vast majority being diagnosed incidentally by routine chest roentgenogram. Symptomatic patients may experience vague gastrointestinal complaints, depending mostly on the mass of abdominal organs that herniate into the thorax.

The use of laparoscopy in patients known to have a diaphragmatic hernia is relatively contraindicated. It is not an absolute contraindication because with appropriate precautionary measures and monitoring laparoscopy can be safely accomplished. Precautionary consideration should focus on the type of anesthesia, the degree of Trendelenburg tilt, and the amount of gas insufflated to create the pneumoperitoneum.

Type of Anesthesia. The potential for herniation of abdominal organs into the thorax is directly related to the size of the diaphragmatic defect and the increment in intra-abdominal pressure. Ectopic protrusion of organs into the thoracic cavity will result in respiratory distress which may reach life-threatening proportions. Controlled ventilation with an endotracheal cuffed tube may be needed to help correct the respiratory difficulties. An increase in the inspiratory pressure required to expand the lungs is a reliable indicator of excessively elevated intra-abdominal pressure. Additional insufflation of gas into the abdomen is inadvisable since it would enhance organ herniation into the thorax and magnify respiratory compromise.

Trendelenburg Tilt. The Trendelenburg position is used in laparoscopy to displace the intra-abdominal organs into the upper abdomen, thus facilitating visualization of the pelvic structures. Adoption of the head-down position places undue pressure on the diaphragm by the displaced abdominal contents. This effect may be counterproductive in patients with a diaphragmatic hernia. Therefore, if possible, it is prudent to avoid the Trendelenburg position in these cases. Whenever this cannot be accomplished, the degree of Trendelenburg tilt must not exceed a 15° angle. This keeps the pressure on the undersurface of the diaphragm relatively low.

Volume of Gas Insufflated. The amount of gas insufflated to produce an adequate pneumoperitoneum varies from patient to patient. The patient's size and weight and the elasticity of her abdominal wall are the factors principally responsible for these variations. As described in Chapter 2, it is the elevation in intra-abdominal pressure rather than the total volume of insufflated gas that produces respiratory embarrassment and circulatory difficulties.

Undesirable complications resulting from increased intra-abdominal pressure in patients with a diaphragmatic hernia include respiratory distress by protrusion of the hernia sac and/or abdominal contents into the thoracic cavity;

gastric regurgitation is a complication in those with esophageal hernias. Intrusion of the hernial sac, with or without abdominal contents, reduces the lung capacity and impinges on normal expansion. If the esophageal-gastric junction is displaced into the thoracic cavity, pressure on the stomach wall increases. Significant regurgitation of gastric contents into the esophagus can then occur. If the protective gag reflexes are abolished by general anesthesia, it becomes mandatory to utilize endotracheal cuffed intubation to prevent the serious complications resulting from aspiration of gastric material.

Severe Cardiac Disease

It is repeatedly stated that an absolute contraindication to laparoscopy is severe cardiac disease. The reasons given for such a dogmatic recommendation are not always clear. The benefits of laparoscopy ought not to be traded for those of a procedure such as laparotomy, which may invoke still greater risks. A decision should not be based on unwarranted fears, but rather on carefully documented objective considerations.

A thorough evaluation of the need for surgery is essential. Categorization of patients according to their functional status bears special relevance with respect to their preoperative preparation and monitoring during the procedure. Categorization does not affect the indication or the need for that diagnostic or therapeutic procedure, but it may influence the risk/benefit relationship. To this end, the classification of risk status proposed by the American Society of Anesthesiology (ASA I to ASA V for increasing degrees of risk) should be applied to all patients.

The surgeon must differentiate the risk associated with the endoscopic portion of the procedure from the risks attributable to the anesthesia used to carry out the operation. Limitations to the use of general anesthesia can be overcome be performing a laparoscopy under local anesthesia with or without adjunctive sedation. However, use of local anesthesia does not eliminate the risk entirely. Even if one selects local infiltration for the procedure, participation of a fully trained anesthetist to assist in the monitoring of these potentially sick patients is critical. The choice of local or regional anesthesia instead of general inhalation anesthesia should be made in consultation with the anesthesiologist.

The risk of laparoscopy in women with a preexistent cardiac condition is different in patients requiring upper abdominal endoscopy from the risk in those requiring pelvic endoscopy. The former do not require the patient to be placed in the Trendelenburg position, thus reducing the stress on the cardiovascular system. In patients requiring pelvic laparoscopy, in whom some degree of head-down tilt is required, the incline should be limited to no more than 15° from the horizontal. Positioning the patient also affects the amount of insufflated gas needed to achieve good pelvic visualization. The amount of gas to be insufflated is inversely proportional to the degree of Trendelenburg tilt which can be safely achieved.

As will be discussed in Chapter 9, circulatory changes are affected by the intra-abdominal pressure reached at maximum peritoneal distention. Open laparoscopic technique, which permits the insufflation of gas with the laparoscope in place, limits the size of the pneumoperitoneum to the smallest amount required to carry out the procedure. This usually totals no more than 2 L of gas to achieve an intra-abdominal pressure of less than 10 mm Hg.

At the present time, the accumulated experience with laparoscopy supports its use in patients with preexisting cardiac disease provided it is done under closely monitored conditions. With appropriate careful surveillance of cardiac and respiratory functions, it is difficult to envision a situation in which laparotomy can be favored over laparoscopy. Furthermore, the degree of postoperative discomfort and anticipated complications have to be taken into account when deciding between laparoscopy and laparotomy.

Chronic Obstructive Pulmonary Disease

Chronic obstructive pulmonary diseases encompass a variety of respiratory disorders. Their common denominator is a limitation to the expiratory flow of air due to airway narrowing. Chronic bronchitis, bronchial asthma, and emphysema are the most frequently encountered entities presenting with manifestations of expiratory flow obstruction.

The relative contraindication to laparoscopy in patients with chronic obstructive pulmonary disease stems from their susceptibility to anesthetic complications, especially if they require a general anesthesia. Even with local or regional anesthesia, the restrictive ventilatory alterations imposed by the increased intra-abominal pressure and Trendelenburg position (see Chapter 10) may interfere with compensatory ventilatory responses. A complete assessment of the respiratory function in these individuals is advisable. Similar to patients with preexisting severe cardiac disease, women with chronic obstructive pulmonary disease will benefit both during surgery and postoperatively when laparoscopy is chosen in lieu of laparotomy. Regardless of the anesthetic technique employed to provide pain relief for the laparoscopic procedure, an experienced anesthesiologist must be a member of the surgical team.

Intolerance to Trendelenburg Position

Albeit not always essential, the Trendelenburg position is almost universally used in the course of laparoscopy. Circulatory and respiratory changes associated with this position will be described in Chapters 9 and 10, respectively. Circulatory changes occur as a result of altered venous return, cardiac output, and blood pressure. These are usually mild and of limited consequence in the young, healthy adult female. This is not the case in a patient with a preexistent cardiovascular problem in whom Trendelenburg position may aggravate the condition or precipitate a crisis.

The head-down position may affect the cerebral circulation in a significant fashion. Jugular vein pressure can increase 3- to 4-fold over baseline levels. Resulting intracranial blood stasis may also decrease carotid blood flow, further compromising a patient with reduced cerebral circulation. Elevation of cerebral venous pressure may also enhance the increased intracranial pressure that trauma victims tend to develop. This should be kept in mind when laparoscopy is being considered for the evaluation of occult intra-abdominal injury in accident victims. Changes in intracranial pressure can be accompanied by marked increases in intraocular tension. If this occurs, it can cause acute glaucoma in a susceptible patient. In the normal patient, intraocular pressures show little variation in response to the head-down position.

Respiratory changes also take place as a consequence of placing a patient in the Trendelenburg position. It is common to find reduction in the vital capacity of the lung resulting from the abdominal viscera pressing on the undersurface of the diaphragm (see Chapter 10). Nevertheless, no changes in blood gases or minute volume determinations have been reported in patients placed in the head-down position during a laparoscopy. Some of the changes attributable to position are similar to those resulting from the pneumoperitoneum. It is difficult to distinguish which is causative in a given case, and their effects may be additive.

Other Relative Contraindications

Laparoscopy is contraindicated in patients in whom changes in cerebral circulation can be expected to aggravate a preexisting condition or cause a serious problem. One must be alert to the special needs of women with glaucoma and/or marginal cerebral circulation.

Obesity, which was previously considered a relative contraindication to a laparoscopic investigation, is now acceptable. Actually, less morbidity and lower mortality rates are seen in obese patients undergoing diagnostic laparoscopy than in those subjected to exploratory laparotomy.[7] In the past, creation of the pneumoperitoneum seemed to be the most troublesome obstacle to laparoscopy. Failure to attain a suitable pneumoperitoneum was thought to be due to the shortness of the standard size Verres needle. However, development of a longer Verres needle did not prove to be universally successful in solving this problem.

As described in Chapter 2, little variation is encountered in the anatomical configuration of the umbilicus and periumbilical area irrespective of the patient's weight. All layers of the abdominal wall (skin, fascia, and peritoneum) are fused at the umbilicus into a single fibrotic layer without any intervening subcutaneous tissue. Thus, the umbilicus and its inferior border rarely exceed 1 cm in thickness.

Toth and Graf reported no failures to obtain an adequate pneumoperitoneum in 217 patients when using the center of the umbilicus as the entry site for the Verres needle.[11] Personally, I prefer to avoid the umbilicus itself because of the difficulty in cleansing the area adequately. Insertion of the Verres needle at the lower border of the umbilical fossa perpendicular to the fascial layer is just as effective. The laparoscope trocar must also be inserted in an analogous way. The technical challenge these patients present can be easily overcome by adhering strictly to all appropriate methodological details in the performance of the laparoscopy (see Chapters 2 and 13).

Ascites was also once thought to be a relative contraindication to laparoscopy. Experience gathered by gastroenteroscopists proved this to be unfounded. At times, evacuation of the ascitic fluid may be required prior to the insufflation of gas for the pneumoperitoneum, especially if the abdomen is markedly distended. Removal of the ascitic fluid must be performed just prior to the insufflation of the distending gas to preclude reaccumulation of newly formed peritoneal transudate.

References

1. Ahn YW, Owens B. Techniques for laparoscopy on patients with previous abdominal surgery. Int J Fertil 1979; 24:264-266.
2. Berek JS, Griffiths CT, Leventhal JM. Laparoscopy for second-look evaluation in ovarian cancer. Obstet Gynecol 1981; 58:192-198.
3. Chi I, Feldblum PJ, Balogh SA. Previous abdominal surgery as a risk factor in interval laparoscopic sterilization. Am J Obstet Gynecol 1983; 145:841-846.
4. Cook WA. Needle laparoscopy in patients with suspected bowel adhesions. Obstet Gynecol 1976; 49:105-106.
5. Frenkel Y, Oelsner G, Ben-Baruch G, Menczer J. Major surgical complications of laparoscopy. Eur J Obstet Gynaecol Reprod Biol 1981; 12:107-112.
6. Ivankovich AD, Miletich DJ, Albrecht RF, Heyman HJ, Bonnet RF. Cardiovascular effects of intraperitoneal insufflation with carbon dioxide and nitrous oxide in the dog. Anesthesiology 1975; 42:281-287.
7. Loffer FD, Pent D. Laparoscopy in the obese patient. Am J Obstet Gynecol 1976; 125:104-107.
8. Scott DB, Julian DG. Observations on cardiac arrhythmias during laparoscopy. Br Med J 1972; 1:411-413.
9. Smith I, Benzie RJ, Gordon NLM, Kelman GR. Cardiovascular effects of peritoneal insufflation of carbon dioxide for laparoscopy. Br Med J 1971; 3:410-411.
10. Taylor J, Weil MH. Failure of the Trendelenburg position to improve circulation during clinical shock. Surg Gyn Obst 1967; 124:1005-1010.
11. Toth A, Graf M. The center of the umbilicus as the Verres needle's entry site for laparoscopy. J Reprod Med 1984; 29:126-128.

7 NONGYNECOLOGIC INDICATIONS

Laparoscopy, albeit well established as a diagnostic and operative tool in the field of gynecology, has not yet gained universal acceptance among general surgeons and internists. This is in marked contrast with its original application at the turn of the twentieth century. Reported independently by Kelling and Jacobeus as a method to visualize the peritoneal cavity, it was then called celioscopy or peritoneoscopy. Primitive instrumentation and unexpected complications relegated this technique to a limited number of investigational centers.

Following the reintroduction of laparoscopy into the routine practice of gynecology, which occurred in the 1960s, interest among other specialties has been growing. It was initially reserved for the unexplained and difficult diagnostic dilemma, but it was soon found to provide essential information for the workup and differential diagnosis of more common conditions. Recently, studies comparing the accuracy and specificity of various diagnostic modalities demonstrated laparoscopy to be the most reliable tool in the diagnosis of widespread liver disease.[20] This has encouraged the routine use of laparoscopy by hepatologists and has stimulated utilization by internists in cases of unresolved intra-abdominal disease.

Contrary to logical expectations, general surgeons have been reluctant to incorporate laparoscopy into their diagnostic armamentarium. Its proven value in the diagnosis and staging of intra-abdominal pathological conditions has yet to receive adequate recognition.[7] Reports about successful avoidance of major surgery by preliminary endoscopic evaluation of the peritoneal cavity have not been fully appreciated.[23] Judicious use of laparoscopy as an aid in the diagnosis of abdominal trauma has been shown to reduce the need for a great number of exploratory laparotomies.[15] Most hospitals have the required laparoscopic instrumentation since it is universally employed by gynecologists today. The wide variety of nongynecologic conditions in which laparoscopy can be applied will be described in this chapter.

THE APPENDIX

The appendix can usually be visualized without difficulty during diagnostic laparoscopy. Its location, configuration, and relationship to other abdominopelvic organs are important pieces of information that can be obtained during a laparoscopic evaluation irrespective of the primary indication for the procedure. With the exception of the retrocecally located appendix, a minimal amount of manipulation with a solid probe is generally needed to find the appendix and to visualize it completely (Figure 7.1). This operative step does not prolong the duration or increase the risk of a laparoscopy. Laparoscopists in general and gynecologists in particular should be encouraged to explore for the appendix and describe it in detail as an integral part of their operative note.

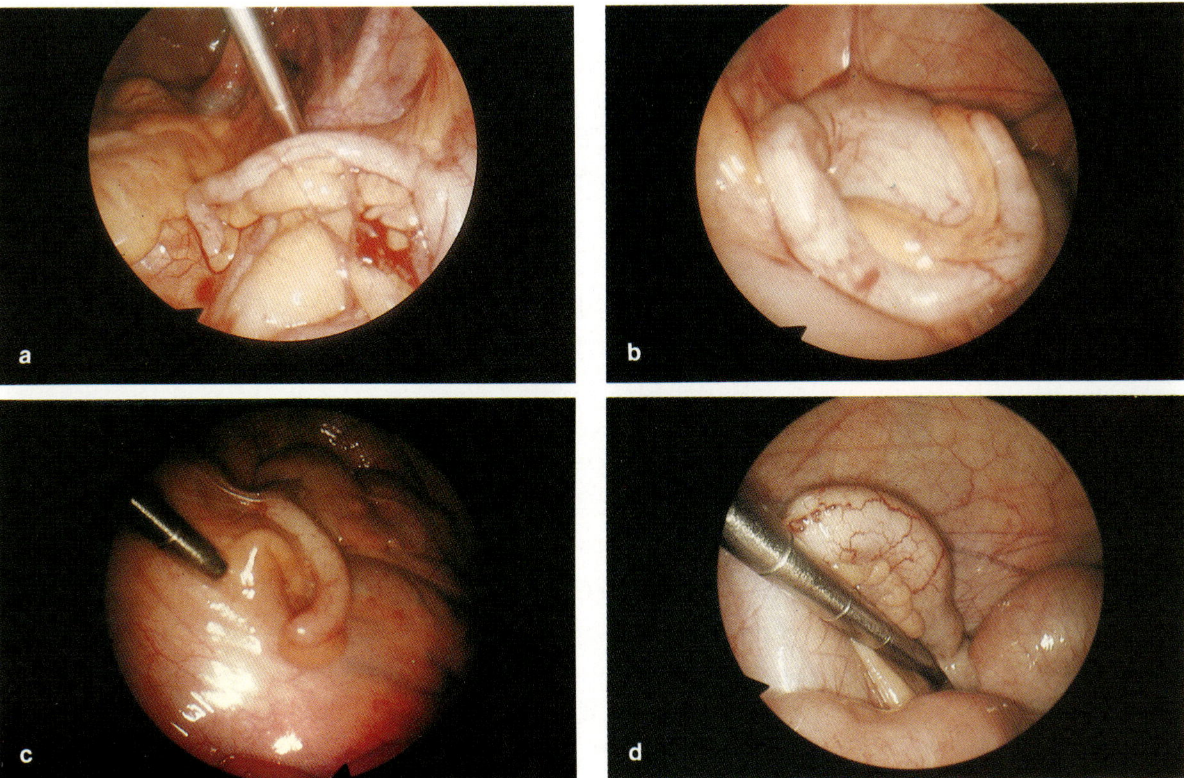

Figure 7.1 Visualization of the appendix. *a*. Minimal manipulation is required to locate and visually explore the entire appendix. Gently touching the appendix with the probe gives the operator a feel of its consistency. *b*. Induration felt at any level is a positive sign of inflammation. *c*. The appendix ought to be able to be moved freely when displaced by the probe. *d*. Fixation to any adjacent structure may require surgical definitive therapy by laparotomy.

The overall error rate in diagnosis of acute appendicitis varies from 5 to 30 percent. This has led to the performance of unnecessary laparotomies and appendectomies. Such procedures are said to be justified in order to avoid exposing the unoperated patient with suspected appendicitis to the more serious complications of rupture. It is generally acceptable for surgeons to remove 10 to 20 percent of normal appendices. Indeed, this condition is considered to be underdiagnosed if the rate falls below this range. This is a concept that has been handed down among surgeons for several generations.

Appendicitis may present in a variety of ways. Typically, it is progressive with worsening signs and symptoms. Diagnostic difficulties arise when other concomitant medical conditions are present (such as salpingitis, adnexal torsion or ureteral stone) (Figures 7.2 to 7.4) or when certain medications are being taken (such as steroids or antibiotics). These complicating factors are more preponderant in women during reproductive years.[9] The type of complications one may encounter by resecting a normal appendix range from mild wound infection to death; the latter is reported to occur about once in every 1,538 operations. Even in the absence of postoperative complications, the performance of an unnecessary laparotomy for appendectomy requires prolonged hospitalization and serious economic loss to the patient.

Leape and Ramenofsky performed 32 diagnostic laparoscopies in patients with suspected appendicitis whose clinical findings were equivocal or insufficient to establish the diagnosis.[17] Appendicitis was confirmed in 17; an unrelated diagnosis was made in eight; and seven were found to have no pathologic abnormalities. Thus laparotomy was spared in 37.5 percent of their patients and the rate of appendectomy for normal appendix decreased from 10 to 1 percent.

Deutsch et al reported a prospective study of 36 women, aged 18 to 50 years, in whom diagnostic laparoscopy was performed for a diagnosis of appendicitis.[9] Laparoscopy interdicted further surgery in one-third, on the basis of the findings of acute gynecologic disease not requiring surgical correction. Laparoscopy in this series was performed through a right lower paramedian incision, which could be enlarged if appendectomy was required. In one case, the appendix was under the liver; it was removed by way of a right subcostal incision. Laparoscopy was thus useful for helping to establish the most appropriate incisional site.

The advantages of performing a laparoscopy in all cases in which appendicitis is suspected, but not fully substantiated are obvious. They include avoidance of unnecessary surgery and postoperative complications, reduced hospitalization and use of health resources, and, not the least important, diminished overall cost. If laparotomy has to be done after the laparoscopy, neither hospitalization nor cost should be substantially increased.

Nevertheless, some precautions have to be kept in mind. In 10 to 20 percent of patients, the appendix is retrocecal in location, thereby precluding com-

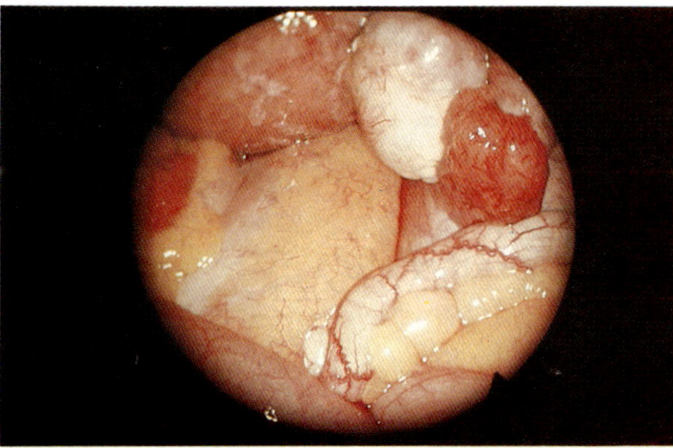

Figure 7.2 Anatomical proximity of appendix, fallopian tube, and right ovary. Inflamed fimbrial end of the tube suggests salpingitis as the source of pain in this case. Signs of appendiceal inflammation are probably reactive rather than primary in nature.

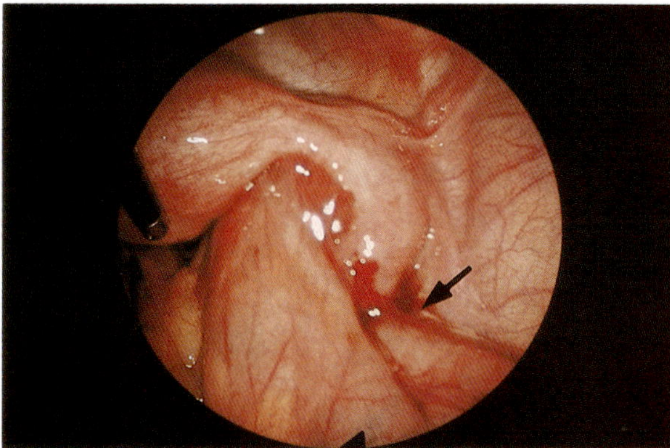

Figure 7.3 Appendiceal abscess. Appendix is seen dipping into the pelvis (arrow) out of sight. Bowel, fallopian tube, and appendix appear to be components of a single abscess formation. Inability to visualize the appendix in its entirety makes the laparoscopy inconclusive. The risk of overlooking an appendiceal abscess requires laparotomy for definitive diagnosis and therapy.

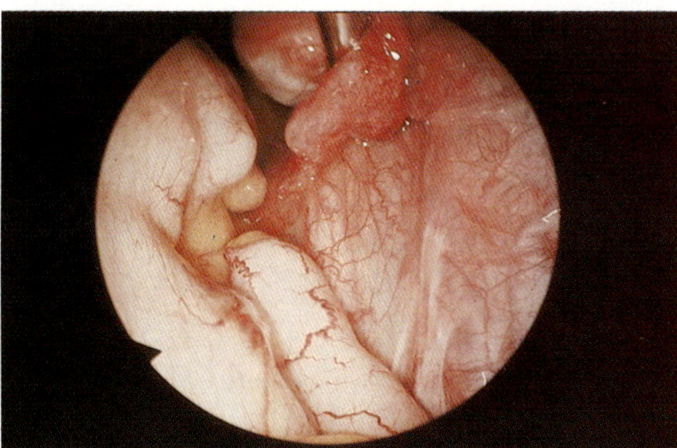

Figure 7.4 Appendicitis. Edematous appendix is seen lying over the pelvic brim. Palpation with a probe revealed it to be indurated. Diagnosis was confirmed by subsequent histologic evaluation following appendectomy.

plete visualization. These patients may need a laparotomy (and appendectomy) since a satisfactory diagnosis cannot be made through the laparoscope. A similar situation exists in patients who have intraperitoneal adhesions or whose omentum is attached to the appendix. Some of them may have an inflamed appendix. As a rule, whenever the appendix cannot be entirely visualized, laparoscopy must be considered ineffective for ruling out a diagnosis of appendicitis (Figure 7.5). Surgical intervention by laparotomy is indicated under these circumstances.

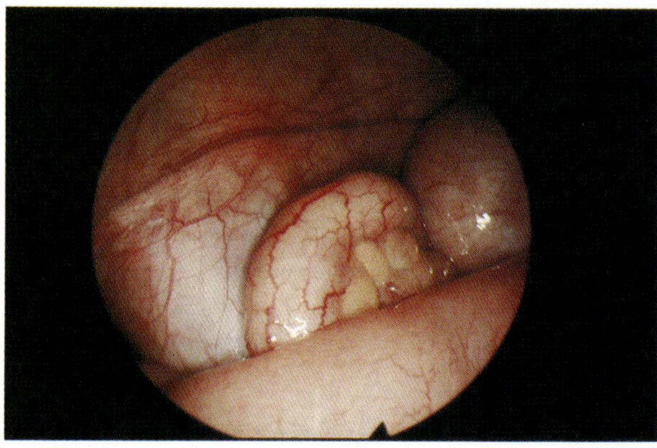

Figure 7.5 Incompletely visualized appendix. Inability to visualize the entire appendix must be considered an incomplete laparoscopic evaluation to rule out appendicitis. Laparotomy is required for definitive diagnosis and therapy. A similar situation exists for a partial or total retrocecal appendix.

LIVER DISEASE

Except for liver biopsy (see p. 161), the diagnosis of liver disease has heretofore been based mainly on noninvasive tests. Radioisotopic scanning of the liver is supplemented by ultrasonography and more recently by computed tomography. These constitute the screening tests of choice for diffuse and focal liver abnormalities. Although they prove valuable for gross disease, small lesions (especially those less than 1 cm in diameter) still escape detection by these modalities.

Laparoscopy has gained wide acceptance in Europe as a means for diagnosing liver disease. The ability to visualize the external hepatic surface allows morphologic evaluation. Organ density can be assessed by direct palpation with a probe. Positioning of the patient on his or her left side in reversed Trendelenburg position (Fowler's position) permits one to inspect as much as 80 to 90 percent of the liver surface.

Normally, the liver has distinctive characteristics. When these features are absent, one should suspect organic disease. The surface color is reddish brown and may vary with the amount of blood perfusion (Figure 7.6). Significant departure from normal coloration indicates the presence of an abnormality. The liver edge should have an acute angle; loss of angulation suggests liver enlargement (Figures 7.7 and 7.8). The consistency is normally soft; the tissue can be indented with gentle pressure of the probe. Induration of the liver indicates an increased degree of tissue density suggestive of a parenchymal disorder (Figure 7.9). Under normal conditions, the liver surface is smooth and shiny because its capsule reflects the illuminating optical light source. Some wrinkling is seen with age, but this has no pathological significance.

Laparoscopy is indicated to evaluate the liver in patients with suspected liver disease in whom no diagnosis has been reached by the use of noninvasive tests or in whom blind liver biopsy is unlikely to be beneficial. Direct visualization of the hepatic surface is indicated in patients with suspected cirrhosis, unexplained hepatomegaly, or chronic liver disease. It may be helpful if transformation of chronic hepatitis into cirrhosis or of cirrhosis into neoplasia is believed to have taken place.

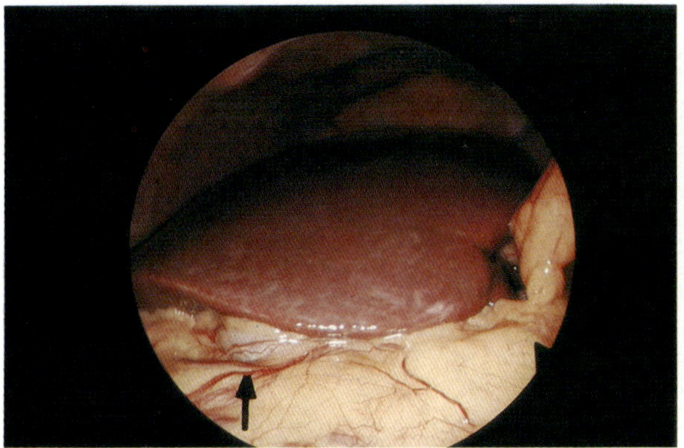

Figure 7.6 Normal liver. Smooth surface, reddish-brown color and sharp edges characterize the appearance of a normal liver. A normal gallbladder is also seen (arrow).

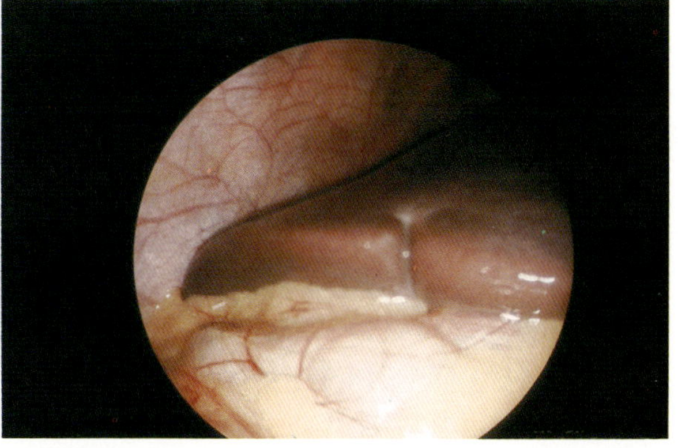

Figure 7.7 Congested liver. Loss of the sharp angulation seen in the normal liver (compare Figure 7.6) suggests liver enlargement. The consistency is soft and the surface is easily indented with a probe.

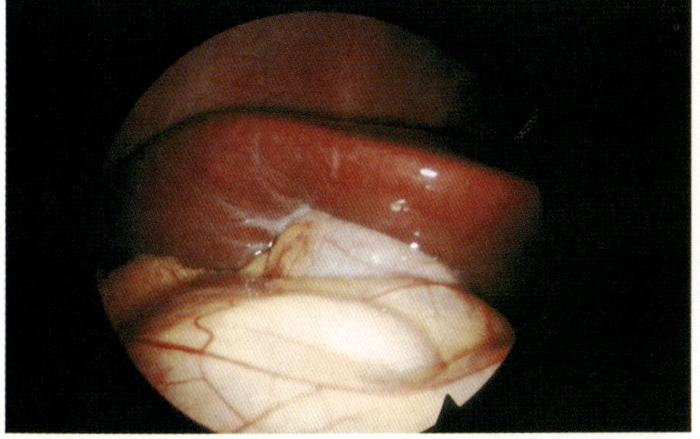

Figure 7.8 Hyperemic liver. Loss of normal liver angulation suggests a congestive process. Loss of translucency of the gallbladder wall and the appearance of fibrinous exudate between the liver and gallbladder suggests cholecystitis as the underlying cause.

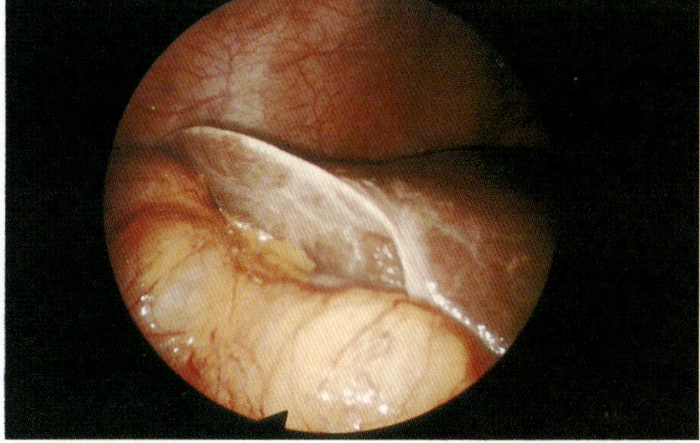

Figure 7.9 Cirrhosis of the liver. Induration of the liver parenchyma can be assessed by palpation with a probe. White fibrotic edge reveals chronic changes. Histologic evaluation of a liver biopsy may be required for a definitive diagnosis.

Detection, localization, and determination of the extent of liver metastases prior to surgery or chemotherapy for a malignancy are perhaps the most important indications for laparoscopic assessment of the liver. Laparoscopic evaluation is recommended for possible liver metastases prior to surgical resection of a primary carcinoma of the lung or breast. As many as 20 percent of patients undergoing thoracotomy for malignant pulmonary lesions have infradiaphragmatic metastases at the time of surgery.[10] Nearly 70 percent of these intra-abdominal metastases are located in the hepatic parenchyma. Laparoscopic identification of liver metastases in these patients would spare them needless surgery.

In a patient suspected clinically of having cirrhosis, laparoscopy provides direct visualization of the hepatic surface. The color of the liver, the appearance of the capsule, and the finding of nodularity supply the endoscopist with information about the existence of cirrhosis as well as its type and etiology. Assessment of the status of the left lobe (which is not accessible to blind percutaneous biopsy) and preselection of the most appropriate site for visually directed biopsy are additional advantages of laparoscopy in these cases.

Enlargement of the liver (hepatomegaly) may be due to a variety of underlying processes. Laparoscopic evaluation of an enlarged liver is of proven value for obtaining a proper biopsy sample, especially when the growth is localized rather than diffuse. Coupland et al reported that laparoscopy allowed identification of the cause of hepatomegaly in 91 percent of patients.[7] Biopsy was not required in more than 20 percent, usually because the liver appeared grossly normal or there was obvious cancer. In patients with known hepatoma, laparoscopy also allows one to assess the ostensibly normal lobe. Without doubt, the most important role of laparoscopy in patients with hepatomegaly is the assurance it gives that representative biopsy sampling has been done. This applies most in those cases in which normal histology is found. Exploratory laparotomy is thus avoided.

Noninvasive techniques for the diagnosis of liver metastases have low specificity. They are often unable to distinguish between benign conditions—such as cysts, cirrhosis, and fatty liver—and metastatic nodules. Laparoscopic confirmation of the presence or absence of liver metastases obviously influences management. When laparoscopy is used for staging a primary cancer of lung or breast, the documentation of liver metastases may preempt the use of radical surgery, as previously mentioned.

Laparoscopy is highly effective in the evaluation of patients with liver cancer. Its greatest advantage is its ability to identify small lesions on the liver surface. Autopsy evaluation of patients with metastatic liver disease reveals metastases on the liver surface in about 90 percent of cases. Noninvasive techniques, such as radionuclide scans, ultrasonography and computed tomography, require the metastatic lesion to be at least 1 cm in diameter for consistent detection.

In an attempt to overcome complications related to the technique for obtaining liver tissue by biopsy, Lightdale et al evaluated a translaparoscopic sheathed cytology brush.[18] Cells obtained by brushing the liver, spleen, and peritoneum proved diagnostic for malignancy even when a biopsy failed to show neoplastic tissue. This method caused negligible trauma and was quick and simple to perform. Therefore, brushing the suspected surface area may be considered a useful laparoscopic supplement to needle and forceps biopsies.

Under certain conditions, particularly if liver adhesions are present, the posterior and inferior surfaces of the liver may not be amenable to biopsy. Sugarbaker reported a double telescope technique which expands the visual field, thereby allowing more of the liver surface to be inspected.[26] After insertion of the first laparoscope at the level of the umbilicus, a second endoscope is inserted under direct vision substernally in the midline at a point approximately one-third the distance between the xiphoid and the umbilicus. The use of two laparoscopes permits one to examine the superior and inferior liver surfaces as well as the entire left hepatic lobe.

LIVER BIOPSY

Since its introduction in the late 1950s, percutaneous liver biopsy has remained a cornerstone in the diagnosis of hepatic diseases. Because it provides histologic identification, liver biopsy is an integral component of the diagnostic work-up in cases with focal and diffuse hepatic disorders. The procedure is short and requires neither general anesthesia nor specialized facilities.

The widespread use of percutaneous liver biopsy has disclosed some shortcomings and limitations. The procedure is not risk free. Moreover, the tissue sample obtained is only 1/50,000 to 1/100,000 the size of the entire organ; all too often, it may not be an accurate representation of the liver as a whole. Estimates of false-negative biopsy rates in cirrhosis range from 10 to 50 percent. This sampling error may even be higher in cases with less diffuse, more focalized disease such as metastatic liver neoplasia. False-negative rates as high as 40 to 60 percent have been reported in patients with proven hepatic cancer.

The accuracy of blind percutaneous liver biopsy improves with multiple sampling and with use of ultrasonographic guidance. Nevertheless, sampling errors remain unacceptably high. Technical limitations include difficulty in identifying small solitary nodules. The commonly used Menghini needle tends to be deflected away from hard fibrous tissue; it thus samples the softer surrounding liver parenchyma. The risk of hemorrhagic diathesis increases proportionally with the number of samples obtained.

Laparoscopy overcomes most of the shortcomings and limitations of blind percutaneous liver biopsy. Although risks are not completely eliminated, control and correction of complications are facilitated by their early recognition. Laparoscopy permits visualization of more than 80 percent of the liver surface. Small changes in liver contour are fully appreciated and accurately localized. Hepatic consistency can be evaluated by palpation with a probe. Color changes of the liver parenchyma near the surface are seen at first glance. One can sometimes see pathognomonic signs of a condition that clearly contraindicates a biopsy, such as those of an hepatic hemangioma.

The most important feature laparoscopy offers in the evaluation of hepatic disorders is its ability to guide one in obtaining an optimal liver biopsy. Visualizing the area under surveillance reduces the number of biopsies required for correct diagnosis. Furthermore, laparoscopy allows utilization of larger biopsy instruments, thus providing a more representative tissue sample for histologic evaluation.

Laparoscopically guided biopsy of the liver has served for diagnosis of benign and malignant conditions. In the evaluation of benign hepatic disorders, Mansi et al showed laparoscopy to be more reliable diagnostically than ultrasonography and computed tomography.[20] Its diagnostic superiority persisted even when compared with liver scanning techniques (^{99}Tc-sulfur colloid). Blackwell et al compared laparoscopy and radioisotope imaging for the investigation of suspected liver disease.[2] Laparoscopy and ^{99}Tc-sulfur colloid liver imaging, assessed independently, failed to detect hepatic malignancies in a few cases; none was missed when both investigational methods were used concomitantly. The high sensitivity and specificity of laparoscopically guided biopsy for benign hepatic disorders support recommendations for more widespread use of this technique.

As part of the evaluation program for patients with malignant liver disease, laparoscopy has proven to be highly effective. In primary hepatic carcinoma, it ensures that the most representative area is sampled; moreover, it aids in the staging of the neoplastic process. Detection of bilobular involvement averts the need for a laparotomy to diagnose multifocal disease. Confirmation of local peritoneal dissemination shows the primary tumor to be unresectable. Visual and histologic documentation of a concurrent severe cirrhotic process precludes major hepatic resection. In experienced hands, laparoscopically guided liver biopsies for the diagnosis of early hepatic neoplasias has replaced open biopsy at laparotomy.

Laparoscopy is similarly useful in the diagnosis of metastatic disease. Finding liver metastases from a primary neoplasia elsewhere carries enormous clinical significance. It usually implies incurability and poor short-term prognosis. Differentiation from a benign condition such as cirrhosis or fatty degeneration, which may mimic liver metastasis, is essential. Lightdale reported more than 90 percent sensitivity and nearly 100 percent specificity for laparoscopically guided liver biopsies in the diagnosis of metastatic liver disease.[19] Detection of small nodules under the liver capsule seems to suggest that the peripheral liver substance is the most likely area for initial metastatic implantation. Bleiberg et al found that increasing the number of deep blind biopsies did not increase the yield of metastatic tumor in cases in which the surface of the liver was apparently free of disease.[3]

Bleeding from the biopsy site following a blind percutaneous liver biopsy is a much feared complication. At times, it may be so significant as to require laparotomy for hemostasis. Patients with a known bleeding diathesis are not well suited for any type of blind biopsy because it is difficult to ensure appropriate hemostasis following the procedure. This is particularly the case for liver biopsy since a large amount of blood can extravasate slowly into the peritoneal cavity before the patient experiences any systemic signs of hypovolemia.

Friedman and Wolff reported the use of laparoscopically guided liver biopsy in high-risk patients, including some with coagulation disorders.[12] Direct observation of firm clot formation and absence of oozing from the biopsy site is indispensable in all patients, most particularly in those with an underlying clotting abnormality. If bleeding persists, the site can be tamponaded by pressing the abdominal wall against the liver surface. Contact electrocoagulation or application of local hemostatic agents, such as microfibrillar collagen, may also be employed. A review of the literature fails to disclose any cases in which bleeding at the site of a translaparoscopically guided liver biopsy required major surgery for hemostatic purposes.

Laparoscopy is also useful for preventing other complications resulting from blind percutaneous liver biopsies. Inadvertent perforation of the gallbladder is an example of a potentially serious problem, that can cause bile leakage and subsequent peritonitis. Guiding the biopsy instrument under direct vision eliminates this complication. Intrathoracic complications reported to occur with the blind percutaneous approach are also averted when the procedure is visually controlled.

PERIHEPATIC ADHESIONS

Peritonitis of the upper abdomen (including perihepatitis) associated with pelvic inflammation was originally described by Stajano in 1920; he called it "phrenic reaction in gynecology."[25] In the early 1930s, Fitz-Hugh and Curtis independently described the cause and effect relationship between acute gonococcal peritonitis of the upper quadrant and the perihepatic violin-string adhesions left as its sequelae.[8,11] The right hemidiaphragmatic lymphatics are the main site of reabsorption of particles and bacteria from the peritoneal cavity.[8] This observation helps explain the pathophysiology of such observations. Grossman et al reported a 27 percent incidence of chronic perihepatic adhesions in infertility patients with hydrosalpinx.[16] There may thus be a correlation between right hemidiaphragmatic adhesions and pelvic inflammatory disease. It is now recognized they can develop without any prior association with gonococcal infection (Figures 7.10 and 7.11).

Persistent right upper quadrant pain, in the absence of any evidence of organic disease, should raise the suspicion of perihepatic adhesions as a causative factor. Laparoscopy offers the opportunity to obtain a definitive diagnosis in patients in whom extensive medical evaluation has proved inconclusive. Although the presence of perihepatic adhesions is an incidental finding in asymptomatic patients, Reichert and Valle reported several with classical Fitz-Hugh-Curtis syndrome, which consisted of persistent right upper quadrant pain; their symptoms resolved completely following translaparoscopic fulguration and lysis of the violin-string perihepatic adhesions.[22]

Laparoscopy need not be restricted to cases that are chronic in nature. Acute perihepatitis must be differentiated from acute cholecystitis, perforated peptic ulcer, or subphrenic abscess. This can be done by laparoscopy. If needed, drainage

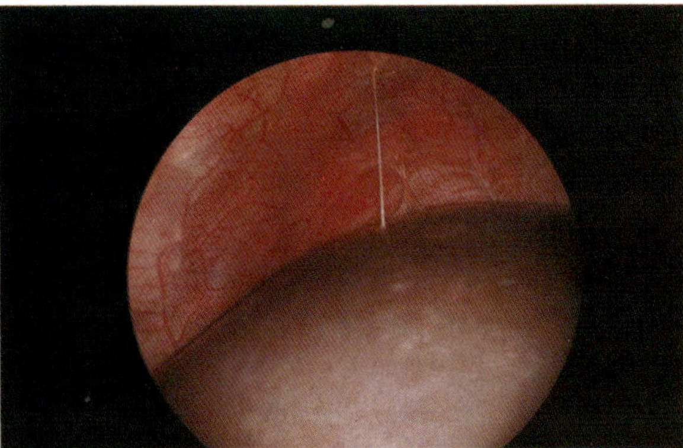

Figure 7.10 Violin-string adhesions between the right lobe of the liver and the undersurface of the right hemidiaphragm. They are usually asymptomatic. Adhesions of this type are usually seen following a transparietal needle liver biopsy.

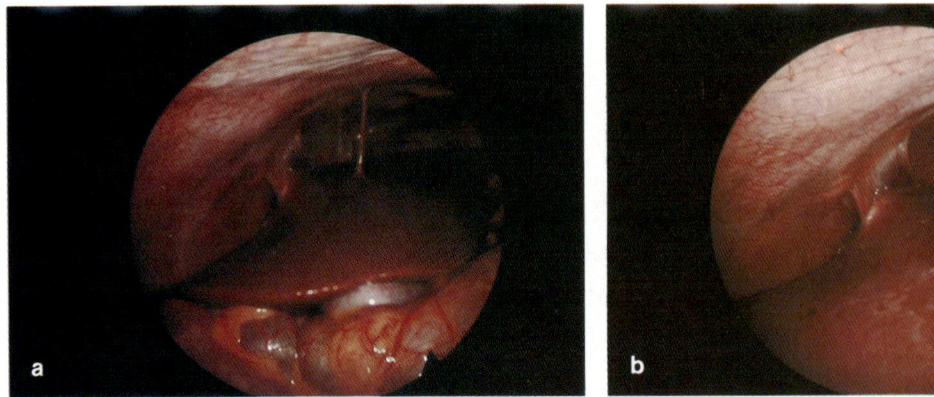

Figure 7.11 Fitz-Hugh-Curtis syndrome. *a*. Thick, fibrotic perihepatic adhesions following an infectious pelvic process. Right upper abdominal quadrant pain is often the presenting symptom. *b*. A closer view reveals tenting of the liver surface. Stretching of the liver capsule (Glisson's capsule) is the source of pain.

is achieved under direct visualization through an accessory puncture. Alternatively, accurate placement of transcutaneous subphrenic drains can be accomplished without injuring the liver parenchyme. This enhances both the diagnostic accuracy and the therapeutic safety.

GALLBLADDER AND BILIARY TREE

Visualization of the gallbladder during laparoscopy is not difficult. The distinctive shape and subhepatic location make its identification relatively easy (Figures 7.12 and 7.13). It is usually partially covered by the omentum and the anterior liver margin. Complete visualization of the gallbladder may require displacement of the omentum and elevation of the liver edge with a blunt probe.

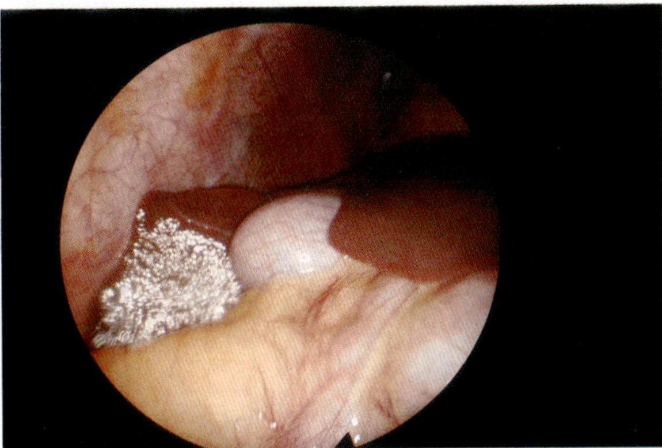

Figure 7.12 Normal gallbladder. The wall of the gallbladder contains many vessels that crisscross its surface without a particular pattern. Parenchymatous liver atrophy seen over the gallbladder (so-called monkey fissure pattern) is of little significance.

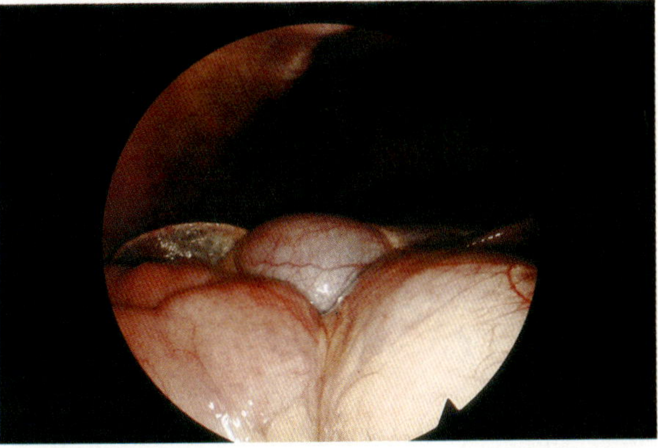

Figure 7.13 Functional vesicular distention of gallbladder. The bile within gives the wall its greenish-blue appearance. When the gallbladder is full, it is easy to evaluate its wall.

Additional maneuvers to facilitate its inspection include placing the patient on his or her left side (or axially rotating the operating table) and in reverse Trendelenburg position (Fowler's position).

Normally, the gallbladder is located under the right lobe of the liver. Its endoscopic appearance is characteristic. The outer wall contains many blood vessels which crisscross its surface without a particular pattern. It is bluish in appearance due to its bile content and has a thin, translucent wall. Anomalies of position, form, and fixation have little clinical importance. The so-called floating gallbladder may be noteworthy because its long, pendulous mesentery may allow it to undergo torsion on its pedicle, causing pain, ischemia, and necrosis.

Inflammation of the gallbladder (cholecystitis) is usually diagnosed on a clinical basis. Suspicion of cholelithiasis can be confirmed by contrast roentgenograms and/or abdominal sonography. Although these conditions are not primary indications for laparoscopy, the endoscopist ought to be familiar with the fact that they can be diagnosed through the laparoscope.

Visualization of an abnormally enlarged gallbladder with a whitish and thickly edematous wall should alert one to the probability of an underlying inflammatory process. Frequently, the omentum is adherent to the area of inflammation, thereby precluding good visualization of the gallbladder. This finding is significant since it is so frequently present with cholecystitis. As an incidental finding in an asymptomatic patient undergoing laparoscopy for an unrelated condition or in a patient with vague right upper quadrant abdominal symptoms, the aforementioned observations require appropriate follow-up by the gastroenterologist.

Carcinoma of the gallbladder in its early stages is usually diagnosed at the time of exploratory surgery. Laparoscopy offers a viable alternative for direct visualization of this condition in high-risk patients (such as those with chronic recurrent cholecystitis). Circumscribed white nodules with centripetal neovascularization are characteristic of this condition. Local metastatic spread to the liver may precede any visible changes in the gallbladder. Accurate evaluation of the extent and operability of a carcinoma of the gallbladder can be accomplished through the laparoscope. This obviates a major surgical procedure for diagnostic purposes.

Under certain conditions, oral and intravenous cholecystograms fail to outline the gallbladder roentgenographically. The newer forms of intraluminal endoscopic retrograde cholangiography may also fail to delineate the organ in cases with obstruction of the common bile duct. In these special situations, direct translaparoscopic cholangiography may be helpful in diagnosing the extent of the obstruction. This entails injecting contrast dye directly into the gallbladder through its wall under visual control.

JAUNDICE

In approximately one-fifth of patients with hyperbilirubinemia, the underlying cause is unknown and cannot be determined by clinical or laboratory evaluations. Exploratory laparotomy is not well tolerated in instances of nonobstructive jaundice and is usually contraindicated. The current recommendation is to observe patients with jaundice of unknown cause before surgical exploration is undertaken. This leads to costly and needlessly prolonged hospitalizations. Percutaneous cholangiography and operative cholangiogram (at laparotomy) are accompanied by unusually high morbidity.

Laparoscopic evaluation of the patient with jaundice of unknown etiology offers the physician the opportunity to visualize the liver and the extrahepatic biliary tree simultaneously. It has also proved helpful when combined intra- and extrahepatic cholestasis is suspected. More important, it provides the option to inject radiopaque material directly into the gallbladder under vision.

Laparoscopic transhepatic cholecystocholangiography enables the surgeon to obtain an operative cholangiogram without subjecting the patient to an exploratory laparotomy. Visualization of the right lobe of the liver and gallbladder permits one to introduce a 20-gauge needle into the right anterior liver parenchyma. Advancing the needle, one enters the gallbladder lumen through its posterior wall (via the hepatic surface of the gallbladder). This prevents any postoperative bile leakage since the point of entry into the gallbladder is tamponaded by the liver substance.

Using laparoscopic transhepatic cholecystocholangiography in patients with jaundice of undetermined cause, Gaisford reduced prolonged hospitalization by identifying surgically correctable causes in 82 percent of cases.[13] In the remaining 18 percent, confirmation of biliary cirrhosis avoided unnecessary surgical exploration. Direct puncture into the gallbladder is recommended so as to avoid perforating an icteric liver and risking hyperbilirubinemia and bacteremia in infected cases.

The recent advent of endoscopic retrograde cholangiography (via the bowel lumen) has reduced the indications for translaparoscopic cholecystocholangiography. Nevertheless, whenever the possibility of tumor metastasis is suspected, laparoscopic visualization of the liver and peritoneal surfaces offers distinct advantages.

INTRA-ABDOMINAL MALIGNANCY

Diagnostic laparoscopy for the evaluation of patients with malignancy of the fallopian tubes and ovaries is widely practiced in gynecology. Second-look procedures to assess the degree of therapeutic success have been described in Chapter 3. Similar use for the identification of other intra-abdominal primary or metastatic malignancies has failed to gain generalized acceptance. Indications for laparoscopic evaluation of patients with suspected or proved intra-abdominal neoplasms include evaluation of intra-abdominal pathological conditions suspected of being malignant, assessment for intra-abdominal metastases from known primary carcinomas (to determine the degree of operability), and staging lymphomas.

Intra-abdominal Condition Suggestive of Malignancy. Laparoscopy has proved beneficial for evaluation of patients with strong suspicion of neoplasm based on history, physical examination, and laboratory findings. Abdominal pain, unexplained weight loss, abnormal liver function tests, jaundice, and elevated erythrocyte sedimentation rate are collectively very suggestive of malignancy. The presence of an abdominal mass, ascites, hepatomegaly, or an abnormal isotopic liver scan greatly increases the probability that there is an underlying malignant process.

Coupland et al reported the laparoscopic exploration of 103 patients with these characteristics.[7] Cancer was found in 30 of them. Definitive diagnosis averted laparotomy in 75. Failure to carry out a satisfactory laparoscopy in 22 patients was due mainly to intra-abdominal adhesions from previous surgery.

Metastatic Work-up (Assessment for Operability). In many instances it is crucial in the management of a patient known to have cancer to determine whether there is intra-abdominal dissemination. Current noninvasive methods for assessing the stage of intra-abdominal malignancy are notoriously inaccurate. Direct visualization of the liver, spleen, omentum, and peritoneal surface by means of laparoscopy provides much more precise evaluation for staging purposes.

As described in the discussion on liver disease (see p. 160), 90 percent of liver metastases are located on or near the surface. Laparoscopy is capable of visualizing 80 to 90 percent of the hepatic surface, thus offering an adequate method for evaluating dissemination to the liver. Dombernowsky et al found 21 percent of patients with small-cell anaplastic carcinoma of the lung to have biopsy proved liver metastases when staged by laparoscopy prior to thoracic surgery for the primary lesion.[10] An additional 9 percent of their patients had macroscopic signs of hepatic involvement seen at laparoscopy (lesions greater than 10 mm in size). No biopsy was performed in the latter group.

If intra-abdominal dissemination of a neoplastic process is identified, the patients are spared needless exploratory laparotomy. Furthermore, this finding may interdict surgery for resection of the primary tumor. To the contrary, merely because one cannot identify metastatic dissemination by laparoscopy does not give one the assurance they are not present. If there is a high degree of suspicion, exploratory laparotomy is indicated.

As previously described (see Chapter 3), laparoscopy need not be limited to the staging of a neoplastic process. Second-look operations to identify recurrence or to assess the response to chemotherapy have been shown to be beneficial in the follow-up of patients with cancer.

Staging Lymphoma. Accurate staging of a lymphoma remains a crucial step for planning treatment. In most cases, hepatic involvement precludes radiation therapy as the primary therapeutic modality in favor of chemotherapy. Splenic and nodal infiltration are of similar importance. Not unlike other type of tumors, liver function tests, radioisotopic scans, and percutaneous liver biopsies are notoriously inaccurate for determining the degree of liver involvement in a lymphomatous process. Visualization of approximately 90 percent of the liver surface and the spleen make laparoscopy the ideal method for evaluating hepatic and splenic involvement in these cases. Coleman et al found laparoscopy to be highly accurate in staging Hodgkin's disease.[6] They evaluated 35 previously untreated patients with Hodgkin's disease by laparoscopy and laparotomy. In only one of 31 instances did laparotomy fail to confirm the normal findings of laparoscopy. The low morbidity and lack of mortality led them to recommend laparoscopic evaluation for staging patients with Hodgkin's disease.

Castellani et al compared sequential pathologic staging of untreated lymphomas (excluding Hodgkin's disease) by laparoscopy and laparotomy combined with marrow biopsy in 119 patients.[5] Translaparoscopic liver and spleen biopsy specimens were obtained when feasible. They reported that laparoscopy with needle marrow biopsy was able to detect 89 percent of patients who were finally classified as having Stage IV disease. Laparotomy was useful for detecting occult lymphoma in the abdominal lymph nodes. They concluded that laparoscopic liver and spleen biopsies combined with needle marrow biopsy are extremely helpful procedures in the pathologic staging of non-Hodgkin's lymphoma.

ABDOMINAL TRAUMA

Blunt abdominal trauma confronts the surgeon with a serious diagnostic dilemma. Negative findings are encountered in 15 to 20 percent of exploratory laparotomies. This points out the pitfalls in the clinical diagnosis of intra-abdominal injuries. If laparotomies performed for trivial injuries (minor liver laceration and self-limited splenic hemorrhage, for example) are also included, the rate of unnecessary celiotomies rises to more than 50 percent among cases admitted for evaluation of abdominal trauma.

The serious consequences of overlooking active intra-abdominal bleeding or a perforated viscus mandates thorough evaluation of a patient with abdominal trauma. Physical examination, diagnostic paracentesis, and peritoneal lavage with quantitative and qualitative analysis of the fluid obtained generally form the basis for most surgical decisions in these patients. Routine roentgenography has proven of little value in assessing intra-abdominal injuries.

Laparoscopic evaluation of patients with intra-abdominal trauma has been reported to be useful in their management.[21] Nevertheless, laparoscopy has been used sporadically at best and has not even approached its potential. Sherwood et al reported their initial experience in 15 patients admitted for blunt abdominal trauma.[24] Most had been injured in vehicular accidents and presented with multiple system trauma, unexplained hypotension, or equivocal abdominal manifestations. Laparoscopic findings were normal in six of these patients; limited hemoperitoneum with no active bleeding was identified in seven others. Only two required immediate laparotomy following endoscopic examination of the peritoneal cavity.

Carnevale et al evaluated patients with abdominal stab wounds or blunt abdominal trauma.[4] All these patients would have been subjected to an exploratory celiotomy had they not had a preoperative laparoscopy first. Laparotomy was avoided in 12 (60 percent); either no visceral injury or only self-limiting intraperitoneal bleeding due to hepatic laceration was found among them. The remaining eight patients (40 percent) required laparotomy for repair of the intra-abdominal injuries identified at the laparoscopy. The average hospitalization period for the patients not subjected to laparotomy was 4.5 days, while it was 16 days (range 7 to 28 days) for those requiring an exploratory celiotomy.

Berci et al used laparoscopy instead of peritoneal lavage in patients admitted to the emergency room with abdominal trauma.[1] Most of the laparoscopic procedures were performed in the emergency unit under local anesthesia with supplementary intravenous sedation (diazepam, meperidine) as required. In 53.5 percent of their patients, the laparoscopic findings were negative; 25.4 percent had minimal to moderate hemoperitoneum which was managed nonoperatively by expectancy. Laparotomy was required in only 21.1 percent. Performing the procedure under local anesthesia in an emergency room setting, demonstrated by Berci et al to be feasible, permits rapid identification of the patient who requires immediate exploratory laparotomy. In the remainder, it not only averts unnecessary surgical explorations, but also results in shorter hospitalization, thus lowering costs.

Laparoscopy is clearly not recommended for patients with obvious indications for laparotomy, such as hypotension and shock. These pressing manifestations are present in less than one-third of patients who have had blunt abdominal trauma or stab wounds. Identification of blood by peritoneal lavage is not an indication for immediate laparotomy by itself. Nearly 20 percent of patients with overt hemoperitoneum on lavage were found to have no evidence of visceral injury or source of active bleeding at exploration.[21]

PEDIATRIC LAPAROSCOPY

The use of laparoscopy in children was essentially unknown until Gans and Berci reported their initial experience in 1971.[14] With minor modifications (involving anesthesia, degree of pneumoperitoneum and size of instruments), it has since become evident that extremes of age or body size are not contraindications to diagnostic or operative laparoscopy. Indications and contraindications are similar in children to those in the adult (see Chapter 6).

Leape and Ramenofsky reported results in 120 infants and children who underwent diagnostic laparoscopy for a variety of indications.[17] These included chronic abdominal pain, question of appendicitis, liver biopsy, biliary atresia, and abdominal trauma. They obtained a specific diagnosis in 71 percent of their patients; 59 percent of them were spared a laparotomy. Their conclusion mirrored the recommendations for the use of laparoscopy in adults. The significant decrease in exploratory laparotomies circumvents the discomfort and potential complications of a major surgical procedure. The low morbidity associated with laparoscopy also results in a marked reduction in the length of hospitalization.

The need for general anesthesia for laparoscopy in infants and children means that this procedure has to be reserved for patients who would otherwise require a laparotomy. Laparoscopy cannot and should not be substituted for less hazardous noninvasive tests. Nevertheless, if the procedure were used appropriately it would limit major surgical operations to those deemed necessary for therapeutic purposes.

References

1. Berci G, Dunkelman D, Michel SL, et al. Emergency minilaparoscopy in abdominal trauma: An update. Am J Surg 1983; 146:261-265.
2. Blackwell JN, Dean ACB, MacLeod IB, Sumerling MD, Finlayson NDC. Laparoscopy and radioisotope imaging in the investigation of suspected liver disease. Digest Dis Sc 1981; 26:507-512.
3. Bleiberg H, Rozencweig M, Mathieu M, et al. The use of peritoneoscopy in the detection of liver metastases. Cancer 1978; 41:863-867.
4. Carnevale N, Baron N, Delany HM. Peritoneoscopy as an aid in the diagnosis of abdominal trauma: A preliminary report. J Trauma 1977; 17:634-641.
5. Castellani R, Bonadonna G, Spinelli P, et al. Sequential pathologic staging of untreated non-Hodgkin's lymphomas by laparoscopy and laparotomy combined with marrow biopsy. Cancer 1977; 40:2322-2328.
6. Coleman M, Lightdale CJ, Vinciguerra VP, et al. Peritoneoscopy in Hodgkin disease: Confirmation of results by laparotomy. JAMA 1976; 236:2634-2636.
7. Coupland GAE, Townend DM, Martin CJ. Peritoneoscopy: Use in assessment of intra-abdominal malignancy. Surgery 1981; 89:645-649.
8. Curtis AH. Cause of adhesions in right upper quadrant. JAMA 1930; 94:1221-1222.
9. Deutsch AA, Zelikovsky A, Reiss R. Laparoscopy in the prevention of unnecessary appendectomies: A prospective study. Br J Surg 1982; 69:336-337.
10. Dombernowsky P, Hirsch F, Hansen HH, Hainau B. Peritoneoscopy in the staging of 190 patients with small-cell anaplastic carcinoma of the lung with special reference to subtyping. Cancer 1978; 41:2008-2012.
11. Fitz-Hugh T Jr. Acute gonococcic peritonitis of right upper quadrant in women. JAMA 1934; 102:2094-2096.
12. Friedman IH, Wolff WI. Laparoscopy: A safer method for liver biopsy in the high risk patient. Am J Gastroenterol 1977;67:319-323.

13. Gaisford WD. Peritoneoscopy: A valuable technique for surgeons. Am J Surg 1975; 130:671-678.
14. Gans SL, Berci G. Peritoneoscopy in infants and children. J Pediatr Surg 1973; 8:399-405.
15. Gomel V. Laparoscopy in general surgery. Am J Surg 1976; 131:319-323.
16. Grossman MJ, Rosenfeld DL, Bronson RA. Perihepatic adhesions in infertility patients with prior pelvic inflammatory disease. J Reprod Med 1981; 26:625-626.
17. Leape LL, Ramenofsky ML. Laparoscopy for questionable appendicitis: Can it reduce the negative appendectomy rate? Ann Surg 1980; 191:410-413.
18. Lightdale CJ, Hajdu SI, Luisi CB. Cytology of the liver, spleen and peritoneum obtained by sheathed brush during laparoscopy. Am J Gastroenterol 1980; 74:21-24.
19. Lightdale CJ. Laparoscopy and biopsy in malignant liver disease. Cancer 1982; 50:2672-2675.
20. Mansi C, Savarino V, Picciotto A, et al. Comparison between laparoscopy, ultrasonography, and computed tomography in widespread and localized liver diseases. Gastrointest Endosc 1982; 28:83-85.
21. Morgenstern L, Uyeda RY. Nonoperative management of injuries of the spleen in adults. Surg Gynecol Obstet 1983; 157:513-518.
22. Reichert JA, Valle RF. Fitz-Hugh-Curtis syndrome: A laparoscopic approach. JAMA 1976; 236:266-268.
23. Robinson HB, Smith GW. Applications for laparoscopy in general surgery. Surg Gynecol Obstet 1976; 143:829-834.
24. Sherwood R, Berci G, Austin E, Morgenstern L. Minilaparoscopy for blunt abdominal trauma. Arch Surg 1980; 115:672-673.
25. Stajano C. La reaccion frenica en ginecologia. Semana Med Buenos Aires 1920; 27:243-248.
26. Sugarbaker PH. Optimizing peritoneoscopic visualization of the liver utilizing a double telescope technique. Surg Gynecol Obstet 1981; 152:655-657.

8 CHOICE OF ANESTHESIA

Choosing the most appropriate type of anesthesia for a laparoscopy has to take into account the patient's condition, the indications for the procedure, and the goals of the operation. By virtue of the variable requirements for pneumoperitoneum, lithotomy and extreme Trendelenburg position, and electrocautery, anesthetic needs for gynecologic laparoscopy differ from those of upper abdominal endoscopy. Adequacy of the patient's respiratory function has to be weighed as an especially critical factor. The decision to utilize one anesthetic technique over another should be made in collaboration with the anesthesiologist. Patient safety must prevail above all.

It is more important to optimize the anesthetic considerations in most cases than to compromise them in order to undertake a standardized endoscopic procedure. Therefore, it is necessary for the experienced laparoscopist to be capable of performing the operation under diverse conditions. Appropriate knowledge of the advantages and limitations of each anesthetic modality is essential so that he or she can counsel and prepare the patient accordingly. Physiologic changes inherent in laparoscopy will be discussed in Chapters 9 and 10, whereas those related to the anesthesia will be described here.

ANATOMIC ASPECTS OF PAIN

Provision of analgesia and/or anesthesia to a patient undergoing laparoscopy requires a thorough understanding of the underlying pathophysiologic process that causes the pain of the procedure. In order to provide adequate pain relief for this operation, it is necessary to know about the sensory innervation of the anterior abdominal wall, the peritoneum, and the abdominal organs. Pain control amnesia is detailed in the section on perioperative premedication (see p. 176). Here we will just detail the neuroanatomy relevant to laparoscopy.

The nerve supply to the anterior abdominal wall arises from the five lowest intercostal (thoraco-abdominal) and the three uppermost lumbar nerves (T8 to L3). The umbilicus and the periumbilical area are innervated by the tenth thoracic nerve; the eleventh and twelfth thoracic nerves supply the subumbilical-suprapubic area. A portion of the twelfth thoracic nerve joins the first lumbar nerve to form the iliohypogastric nerve. The anterior cutaneous branch of the iliohypogastric nerve also innervates the skin of the hypogastric region.[6]

The peritoneum is innervated by the six lowest thoracic nerves (T7 to T12). With the exception of the mesenteric root, which is quite sensitive to traction, the visceral peritoneum is relatively insensitive to most pain stimuli. This low sensitivity is the reason an injury to an intraperitoneal organ is not perceived immediately. Pain accompanying perforation of a loop of bowel or a blood vessel does not usually become apparent until free spillage of intestinal contents or blood causes chemical inflammatory response by the peritoneum. By contrast, the parietal peritoneum is richly supplied with somatic afferent nerves and is extremely sensitive to all forms of stimuli, especially the stretching produced by the distending pneumoperitoneum.[6] It is generally not possible to anesthetize the peritoneal layer by local injections of an anesthetic agent. This explains the frequent need for supplementary administration of systemic medication to patients who are undergoing laparoscopy under local anesthesia.

The diaphragm is innervated by the phrenic nerves which originate mainly from the fourth cervical nerve with accessory fibers from the third to the fifth cervical nerves (C3 to C5). The cervical root origin of the diaphragmatic innervation reflects its embryological location. The phrenic nerve, although recognized as the motor nerve to the diaphragm, also contains sensory fibers. Sympathetic fibers join the nerve at the root of the neck. Terminal branches of the phrenic nerve provide sensory fibers to the peritoneum.

When the patient is placed in the Trendelenburg position, irritation of the undersurface of the diaphragm during laparoscopy may be the result of direct pressure caused by the intraperitoneal organs. It may also be caused by accumulation of gas in the subphrenic area. Irritation of the subdiaphragmatic region usually produces pain referred to the shoulder. This referred pain is believed to arise from sensory transmission through the phrenic nerve to the fourth and fifth cervical nerves. These nerves share afferent fibers from the brachial plexus which innervates the shoulder.

In the course of gynecologic laparoscopy, one often has to apply a tenaculum to the uterine cervix and insert a uterine mobilizer to manipulate the uterus. Therefore, it is necessary to have some knowledge of the innervation of the uterus and cervix. Most of the sensory innervation of the uterus derives from the sympathetic nervous system. Sensory afferent fibers run through the hypogastric and aortic plexuses to reach the eleventh and twelfth thoracic nerve ganglia. Sensory innervation of the cervix includes both parasympathetic and sympathetic fibers. They derive from the second, third, and fourth sacral nerves (S2 to S4) and merge to lose their identity in the cervical ganglion of Frankenhäuser. Fibers from this ganglion reach the cervix through the uterosacral ligaments.[6]

A translaparoscopic operative procedure must take into account the innervation of the particular organ to be operated upon, as well. Anesthesia of some viscus organs can be achieved by local infiltration of the relevant area or by contact anesthesia (surface drop technique). Topical anesthesia suffices for procedures involving superficial tissues, but is not adequate for more because it cannot anesthetize the deeper layers.

PREMEDICATION

Most diagnostic and operative laparoscopies are performed as outpatient procedures. Convenience to the patient and economic factors are the main reasons for this practice. Anesthesia for day-care surgery must ensure that the patient will recover quickly and that she will be well enough to leave the surgical center within a few hours after the operation. Preoperative medication includes drugs to help reduce presurgical anxiety.[8] A restful night preceding the day of surgery is clearly advantageous to the patient. Prescribing a fast-acting, short-duration hypnotic drug, such as flurazepam (Dalmane, one dose of 15 to 30 mg according to age and weight), taken orally at bedtime is usually successful for inducing restful sleep. Benzodiazepines are contraindicated in patients who may be pregnant because of the increased risk of congenital malformations if given in first trimester. In these cases, secobarbital sodium (50 to 100 mg by mouth at bedtime) has a similar sedative and hypnotic effect with no known teratogenic risk.

Medication administered just prior to the anesthesia (premedication) has been shown to reduce the dosage of anesthetic agent required for satisfactory induction. The aim of premedication is to obtain mental and emotional relaxation, reduce sensory input, and counteract adverse autonomic nervous reaction.[5] Opponents of routine use of premedication stress the resulting prolongation of the recovery period and increased postoperative nausea and vomiting. For patients undergoing laparoscopy under regional or general anesthesia, the decision as to whether to use premedication or not generally rests with the anesthesiologist. Nevertheless, it is obviously important for the surgeon to be familiar with the method that the anesthesiologist will be using; this allows him or her to counsel the patient properly prior to the procedure.

If laparoscopy is to be done under local anesthesia, light sedation given intravenously has proved beneficial. Advantages to the patient include amnesia and increased analgesia which facilitates the surgery. Combinations of drugs, such as ketamine and diazepam, have been shown to provide good sedation and supplemental analgesia.[7] However, they are associated with a prolonged sedative period postoperatively. This makes them unsuitable for use in outpatient procedures. Short-acting analgesics, such as fentanyl citrate, have gained increased acceptance for many types of surgical procedures performed under local anesthesia. Penfield reported 1,200 cases where fentanyl 0.1 mg was administered intravenously to supplement local anesthesia and found it to be quite satisfactory for outpatient surgery.[9]

Use of intravenous sedation for laparoscopy, without constant attendance by trained personnel to help maintain and monitor the patient's airway and ventilation, is dangerous. It must be discouraged. Fentanyl citrate is a significant respiratory depressant. Diazepam and morphine, also used to achieve mild preoperative sedation, possess similar depressing effects. Whereas the alert patient may respond to and communicate her pain, she is incapable of monitoring her level of respiratory depression, acid-base imbalance, or peripheral circulatory collapse. If a patient experiences respiratory depression while undergoing surgery in a darkened room, without adequate surveillance other than by the operating surgeon, there may be serious delay in diagnosing the complication. Sedation should be light and not exceed a state of drowsiness or slurred speech. The patient should be able to talk and take deep breaths on command.

Surgeons using diazepam, morphine, or fentanyl must be familiar with their biphasic mode of action.[10] This pharmacologic characteristic makes them dangerous when they are given in doses that exceed light sedation. In the case of diazepam, when the initial sedative effect wears off, an active metabolite, oxazepam, is formed. Oxazepam produces a secondary sedative effect 5 to 7 hours after the initial dose of diazepam was given. This effect may not become apparent until the patient has already left the surgical facility. When morphine is administered a secondary sedative effect may develop, as well. It is probably due to a process of internal recirculation. The drug is cleared from the blood by the liver and excreted in the bile. It is then reabsorbed in the intestinal tract to produce the secondary peak effect. Apnea, severe respiratory depression, and even cardiac arrest may occur. These effects have been documented in patients who have apparently recovered fully from the initial sedative effect of the narcotic medication. Such individuals may find themselves in difficulty several hours later, following their discharge.

Atropine sulfate has gained wide acceptance as an agent to be given prior to the administration of the anesthetic medication for a laparoscopy.[4,8] In patients who are to have the procedure under local anesthesia, atropine averts undesirable vasovagal reactions from uterine manipulation and cervical stimulation. When used for premedication in patients receiving general anesthesia, atropine decreases the amount of tracheobronchial secretions. Surgeons would be well advised to inform the patient undergoing a laparoscopy that, if small amounts of sedative drugs do not achieve the desired effect, it is much safer to administer a light general anesthesia than to increase the dosage of narcotic medication.

LOCAL ANESTHESIA

Local anesthesia for laparoscopy offers distinct advantages and just a few counterbalancing limitations. Its advantages include reduced anesthesia time, faster postoperative recovery from anesthesia with less nausea and vomiting, fewer postoperative complications, and lower cost. In addition, one is able to maintain verbal contact with the patient.

The main disadvantage of local anesthesia is the limitation it imposes on the manipulation of pelvic organs because pain and discomfort are produced by peritoneal stretching. Although considered by some as a disadvantage, local anesthesia demands precise and gentle surgical technique by the operator. This is obviously beneficial for reducing both early and late complications. Experience shows that local anesthesia is generally adequate for short translaparoscopic procedures, but it may not always be possible to complete a prolonged diagnostic laparoscopy in a satisfactory manner. Pain of peritoneal origin and visceral manipulation can be controlled by supplemental systemic sedation and analgesia, as discussed earlier. It is strongly recommended that appropriate anesthesiologic backup be available in case general anesthesia should be required.

Blood gases obtained during laparoscopy under local anesthesia reveal a marked fall in arterial PaO_2 and an increase in the arterial $PaCO_2$ (see Chapter 10). The absence of any significant change in the level of bicarbonate or buffer base in these patients shows that the acidosis is respiratory rather than metabolic in nature. These changes are observed in patients in whom carbon dioxide is insufflated for the pneumoperitoneum. Transperitoneal absorption of carbon dioxide augments the hypercarbia and the consequent respiratory acidosis. Rather than carbon dioxide, nitrous oxide is recommended to produce the pneumoperitoneum if general anesthesia is not being given because uncontrolled ventilation does not provide for compensatory hyperventilation to counteract the expected respiratory acidosis. The relative hazards of the several available gases are discussed in Chapter 17.

Preparation of the patient for the procedure should include a step-by-step explanation of the technique and a description of what the patient is most likely to experience. Voluntary preoperative emptying of the urinary bladder should be encouraged in lieu of catheterization because it reduces the risk (albeit small) of an iatrogenic urinary tract infection. Following a pelvic examination to ascertain size and position of the uterus and the adnexa, paracervical anesthesia is given. This is done before attaching the tenaculum to the cervix and inserting the uterine mobilizer into the endometrial cavity. A minimal amount of anesthetic is required for the purpose of applying these instruments. If dilatation and curettage is planned to follow the laparoscopy, a vasoconstrictor should be added to the anesthetic solution to prolong its effect. The combination of lidocaine and epinephrine provides a paracervical block of sufficient duration to permit one to dilate the cervix for the endometrial curettage without the need for any additional anesthesia.

The abdominal portion of the technique requires the infiltration of the abdominal wall layers with a local anesthetic agent (such as 0.5 percent lidocaine with 1:200,000 epinephrine). Because the fibrotic nature of the umbilicus makes infiltration more difficult (see Chapter 2), a midline subumbilical site is preferable. Most of the discomfort related to insertion of the Verres needle is due to the digital pressure required to lift the abdominal wall. The amount of gas insufflated to produce the pneumoperitoneum in the patient being operated on under local anesthesia should be limited to 2 to 3 L. This is done to avoid excessive intra-abdominal pressure which limits diaphragmatic excursion and makes spontaneous respiration difficult.

The use of the single-puncture operative laparoscope is advisable (within its constraints). It does not preclude resorting to a secondary puncture site for auxiliary instruments. If additional puncture sites are required, the midline suprapubic area is chosen. Its avascularity prevents formation of an abdominal wall hematoma from inadvertent injury to a tegumentary vessel.

Translaparoscopic surgery should be preceded by local application (drip or flow-over technique) of lidocaine to the area to be operated upon; alternatively, the structure can be infiltrated. Pharmacokinetic and pharmacodynamic studies of local anesthetic agents show that one can give them safely and yet keep well below convulsive or toxic levels (for lidocaine the convulsive blood level is 18 to 26 μg/ml; for bupivacaine, 4.5 to 5.5 μg/ml).[11]

Local anesthesia has proved to be effective for laparoscopic procedures. It was initially recommended for use in patients in whom general anesthesia was contraindicated. It is now recognized that respiratory and cardiovascular changes are about the same in patients who are awake as in those who are anesthetized. Familiarity with these changes is essential for appropriate preselection of patients for local anesthesia. In addition, good surgeon-patient rapport demands thorough understanding of the procedure by the patient before a laparoscopy under local anesthesia is undertaken.

SPINAL ANESTHESIA

Attempts to achieve adequate pain relief for laparoscopy in a patient who remains conscious throughout led to the evaluation of regional anesthesia. Spinal anesthesia for laparoscopy has been shown to be safe and quite satisfactory for the successful performance of laparoscopy. Disadvantages sometimes associated with this type of anesthesia include incomplete relaxation, respiratory and circulatory disturbances, discomfort due to diaphragmatic irritation by the distending gas, excessive increase of arterial $PaCO_2$ and fall in arterial pH, postspinal puncture syndrome (spinal headache), possible neurological sequelae (such as cranial nerve disturbances and delayed sympathetic recovery), and prolongation of the postoperative recovery period.

Patients who have had laparoscopy under spinal anesthesia generally take some time before motor function is fully recovered. Therefore, they are unsuitable for early discharge. Except for the longer postoperative recovery period, no significant differences have been encountered among patients who had spinal as compared with other types of anesthesia. Burke reported more than 1,000 laparoscopies performed under spinal anesthesia; he found that most of the aforementioned liabilities occurred infrequently, if at all.[2] Abdominal relaxation was adequate for both diagnostic and operative laparoscopy (including sterilization procedures). Patient discomfort was minimal and limited to mild neck and shoulder pain attributed to subdiaphragmatic irritation. The incidence of spinal headache was less than 1 percent. Fewer than 23 percent could be discharged on the same day as the laparoscopy because of the longer postoperative recovery period.

In another study, Caceres and Kim evaluated blood gas effects of laparoscopy under spinal anesthesia.[3] These patients breathed room air. The amount of carbon dioxide insufflated to create the pneumoperitoneum was 3.5 $\pm$ 1.2 L. Trendelenburg tilt was limited to no more than 15° from the horizontal. PaO_2 was found to be significantly increased from a mean preoperative value of 77.4 mm Hg to 90 mm Hg at 5 minutes and 93.3 mm Hg at 15 minutes after an adequate pneumoperitoneum was established. $PaCO_2$ remained stable and pH values varied only slightly ($\pm$ 0.03 units). These changes are explained by hyperventilation occurring in response to increased carbon dioxide. The respiratory center is able to react because it is not depressed at all.

It is obvious that, in patients undergoing laparoscopy under spinal anesthesia, the degree of pneumoperitoneum is limited by the discomfort due to increased intra-abdominal pressure. This is analogous to the situation in those given local anesthesia (discussed earlier). Sensory block at the T4 or T5 level does not relieve pain that originates in the upper abdomen or the diaphragm. The degree of Trendelenburg incline is limited to avoid undesirably high anesthetic levels and increased pressure on the diaphragm by the abdominal contents. Whereas it is feasible to visualize the upper abdomen with laparoscopy under spinal anesthesia, the use of spinal anesthesia is not indicated for the sole purpose of upper abdominal endoscopy. Exposing the patients to its potential risks and side effects without the benefit of upper abdominal pain relief seems unwarranted.

EPIDURAL ANESTHESIA

Lumbar epidural block anesthesia also provides satisfactory pain relief for a laparoscopic procedure. It has technical limitations similar to those of spinal anesthesia, but it offers some advantages over that technique. If a diagnostic laparoscopy is done for the evaluation of pelvic disease, there is always the possibility that laparotomy will be needed. Unruptured ectopic pregnancy, twisted adnexa, and bleeding corpus luteum are some of the entities that would benefit from immediate surgical correction if encountered at laparoscopy. The continuous epidural technique allows one to prolong the anesthesia by repeated supplementation as required.

Bridenbaugh and Soderstrom reported the use of lumbar epidural block anesthesia for laparoscopic sterilization of outpatients.[1] Arterial blood gases evaluated in the first 15 patients were within normal limits. They found excellent patient acceptance. Only one patient stated she would have preferred to be asleep. One inadvertently received a subarachnoid tap and subsequently developed a spinal headache. The epidural anesthesia was adequate for the surgical procedure. It had the additional advantage of being associated with a short postoperative recovery period, thereby allowing patients to be discharged the same day as the operation.

In general, the use of regional anesthesia has not gained popular acceptance for laparoscopy. Nevertheless, it should be kept in mind for the occasional patient who is not a suitable candidate for a general anesthetic and yet desires more pain relief than can be provided by local anesthesia.

GENERAL ANESTHESIA

Notwithstanding the gain in popularity of local and regional anesthesia for laparoscopy, most of these procedures are still performed using general anesthesia. The advantages of general anesthesia include complete relaxation, greater allowable degree of Trendelenburg tilt, controlled ventilation, elimination of patient anxiety, complete analgesia and amnesia, easier manipulation of intraperitoneal organs, and a quiescent operative field. Disadvantages include complications inherent in general anesthetic, prolonged recovery time, greater postoperative discomfort, and increased cost.

Complete Relaxation. Relaxation of the anterior abdominal wall permits one to insufflate larger amounts of distending gas without causing a marked increase in the intraperitoneal pressure. The creation of an ample pneumoperitoneum under low pressure decreases the cephalad pressure on the diaphragm. It thus reduces the inspiratory pressure required for proper ventilation. Additionally, the larger the intraperitoneal gas chamber developed, the greater the distance between the undersurface of the abdominal wall and the large retroperitoneal vessels. This helps reduce the risk of inadvertent injury to these vital structures.

Degree of Trendelenburg Tilt. In patients undergoing laparoscopy under local or regional anesthesia, the degree of Trendelenburg tilt is limited to not more than 15°. This constraint is imposed to limit the upward pressure of the intra-abdominal organs on the diaphragm, thereby facilitating respiration. The degree of head-down tilt is also limited by the amount of intracranial blood stasis the patient is able to tolerate without major discomfort. During certain types of diagnostic laparoscopy (for example, for pelvic adhesions or large fibroid uterus), one's ability to position the patient in Trendelenburg inclinations of 30° or greater could make the difference between a complete and satisfactory evaluation and an incomplete one. General anesthesia permits use of deep head-down tilt that would not be tolerated or feasible in a patient who is awake.

Controlled Ventilation. One of the main advantages of general anesthesia for a laparoscopic procedure is that it permits ventilation to be controlled by the anesthetist. The vital capacity of the lungs is adversely affected by the cephalad displacement of the diaphragm by the pneumoperitoneum and the Trendelenburg position required for laparoscopy. Manual or mechanically assisted ventilation allows one to compensate for any negative factors affecting respiration.

If carbon dioxide is used to create the pneumoperitoneum, hypercarbia results from absorption of carbon dioxide from the peritoneal cavity. Controlled hyperventilation can be given to patients under general anesthesia. This checks the increase in arterial carbon dioxide partial pressure, thereby decreasing the risk of cardiac arrhythmias and other side effects (see Chapter 10).

Manipulation of Intraperitoneal Organs. Thorough evaluation of the entire peritoneal cavity usually requires instrumental displacement of intraperitoneal organs. In laparoscopy performed as part of an infertility work-up, it is essential to visualize the entire cul-de-sac as well as the posterior aspect of the ovaries. In some cases, this requires extensive manipulation of the uterus and the adnexal structures, all of which can be very sensitive to painful stimuli. At times, mobilizing a small anteverted uterus is all that is needed for adequate viewing. However, the problem is not readily solved if the uterus is retroverted or acutely retroflexed, conditions existing in more than 30 percent of women.

Complete diagnostic laparoscopy should routinely include a description of the appendix, if it is still present (see Chapter 7). This requires moving the ileocecal portion of the intestine which is extremely sensitive to instrumental manipulation. Whenever one suspects intraperitoneal adhesions or organomegaly, one may have to displace intraperitoneal structures; this ordinarily requires the use of a general anesthetic.

Elimination of Patient Anxiety. Some degree of anxiety is experienced by all patients undergoing any form of surgery. Laparoscopy is not an exception. Whereas the use of intravenous sedatives and ataractic medication has proven sufficient at times, these do not compare favorably with general anesthesia. Preoperative management of a person who is to undergo laparoscopy must include a detailed explanation of the mechanics of the procedure. Additionally, she should be given a description of what she is most likely to experience during the operation. Patients prepared in this way will usually require a smaller amount of anesthetic medication and react more favorably than others.

Analgesia and Amnesia. The degree of analgesia obtained with general anesthesia is obviously greater than with any other anesthetic technique. An additional important effect of general anesthesia is the amnesia it provides. Stress before and during the laparoscopy is decreased by providing a pain free operation. One should bear in mind that a proportion of patients undergoing laparoscopy may require another procedure in the future, including second look operations or oocyte harvest for in vitro fertilization. Therefore, unpleasant experiences should be avoided whenever possible.

Quiescent Operative Field. A laparoscopic procedure requires the close coordination of every member of the surgical team. Additionally, the use of multiple electromechanical instruments necessitates intense concentration by the surgeon on the technical aspects of the operation. Therefore, it is in the best interests of both the patient and the surgeon for the operative field to be as tranquil as possible. Although some quick transendoscopic surgical procedures can be safely performed under local anesthesia, diagnostic laparoscopies that may include extensive intra-abdominal manipulations are facilitated by the stillness offered by having the patient asleep under general anesthesia.

Risks of General Anesthesia. The risks of serious complications from general anesthetic have been reduced to a minimum as technical skills have improved and better safeguards have been introduced. Nevertheless, they are still real and the patient should be made aware of their existence. Highly trained personnel in a well-equipped institution is required to ensure the safety of general anesthesia for laparoscopy. Complications related to the type of anesthesia used in laparoscopy are detailed in Chapter 13. Regurgitation and aspiration of gastric contents, gastric distention predisposing to puncture of the stomach with the Verres needle or laparoscopy trocar are some of the complications singularly associated with performing a laparoscopy under general anesthesia.

Prolonged Recovery Time. The use of premedication for analgesia and tranquilization, plus hypnotic drugs and muscle relaxants, requires a longer period of recovery following laparoscopy under general anesthesia. Although the half-life of these medications is short and allows accurate titration during administration, there is a wide range of variation in regard to the time needed for complete excretion. The latter affects the duration of the postoperative recovery. Specific side effects of each of the substances used during a general anesthesia are described in more detail in Chapter 11.

Greater Postoperative Discomfort. Undesirable short- and long-term side effects are more often seen in patients receiving general anesthesia than in those exposed to local infiltration anesthetics. Nausea, vomiting, and sore throat from endotracheal intubation are common among patients given systemic anesthesia. Generalized myalgia is also more frequent as a consequence of the use of muscle relaxant drugs. Additionally, patients often have feelings of easy fatigability for several days following the exposure to a general anesthetic; this is as yet an unexplained phenomenon.

Increased Cost. The need for special equipment, highly trained personnel, and expensive back-up systems, including a fully equipped recovery room, contributes to the increased cost of a laparoscopy performed under general anesthesia. Effective cost reductions have been accomplished by preoperative screening and day-care surgery. Caution should be exercised to ensure against attempting to decrease costs at the expense of patient safety.

References

1. Bridenbaugh LD, Soderstrom RM. Lumbar epidural block anesthesia for outpatient laparoscopy. J Reprod Med 1979; 23:85-86.
2. Burke RK. Spinal anesthesia for laparoscopy: A review of 1,063 cases. J Reprod Med 1978; 21:59-62.
3. Caceres D, Kim K. Spinal anesthesia for laparoscopic tubal sterilization. Am J Obstet Gynecol 1978; 131:219-220.
4. Fishburne JI. Anesthesia for laparoscopy: Considerations, complications and techniques. J Reprod Med 1978; 21:37-39.
5. Forrest WH, Brown CR, Brown BW. Subjective responses to six common preoperative medications. Anesthesiology 1977; 47:241-247.
6. Gray H, Goss CM. Anatomy of the human body. Philadelphia, Lea & Febiger 1970:985-988, 1009-1042.
7. Kleindienst W, Frangenheim H. Ketamine-HCl-diazepam anesthesia for laparoscopy. J Reprod Med 1979; 23:299-303.
8. Korttila K, Aromaa U, Tammisto T. Patients' expectations and acceptance of the effects of the drugs given before anesthesia: Comparison of light and amnesic premedication. Acta Anaesth Scand 1981; 25:381-386.
9. Penfield AJ. Laparoscopic sterilization under local anesthesia. Obstet Gynecol 1977; 49:725-727.
10. Porterfield HW, Franklin LT. The use of general anesthesia in the office surgery facility. Clin Plast Surg 1983; 10:289-294.
11. Spielman FJ, Hulka JF, Ostheimer GW, Mueller RA. Pharmacokinetics and pharmacodynamics of local analgesia for laparoscopic tubal ligations. Am J Obstet Gynecol 1983; 146:821-824.

9 CIRCULATORY CHANGES

Cardiovascular alterations occur often during laparoscopy. Major complications, such as arterial hypotension, shock, cardiac arrest, and sudden death are reported in most published surveys. In addition, minor changes take place in blood pressure, cardiac output, and peripheral venous return. Cardiac arrythmias are also a fairly common occurrence. Cardiovascular derangements accompany the postural changes that are required for positioning the patient properly on the operating room table. They are generally mild and insignificant by themselves. However, they can be superimposed on cardiovascular changes secondary to the increase in intra-abdominal pressure caused by creation of a pneumoperitoneum. Under these circumstances, they can result in serious complications. Patients who have cardiovascular illness are especially susceptible to the major consequences of these changes.

As more experience has accumulated on the safety of laparoscopy, gynecologists have expanded indications for this procedure and liberalized criteria for selection of patients. Critical to this issue is knowledge of the cardiovascular changes that can be expected to occur, about methods to avoid aggravating them, and about the therapeutic measures required to correct serious complications when they arise. Such information is a sine qua non for the safety and success of a laparoscopic procedure.

Most experience with laparoscopy has been gathered in young, healthy women undergoing sterilization or infertility work-up. Currently, laparoscopy is being used more extensively in oncologic cases. This involves an older population of patients many of whom have underlying systemic diseases which may have to be taken into account. It is also not unusual to be confronted with a young woman who has advanced cardiovascular disease and is thus in need of sterilization to avoid pregnancy. Laparoscopically induced cardiovascular changes, which may bear little significance in the healthy population, have to be given proper consideration in these at-risk patients.

POSTURAL CHANGES

Variations in cardiovascular homeostasis result from changing the position of the patient during laparoscopy. Blood pressure, central venous pressure, and pulse pressure change when the patient is moved from supine to the lithotomy and Trendelenburg positions. These effects are due mainly to the redistribution of the blood mass caused by elevating the lower extremities above the level of the heart. In the young, healthy, normovolemic individual, circulatory disturbances are rapidly stabilized by compensatory mechanisms, such as improved myocardial contractility and variations in intrathoracic pressure during respiration. Such compensatory activity may not be fully operational in patients who are under general anesthesia and who may be receiving multiple medications.

Pressure of the abdominal organs on the diaphragm in the Trendelenburg position can, in itself, decrease the stroke volume and the cardiac output. As will be described later, this is further complicated by the increase in intra-abdominal pressure resulting from the pneumoperitoneum. Additionally, evaluation of hypotensive patients in shock shows that the arterial blood pressure decreases rather than increases when they are placed in the head-down position.[14] This is contrary to the long held concept that the Trendelenburg position helps to perfuse vital organs.

The effects on blood pressure and cardiac function become even more critical if the laparoscopy is being done for suspected intra-abdominal bleeding. Compensatory mechanisms may sustain normal or near normal blood pressure and pulse in the face of substantial intra-abdominal bleeding. Superimposed variations in stroke volume and cardiac output as a consequence of the head-down position may overcome these stabilizing effects, thereby placing the patient at risk of severe hemodynamic disruption. Because of these cardiovascular alterations, one should try to minimize the degree and duration of the Trendelenburg position during a laparoscopic procedure.

Additional significant hemodynamic changes take place when the patient is taken out of the lithotomy position at the completion of the procedure. Suddenly lowering the legs may enhance reduction in the blood pressure. These circulatory changes can be minimized by slowly lowering the legs, with both extended simultaneously, after first having returned the patient to the horizontal supine position.

VENOUS RETURN

Acute cardiovascular collapse during laparoscopy is a serious potential hazard. It has been sporadically reported in the literature.[1] The mechanism appears to be reduced venous return created by increased intra-abdominal pressure from the pneumoperitoneum. This in turn reduces cardiac output to yield a shock-like state. It is analogous to the pathogenesis of the supine hypotensive syndrome of pregnancy. Since the heart can only pump as much blood as it receives, impaired venous return is reflected in diminished cardiac function.

Venous return to the heart is determined by three factors, namely the mean systemic venous pressure, the venous resistance, and the intrathoracic pressure. An elevation in the mean systemic venous pressure for a given right atrial pressure proportionally increases the venous return. This situation can be seen in the augumented blood volume that results from the autotransfusion created by elevating the legs to place the patient in lithotomy position. The venous resistance (or resistance to venous return) is determined by the impediment of blood flow through the inferior and superior vena cava. It varies in direct proportion with the intrathoracic and intra-abdominal pressures. An increase in venous resistance reduces the venous return to the heart. When the intrathoracic (pleural) pressure becomes greater than the right atrial pressure, the vena cava is compressed and the venous return thereby reduced. Rising intra-abdominal pressure decreases the venous return from the pelvis and legs by compressing the inferior vena cava and elevating the venous resistance.

Hodgson et al actually found a marked increase in venous return in 18 patients undergoing laparoscopy. He suggested that this might be caused by transfer of blood from the abdominal organs and the inferior vena cava into the thoracic cavity.[5] The observation was subsequently confirmed by others. Enhanced sympathetic activity due to increased arterial pressure of carbon dioxide may be responsible.

Motew et al reported a similar increase in venous return even when intraperitoneal insufflation of carbon dioxide was limited so as to avoid exceeding an intra-abdominal pressure of 20 mm Hg. In cases where intra-abdominal pressure was allowed to rise above 20 mm Hg, there was diminution in central venous pressure, thereby reflecting inhibited venous return.[10] Kelman et al found a similar biphasic change in central venous pressure as the intra-abdominal pressure rose.[6] Moreover, they noted that the central venous pressure did not return to preoperative levels even after the intra-abdominal pressure had returned to zero at the conclusion of the laparoscopy. Sympathoadrenal constriction of the capacitance vessels was felt to be responsible for pooling the blood peripherally in these cases.

There is clear need for a balanced equilibrium between the parasympathetic and the sympathetic systems. This is corroborated by reported cases of severe bradycardia and hypotension developing in the early stages of carbon dioxide insufflation, well before high intra-abdominal pressures are reached. Intravenous atropine sulfate is effective in reversing the condition. This suggests it is caused by increased vagal stimulation. The vagal hyperstimulation in turn is thought to be due to irritation of the peritoneum by carbon dioxide, which occurs even when small amounts of gas are used, and excessive stretching of the peritoneum by insufflation of large volumes of gas.

Experience strongly supports the cautionary advice advanced by Hodgson et al.[5] They considered laparoscopy to be a potential hazard to the patient with preexisting cardiac disability. This is particularly the case if she is marginally compensated and on the verge of congestive heart failure. To avoid a drop in venous return, central venous pressure, and cardiac output, the intra-abdominal pressure during laparoscopy should never exceed 20 mm Hg in such patients. Indeed, this is a reasonable admonition for all patients.

CARDIAC OUTPUT

The effect of laparoscopy on cardiac output has been studied extensively. Both increases and decreases have been reported, depending on the method used to measure it. Marshall et al reported no significant variations following peritoneal insufflation with carbon dioxide despite the significant increases in mean arterial pressure, central venous pressure, and heart rate that were observed by the dye-dilution technique.[8]

Cardiac output is determined by a number of factors, including the contractility of the myocardium, the heart rate, and the preload or venous return. Moreover, increased extracardiac pressure resulting from high levels of intrathoracic pressure may affect it adversely. Cardiac contractility may be affected by the choice of anesthetic used. High concentrations of halothane, for example, may cause severe myocardial depression. In routine laparoscopy, this effect is counterbalanced by the action of the increased $PaCO_2$ resulting from carbon dioxide insufflation. It has an inotropic effect on myocardium and a pressor effect on peripheral vessels. Venous return or preload has been shown to rise provided intra-abdominal pressure does not exceed 20 mm Hg.

Central venous pressure, as an index of venous return, changes as a consequence of the increase in intra-abdominal pressure produced by the pneumoperitoneum. The increment in intra-abdominal pressure in the patient positioned horizontally has two opposing effects on venous return: It forces blood out of the abdominal organs (splanchnic vascular bed) into the inferior vena cava. At the same time, it sequesters blood in the legs to reduce the central or circulating blood volume. The latter plays a minor role if the patient is in the lithotomy position with legs elevated, and it is further reduced in Trendelenburg head-down position.

An increase in extracardiac pressure occurs when the intrathoracic pressure is elevated. This decreases the distending pressure of the right ventricle and impedes systemic venous return. It subsequently lowers the cardiac output. Smith et al reported increased intrathoracic pressure during artificial ventilation, presumably due to an increase in mean airway pressure.[13] If cardiac output has been reduced by elevated extracardiac pressure, it may be compensated for to some extent by gradually increasing blood volume.

Noninvasive impedance cardiographic techniques have been used to measure cardiac output. Lenz et al, for example, reported a fall of 0.5 to 0.6 L per minute in the cardiac output of 20 normal young women undergoing laparoscopy.[7] McKenzie et al demonstrated a consistent fall in stroke volume and cardiac output without significant changes in heart rate.[9] In their series, cardiac output fell to a mean value of 60 percent in 14 anesthetized patients. Both studies showed greater declines in cardiac output with deeper planes of anesthesia.

It should be noted that the routine intraoperative cardiovascular monitoring (blood pressure, pulse rate, and the clinical assessment of peripheral circulation) may not show any indication of a drop in cardiac output because compensatory mechanisms are usually operating effectively. Whereas such compensatory effects are fully operational in the average young, healthy patient undergoing nonemergency laparoscopy, they do not necessarily apply to patients with acute intra-abdominal hemorrhage, for example.

Diamant et al studied the interaction between acute hypovolemia and halothane anesthesia in dogs with increased intra-abdominal pressure caused by gas insufflation.[2] They found that inhalation anesthesia and intravascular volume depletion accentuated the deleterious hemodynamic effect of the high intra-abdominal pressure. This was true irrespective of the type of gas used. In this regard, they studied nitrogen, nitrous oxide, and carbon dioxide.

In gynecological practice, ruptured tubal pregnancy, bleeding corpus luteum, and uterine perforation are some of the conditions that may require laparoscopic evaluation in a hypovolemic patient. It is essential to reexpand the depleted intravascular volume in these cases before proceeding with the laparoscopy. In this way, the cardiac preload (venous return) is increased. This should not be done for patients who have some preexisting heart disease and in whom cardiac afterload is increased. These women need to have their cardiac contractility improved pharmacologically before a laparoscopy can be safely attempted.

HEART RATE

In the normal individual, the heart beats approximately 70 times per minute. Each beat originates in the sinoauricular node, producing what is known as a normal sinus rhythm. In the young, healthy individual, the heart rate varies with the phases of respiration (producing an inspiratory tachycardia), but these changes are of little clinical significance.

In a patient undergoing a laparoscopic procedure, the heart rate is affected by many factors. Some effects are stimulatory and some are depressive. Any imbalance in the compensatory mechanisms, such as may result from hyperstimulation of one over another, may trigger a response capable of producing serious consequences.

Carmichael reported severe bradycardia during the insufflation of carbon dioxide for pneumoperitoneum.[1] He attributed it to reflex vagal stimulation created by peritoneal stretching. Excessive vagal stimulation is capable of inhibiting the sinoauricular node and slowing the pulse. If severe enough, it can result in sudden loss of blood pressure. By giving 0.4 to 0.8 mg atropine intravenously just prior to the intraperitoneal gas insufflation, he was able to prevent the fall in heart rate. This confirmed that the bradycardia resulted from excessive vagal stimulation.

Fear and anxiety preceding the surgical procedure may enhance the response to moderate vagal stimulation. This unquantified factor might explain the wide range of responses observed by different investigators. Needless to say, it is difficult to assess and control. In this regard, it should be noted that most investigators who have studied the cardiovascular effects of increased intra-abdominal pressure from the pneumoperitoneum actually report a consistent increase in heart rate.

Smith et al reported a 10 percent increase in heart rate and mean arterial blood pressure in the population they studied.[13] El-Minawi et al showed a similar effect in a larger group of patients undergoing laparoscopy.[3] They compared the effects of carbon dioxide and nitrous oxide as insufflating gases. There were significant increases in heart rate in both groups of patients. The increase began at the beginning of the insufflation and reached its maximum when maximal distention was achieved. A return to normal values followed deflation.

The increase in heart rate was greater in patients given carbon dioxide to distend the abdomen. Furthermore, these patients took much longer to return to their preinsufflation heart rate level following deflation than those in whom nitrous oxide had been used. This suggests that the hypercarbia resulting from the carbon dioxide was itself a factor responsible for the increase in heart rate.

In general, stimuli that increase the heart rate also increase the blood pressure. The reverse is also true. The dynamic interactions of the many operating factors make it difficult to establish the reason for the observed tachycardia accurately. Hypercarbia produces an increase in blood pressure and heart rate, as mediated by the hyperactive sympathetic system. High intra-abdominal pressure also enhances peripheral arterial resistance. This raises the blood pressure and subsequently elevates the heart rate. The heart rate comes back to preinsufflation levels following release of intraperitoneal gas. This prompt return lends support to the concept that external pressure on the abdominal portion of the aorta is partially responsible for the tachycardia.

To repeat, these changes have little clinical significance in the young, healthy patient undergoing nonemergency diagnostic or operative laparoscopy. By contrast, they may be important in older patients or in women with preexisting cardiovascular impairment. Special attention is needed for those whose compensatory mechanisms may be impaired or absent.

BLOOD PRESSURE

Smith et al noted a 10 percent increase in the mean blood pressure in patients undergoing carbon dioxide insufflation for pneumoperitoneum in the horizontal position.[13] Motew et al observed a 20 percent increase when the legs were elevated for the lithotomy position. The levels reverted to normal when the patient was placed in a 20° Trendelenburg position.[10] During intra-abdominal insufflation, they found significant rises in both systolic (from 105 to 118 mm Hg) and diastolic pressures (from 67 to 82 mm Hg). Only when the intra-abdominal pressure was greater than 20 mm Hg, with resulting impairment in venous return, was a drop in mean blood pressure seen.

Groover and Bierfeld evaluated sedated patients subjected to laparoscopy under local anesthesia (lidocaine plus diazepam).[4] They reported significant hypertension (diastolic pressures ranging from 100 to 140 mm Hg) in 6 of 19 patients. No correlation was found between any hypertensive effect and any change in blood gases. Preexisting hypertension did not predispose to either.

Blood pressure increases are thought to be due to the transitory hypercarbia resulting from the peritoneal absorption of carbon dioxide. Elevated carbon dioxide acts as a myocardial depressant that stimulates a sympathoadrenal response. This in turn raises the systemic blood pressure. This mechanism does not explain the rise in mean arterial blood pressure seen in patients undergoing a laparoscopic procedure under general anesthesia. The lack of correlation found by Groover and Bierfeld between hypertension and blood gas changes led them to postulate that the peritoneal pain caused by carbon dioxide triggered the increase in blood pressure.[4]

Punnonen and Viinamaki studied the plasma vasopressin concentration in several time frames, namely before general anesthesia was administered, just prior to the insufflation of carbon dioxide, and after adequate pneumoperitoneum was achieved.[11] They reported a significant increase in vasopressin levels at maximum pneumoperitoneum. On this basis, they concluded that increased intra-abdominal pressure and peritoneal distention have a direct stimulating effect on vasopressin release. Elevation in circulating vasopressin may also be responsible for elevation in peripheral blood pressure.

CARDIAC ARRHYTHMIAS

Cardiac arrhythmias are fairly common during a laparoscopic procedure. Scott and Julian reported a 17 percent occurrence rate when carbon dioxide was used to produce the pneumoperitoneum.[12] Only 5 percent of patients showed similar alterations of the cardiac rhythm when nitrous oxide was used for this purpose. Most arrhythmias were ventricular extrasystoles occurring immediately after the electrocardiographic P-wave. They thus fused with the normally conducted impulse. This type of arrhythmia (fusion beats) is almost impossible to diagnose by palpation or auscultation. They are believed to produce little hemodynamic variation.

Carmichael reported two cases of bigeminal rhythm.[1] They required administration of intravenous lidocaine and the procedure was discontinued. These changes were attributed to insufficient ventilation by the anesthetist, although no substantive data were offered to support this contention. Nevertheless, these arrhythmias may play an important role in patients with underlying cardiac abnormalities. Therefore, the laparoscopist must know that they can occur and he or she must understand their pathophysiology so as to be able to take measures to avoid them.

Factors influencing the appearance of cardiac arrhythmias are (a) type of gas used to produce the pneumoperitoneum and (b) choice of anesthesia.

Type of Gas Used For Insufflation

Distention media for laparoscopy include room air, carbon dioxide, and nitrous oxide. Although each has advantages, shortcomings of some necessitate selection of one over another for specific cases. Room air has been discontinued except if needed to help overcome occasional insufflation equipment failure.

Carbon dioxide is used mainly because it is safe. Even when inadvertently insufflated extraperitoneally, it is rapidly absorbed. The risk of gas embolism under these circumstances is negligible (see Chapter 15). Its main disadvantages relate to the hypercarbia it produces from transperitoneal pressure-gradient diffusion into the blood stream. In addition, it causes local peritoneal irritation in the conscious patient. To the contrary, nitrous oxide produces little variation in blood gas homeostasis and little or no peritoneal irritation. Its major drawbacks are its slower reabsorption and excretion. Moreover, it can sustain combustion in a closed space if spark-producing current has to be applied during the procedure. Its use should be encouraged for diagnostic laparoscopies.

Choice of Anesthesia

The anesthesia selected (Chapter 8) may not only influence which gas to give for pneumoperitoneum, but also affect the type and frequency of side effects. General anesthesia overcomes the risk of cardiac arrhythmias from carbon dioxide. Controlled hyperventilation reduces the resulting hypercarbia, decreasing the impact of the factor that precipitates cardiac rhythm disorders. Peritoneal irritation is not a relevant factor under general anesthesia.

If local or regional anesthesia is given, carbon dioxide is unsuitable for insufflation because one cannot control hyperventilation and peritoneal pain can be quite troublesome. Groover and Bierfeld reported their experience with peritoneoscopy under local anesthesia.[4] They recommended giving moderately large doses of a sedative (e.g., diazepam intravenously, titrated to the point of slurred speech or drowsiness) and an analgesic agent (meperidine 50 to 100 mg given parenterally) to reduce the peritoneal irritation. In patients undergoing upper abdominal peritoneoscopy with carbon dioxide pneumoperitoneum, they found no serious cardiac arrhythmias.

It is conceivable that carbon dioxide is not the only cause of cardiac arrhythmias appearing during gynecologic laparoscopy. The need for the lithotomy and Trendelenburg positions may also be precipitating factors.

ELECTROCARDIOGRAPHIC CHANGES

Currently, electrocardiographic evaluation of patients undergoing a surgical procedure has become an integral part of the intraoperative monitoring. If general anesthesia is utilized, cardiac monitoring is under the anesthesiologist's control. This is not always the case when local anesthesia is used. Here the gynecologist carries the responsibility. Therefore, it behooves the gynecologist to become familiar with the electrocardiographic changes that can be expected to occur during the operation.

Alterations in the electrocardiogram do not always indicate the presence of a cardiac abnormality. The electrocardiographic tracing reflects the changing anatomical position of the heart in response to the Trendelenburg position and the elevation of the diaphragm from the pneumoperitoneum. Deviation of the electrical axis to the left, increased amplitude of R-wave, and T-wave inversion can all be produced by excessive distention by the pneumoperitoneum. These changes are uniformly and promptly reversed when the pneumoperitoneum is deflated. Premature supraventricular extrasystoles, aberrant QRS conduction, and sinus tachycardia, all electrocardiographic alterations reported by El-Minawi et al, may belong in this group of benign positional changes.[3]

Altered cardiac rhythm, as discussed, is often impossible to diagnose by palpation and auscultation alone. Ventricular extrasystoles, fusion beats, and the occasional bigeminy become immediately evident by means of continuous electrocardiographic monitoring. These arrhythmias may signal the earliest manifestation of hypoxemia and must be promptly identified and carefully interpreted.

Most electrocardiographic changes reported to occur as a consequence of the pneumoperitoneum required for laparoscopy are not of a serious nature. Nonetheless, the wider use of this form of continuous surveillance is essential in patients who have underlying cardiovascular disease. It should not be taken lightly. Groover and Bierfeld reported 30 consecutive peritoneoscopies done under local anesthesia, using carbon dioxide for insufflation; 16 patients had a history of underlying cardiovascular disease (12 were on maintenance digoxin therapy and 22 were receiving diuretics). They saw no evidence of dangerous cardiac arrhythmias during electrocardiographic monitoring.[4]

Caution should be exercised not to confuse the effects of an upper abdominal diagnostic peritoneoscopy with those of pelvic laparoscopy. Only a small amount of gas is needed to visualize the upper abdominal structures satisfactorily. Much more is needed to study and operate on the lower abdominal and pelvic organs. Not only does pelvic laparoscopy demand larger amounts of gas to obtain a suitable pneumoperitoneum, but it also requires the use of the head-down Trendelenburg position in most cases.

As previously described, abdominal overdistention and shock position elevate the blood pressure, increase the heart rate, and enhance cardiac output. Patients with reduced cardiovascular reserve may not be able to tolerate abdomino-pelvic laparoscopy, although they might accept upper abdominal peritoneoscopy without difficulty. Preselection of patients for laparoscopy is essential to ensure against unexpected catastrophic events.

References

1. Carmichael DE. Laparoscopy: Cardiac considerations. Fertil Steril 1971; 22:69-70.
2. Diamant M, Benumof JL, Saidman LJ. Hemodynamics of increased intra-abdominal pressure: Interaction with hypovolemia and halothane anesthesia. Anesthesiology 1978; 48:23-27.
3. El-Minawi MF, Wahbi O, El-Bagouri IS, Sharawi M, El-Mallah SY. Physiologic changes during CO_2 and N_2O pneumoperitoneum in diagnostic laparoscopy: A comparative study. J Reprod Med 1981; 26:338-346.
4. Groover JR, Bierfeld JL. Cardiac arrhythmias during peritoneoscopy under local anesthesia. Digest Dis 1976; 21:465-467.
5. Hodgson C, McClelland RMA, Newton JR. Some effects of the peritoneal insufflation of carbon dioxide at laparoscopy. Anaesthesia 1970; 25:382-390.
6. Kelman GR, Swapp GH, Smith I, Benzie RJ, Gordon NLM. Cardiac output and arterial blood-gas tension during laparoscopy. Br J Anaesth 1972; 44:1155-1162.
7. Lenz RJ, Thomas TA, Wilkins DG. Cardiovascular changes during laparoscopy: Studies of stroke volume and cardiac output using impedance cardiography. Anaesthesia 1976; 31:4-12.
8. Marshall RL, Jebson PJR, Davie IT, Scott DB. Circulatory effects of carbon dioxide insufflation of the peritoneal cavity for laparoscopy. Br J Anaesth 1972; 44:680-684.
9. McKenzie R, Wadhwa RK, Bedger RC. Noninvasive measurement of cardiac output during laparoscopy. J Reprod Med 1980; 24:247-250.
10. Motew M, Ivankovich AD, Bieniarz J, et al. Cardiovascular effects and acid-base and blood gas changes during laparoscopy. Am J Obstet Gynecol 1973; 115:1002-1012.
11. Punnonen R, Viinamaki O. Vasopressin release during laparoscopy: Role of increased intra-abdominal pressure. Lancet 1982; 1:175-176.
12. Scott DB, Julian DG. Observations on cardiac arrhythmias during laparoscopy. Br Med J 1972; 1:411-413.
13. Smith I, Benzie RJ, Gordon NLM, Kelman GR, Swapp GH. Cardiovascular effects of peritoneal insufflation of carbon dioxide for laparoscopy. Br Med J 1971; 3:410-411.
14. Taylor J, Weil MH. Failure of the Trendelenburg position to improve circulation during clinical shock. Surg Gynecol Obstet 1967; 124:1005-1010.

10 RESPIRATORY CHANGES

In addition to manual dexterity, intraperitoneal endoscopic technique requires an understanding of the interactions between each step of the procedure and its influence on the organism as a whole. The combination of pneumoperitoneum (which elevates the diaphragm and restricts its motion), Trendelenburg position, and absorption of insufflating gas (usually carbon dioxide) produce a sequence of changes which alter the homeostasis and function of both respiratory and circulatory systems.

The respiratory changes occurring during a laparoscopic procedure do not generally present serious hazards to the young, healthy patient. However, similar alterations in patients with an underlying respiratory or cardiovascular disease may lead to catastrophic consequences.

Some derangements of carbon dioxide and oxygen homeostasis are inherent in the technique, whereas others are influenced by the type of anesthesia and/or analgesia used.[5,8] A thorough knowledge of how laparoscopy affects pulmonary function is important for the proper identification and treatment of respiratory complications.

POSTURAL CHANGES

During inspiration, movement of the diaphragm accounts for 75 percent of the variation in intrathoracic volume. Any restriction to diaphragmatic movement impairs the volumetric expansion of the lungs. The lithotomy position, accompanied by some degree of Trendelenburg position, is universally used for the performance of pelvic laparoscopy. Both produce cephalad pressure on the diaphragm.

In addition to the increased pressure of the abdominal organs on the diaphragm produced by these positions, redistribution of the blood mass by the elevation of the lower extremities creates an increase in pulmonary blood volume that further restricts the capacity of the lungs to expand. A decrease of up to

20 percent in the respiratory vital capacity can be seen when a conscious subject is placed in the lithotomy position. A slightly smaller decrease occurs in patients in a moderate Trendelenburg position (20° to 30°). It is fair to assume that a combination of both of these positions would enhance the restrictive action of each on diaphragmatic motion and lung capacity. The need for intra-abdominal insufflation of gas for creating a pneumoperitoneum further increases the subdiaphragmatic positive pressure. This increases the resistance to the inspiratory downward excursion of the diaphragm. In patients receiving spinal or epidural anesthesia for laparoscopy, a further reduction in vital capacity could occur as a result of some intercostal muscle paralysis produced by the regional anesthetic technique.

When laparoscopy is performed under general anesthesia, the respiratory restrictions imposed by interference with the normal mechanics of breathing are compensated for by the use of an endotracheal tube with assisted or controlled ventilation. Increased resistance to the insufflation of gases is mechanically overcome by the ventilator. Inability to properly ventilate the unconscious patient may be an early sign of excessive intra-abdominal pressure due to overdistention by the pneumoperitoneum.

Laparoscopies performed under local or regional anesthesia present additional respiratory changes. The conscious patient responds to the pneumoperitoneum with a reactive hyperventilation, further reducing the tidal volume during inspiration. Increased respiratory frequency partially compensates for this deficiency. To overcome such a deficiency, a thorough explanation of what can be expected during the procedure should be provided for the patient prior to surgery. During the course of the operation, every motion which may affect the patient's response should be anticipated and explained. Creation of the pneumoperitoneum and change in body posture should be performed slowly so as to allow a period of habituation to take place.

The degree and duration of the Tendelenburg position in a patient undergoing a laparoscopy under local or regional anesthesia should be kept to a minimum. It is better not to exceed a 15° to 20° incline. Respiratory changes should be monitored by an assistant and not by the surgeon performing the laparoscopy. Mental concentration on the events occurring in the abdomen may entirely absorb the surgeon's attention, thus making it possible for him or her to overlook variations in the patient's respiratory function.

PNEUMOPERITONEUM

Irrespective of the surgeon's preference for the sequence and timing of the gas insufflation to create a pneumoperitoneum, the gaseous distention of the peritoneal cavity is mandatory for the successful performance of laparoscopy.

The combination of the required postural changes (see above) and the increased intra-abdominal pressure is responsible for a variety of alterations likely to affect respiration. This section will limit itself to the mechanical changes produced by the pneumoperitoneum; biochemical changes resulting from the ventilatory changes and specific distending gases used for insufflation will be discussed in subsequent sections in this chapter.

Mechanical changes in respiration created by the pneumoperitoneum differ in accordance with individual patient characteristics and the type of anesthesia used. Movement of the diaphragm accounts for 75 percent of the change in intrathoracic volume during quiet inspiration. Downward excursion of the diaphragm ranges from 1.5 cm during normal inspiration to 7 cm with deep inspiration. Scott calculated that a pneumoperitoneum which creates an intraabdominal pressure of 25 mm Hg exerts a force of approximately 30 g per square centimeter on the diaphragm; in all, this amounts to a total force of 50 kg or more.[9] The marked elevation of the diaphragm resulting from the increase in intraperitoneal pressure affects ventilation in several ways. Mechanical compression of the lung bases already produced by the Trendelenburg tilt is further aggravated by the elevation of the diaphragm. As a consequence, some perfused areas of the lung do not participate in the oxygenation process. The increase in respiratory impedance, as measured by Alexander et al, results in decreased thoracic compliance and consequent reduction in tidal volume.[1] In the awake patient, such a diminution in lung volume is compensated for by an increase in respiratory frequency. In a patient under general anesthesia, an increase in inspiratory pressure on the ventilator is required to overcome the increment in resistance to diaphragmatic excursion.

The extremely obese patient presents a serious challenge to the surgeon and the anesthesiologist alike. The respiratory physiologic parameters are in the low normal range or even below normal; thoracic compliance and tidal volume are reduced and respiratory frequency increased. The additional challenge of enhanced intraperitoneal pressure may precipitate acute hypoventilation. Hodgson et al found it impossible to maintain controlled ventilation at the prepneumoperitoneum minute volume unless the intra-abdominal pressure is kept below 15 mm Hg.[7] Nulliparous young women or very athletic patients with strongly developed anterior abdominal wall musculature pose a similar problem. Small amounts of gas insufflated intraperitoneally greatly raise the intra-abdominal pressure producing increased pressure on the diaphragm. Some anesthesiologists believe that it is imperative to administer a muscle relaxant to patients undergoing laparoscopy; relaxation of the muscles of the anterior abdominal wall allow the wall to balloon out with an average amount of insufflation while concomitantly avoiding an excessive increase in intra-abdominal pressure.

Under local or regional anesthesia, the degree of peritoneal distention is limited by the discomfort experienced by the patient as a consequence of peritoneal stretching and diaphragmatic irritation. Additionally, the amount of insufflated gas required to reach any given intraperitoneal pressure is reduced by the lack of relaxation of the abdominal wall. Brown et al found an increase in minute ventilation after the pneumoperitoneum was established; the increased ventilation was due to an increase in respiratory rate notwithstanding the diminution in tidal volume.[4] The mean vital capacity was significantly decreased as a consequence of the increased intraperitoneal pressure produced by the pneumoperitoneum.

Caution should be exercised in patients receiving regional anesthesia for laparoscopy. Paralysis of the intercostal muscles seen with regional anesthesia may impair the inspiratory effort in a patient breathing spontaneously.

When general anesthesia is used for laparoscopy, the surgeon should request that the anesthesiologist inform him or her as soon as the inspiratory pressure requirement begins to rise. This can be interpreted as the first sign of increased intra-abdominal pressure; the intraperitoneal insufflation of gas is then reduced to maintenance levels. Any further increment in insufflation results in an additional increase in intra-abdominal pressure not only making ventilation more difficult but also increasing the likelihood of triggering the cardiovascular changes described in the previous chapter. This is the result of aortic and inferior vena cava compression.

With intra-abdominal pressures below 10 mm Hg, the mechanical alterations imposed on the respiratory process are well compensated. If the intra-abdominal pressure is measured while the distending gas is being insufflated at a rate of 1 L per minute, pressures of up to 20 mm Hg are often encountered. These are usually well tolerated. Patients requiring amounts of insufflated gas that exceed this safety threshold should be considered poor candidates for undergoing a laparoscopic procedure.

CARBON DIOXIDE HOMEOSTASIS

Carbon dioxide is the gas most widely used to distend the peritoneal cavity for purposes of creation of a pneumoperitoneum. Its preference over other gases is mainly based on its rapid absorption from closed body cavities (even when misdirected extraperitoneally). Its inability to sustain combustion makes it nonexplosive when diathermy is used. The high level of tolerance when injected intravascularly makes it less likely to be the cause of a serious embolic phenomenon.

Knowledge about what happens to the carbon dioxide after it is insufflated into the peritoneal cavity is important. As the laparoscopic procedure is going on, a constant absorption-exchange process is taking place between the peritoneal cavity and the circulating blood. Variations in carbon dioxide tension in arterial blood ($PaCO_2$) affect not only the respiratory system but the cardiovascular system as well, thereby becoming the potential source of major changes in the patient's homeostatic mechanisms.

Normally, the amount of carbon dioxide in the arterial blood remains constant. The $PaCO_2$ of venous blood is 46 mm Hg, whereas that of alveolar air is 40 mm Hg. Carbon dioxide diffuses by pressure gradient between the alveoli and the circulating blood. The blood leaving the lungs (arterial blood) has a $PaCO_2$ of 40 mm Hg (normal range of $PaCO_2$ is 34 to 44 mm Hg). A rise in $PaCO_2$ stimulates receptors in the carotid and aortic bodies, which in turn increases the level of respiratory center activity to cause hyperventilation. This latter persists until a normal $PaCO_2$ is reached. In addition to the aortic and carotid chemoreceptors, other receptors sensitive to increases in $PaCO_2$ are located in the brain stem near the respiratory center itself; these act in a similar manner.

A further rise in $PaCO_2$ results in an increase in heart rate and blood pressure and also stimulates catecholamine secretion. Additional increases in $PaCO_2$ eventually produce myocardial depression, bradycardia, and a fall in blood pressure.[10] High levels of carbon dioxide have a narcotic effect on the central nervous system. The ability of some inhalation agents to reduce cerebrovascular resistance may potentiate the effect of moderate increases in $PaCO_2$, thereby resulting in increased toxicity. Such high levels are rarely reached as a consequence of reabsorption of carbon dioxide from the peritoneal cavity during a laparoscopy. To the contrary, moderate increases in $PaCO_2$ have a stimulatory effect on the central nervous system and result in an increase in cerebral blood flow and intracranial pressure.

Alexander and Brown in 1969 first reported a significant rise in $PaCO_2$ in patients undergoing laparoscopy under general anesthesia in whom carbon dioxide was used as the distending gas to produce the pneumoperitoneum.[2] Their uncertainty about the cause of the rise in $PaCO_2$ (increased absorption of carbon dioxide from the peritoneal cavity versus hypoventilation) was clarified when they repeated the measurements in patients in whom nitrous oxide was used as the insufflating gas for production of the pneumoperitoneum. The lack of a significant change in $PaCO_2$ in the latter group identified the increased absorption of carbon dioxide from the peritoneal cavity as the source of the relative hypercarbia.

Gases diffuse from areas of high pressure to areas of low pressure; the rate of diffusion is dependent upon the differential in the concentration gradient and the nature of the dividing barrier. When 100 percent carbon dioxide at atmospheric pressure is insufflated into the peritoneal cavity, the gas tension difference across the peritoneal-capillary wall is approximately 660 to 670 mm Hg. During the laparoscopic procedure, the gas mixture in the peritoneal cavity comes into equilibrium with the gases in blood. Thus, carbon dioxide is rapidly absorbed into the circulation and excreted through the lungs.

Hodgson et al studied serial blood gases in two groups of patients undergoing laparoscopy under general anesthesia; one group was allowed to ventilate spontaneously and a second group had their ventilation controlled.[7] Blood samples drawn at 5-minute intervals prior to and following the intraperitoneal insufflation of carbon dioxide revealed a significant increase in mean $PaCO_2$ in both groups. Of significance is the fact that pre- and post-insufflation levels of $PaCO_2$ were lower in the group undergoing controlled ventilation. This was interpreted as a positive effect from the hyperventilation possible when ventilation is controlled. In a similar study, Desmond and Gordon confirmed the higher level of $PaCO_2$ in patients who were allowed to ventilate spontaneously and in whom carbon dioxide was used to produce the pneumoperitoneum.[5] An excessive $PaCO_2$ is considered dangerous when halothane is used as the inhalation agent for general anesthesia. The elevation in $PaCO_2$ may exceed the arrhythmia threshold for halothane. If arrhythmias are triggered, acute hypotension may result. Controlled hyperventilation, even to the degree of producing a moderate respiratory alkalosis, prevents the rise in $PaCO_2$ from reaching the arrhythmia threshold. This practice is recommended to prevent sudden cardiovascular collapse.

Utilization of laparoscopy in patients with underlying pulmonary or cardiovascular disease is on the rise. Because $PaCO_2$ does not change when nitrous oxide is insufflated for the pneumoperitoneum, it is perhaps to be preferred over carbon dioxide in this class of patients.

OXYGEN HOMEOSTASIS

A measure of satisfactory lung function is the maintenance of normal levels of oxygen and carbon dioxide in the arterial blood. Under normal conditions, homeostatic mechanisms ensure that blood gas levels remain within a normal range under varying circumstances. However, during laparoscopy, respiration may be altered in response to fluctuations in oxygen and carbon dioxide tension in blood.

Under normal conditions, the oxygen tension varies according to the site from which it is measured. In ambient air, it is approximately 158 mm Hg; at the alveoli, 100 mm Hg. With no significant alveolar-arterial gradient, the PaO_2 is minimally reduced to 95 mm Hg. Following oxygenation of the tissues by diffusion, the oxygen tension in venous blood decreases to around 40 mm Hg.

Whether the combination of a tensely distended abdomen and the Trendelenburg position adversely affects oxygenation was extensively studied. Alexander and Brown found no significant fall in arterial PaO_2 values in patients undergoing laparoscopy under general anesthesia.[2] Decreases in PaO_2 seen in some subjects during laparoscopy under local anesthesia were attributed to excessive narcotic sedation.

Baratz and Karis compared blood gases in the course of laparoscopy under general anesthesia with those in controlled respiration versus spontaneous breathing.[3] They also reported no significant difference in the arterial oxygen tension.

ACID-BASE CHANGES

The maintenance of a stable acid-base environment depends on the homeostasis of the body's pH. The pH of a solution is the logarithm (to the base 10) of the reciprocal of the hydrogen ion (H^+) concentration. Normally, the pH of the extracellular fluid blood is maintained at 7.40 with minimal range of variation in the order of ± 0.05 pH unit. The body fluids have the capacity to act as buffers to help maintain the pH within such a narrow range of normality. One of the buffer substances in the body is carbonic acid which is only slightly dissociated into H^+ and bicarbonate ($H_2CO_3 \rightleftarrows H^+ \; HCO_3^-$). The carbonic acid level in plasma is in equilibrium with dissolved carbon dioxide; the amount of dissolved carbon dioxide is controlled in turn by respiration. The elevation in $PaCO_2$ results in an increase in H_2CO_3 ($CO_2 + H_2O \rightleftarrows H_2CO_3$) and the pH drops. Any increment in $PaCO_2$ and/or H^+ stimulates respiration in an attempt to eliminate greater quantities of carbon dioxide through the lungs and bring the system back to normality.

Alexander et al found a significant drop in pH in laparoscopy patients in whom CO_2 was used as the distending gas to create the pneumoperitoneum.[1] Failure to show a similar drop in pH when nitrous oxide was used to distend the peritoneal cavity showed quite conclusively that the reduction in pH was due to increased absorption of carbon dioxide from the peritoneal cavity rather than from impaired ventilation as was originally suspected. In a more comprehensive study, El-Minawi et al showed similar alterations in $PaCO_2$ and pH without any significant change in the level of bicarbonate or base excess.[6] This confirms that the acidosis seen when carbon dioxide is used as the distending gas is strictly respiratory in origin and can be corrected by increasing the respiratory minute volume.

While these reported changes in acid-base balance are statistically significant, they are seldom clinically very important. The respiratory acidosis is mild and not the cause of any observable cardiovascular change. The relatively short duration of a laparoscopic procedure limits the degree of acidosis. The pH has been shown to return to a normal level quite promptly upon deflation of the pneumoperitoneum. In patients in whom even slight variations of pH are of concern, the use of nitrous oxide for the creation of the pneumoperitoneum is recommended.

References

1. Alexander GD, Noe FE, Brown EM. Anesthesia for pelvic laparoscopy. Anesth Analg 1969; 48:14-18.
2. Alexander GD, Brown EM. Physiologic alterations during pelvic laparoscopy. Am J Obstet Gynecol 1969; 105:1078-1081.
3. Baratz RA, Karis JH. Blood gas studies during laparoscopy under general anesthesia. Anesthesiology 1969; 30:463-464.
4. Brown DR, Fishburne JI, Roberson VO, Hulka JF. Ventilatory and blood gas changes during laparoscopy with local anesthesia. Am J Obstet Gynecol 1976; 124:741-745.
5. Desmond J, Gordon RA. Ventilation in patients anaesthetized for laparoscopy. Can Anaesth Soc J 1970; 17:378-387.
6. El-Minawi MF, Wahbi O, El-Bagouri IS, Sharawi M, El-Mallah SY. Physiologic changes during CO_2 and N_2O pneumoperitoneum in diagnostic laparoscopy: A comparative study. J Reprod Med 1981; 26:338-346.
7. Hodgson C, McClelland RMA, Newton JR. Some effects of the peritoneal insufflation of carbon dioxide at laparoscopy. Anaesthesia 1970; 25:382-390.
8. Kelman GR, Swapp GH, Smith I, Benzie RJ, Gordon NLM. Cardiac output and arterial blood-gas tension during laparoscopy. Br J Anaesth 1972; 44:1155-1162.
9. Scott DB. Some effects of peritoneal insufflation of carbon dioxide at laparoscopy. Anaesthesia 1970; 25:590.
10. Versichelen L, Serreyn R, Rolly G, Vanderkerckhove D. Physiopathologic changes during anesthesia administration for gynecologic laparoscopy. J Reprod Med 1984; 29:697-700.

11 POSTOPERATIVE RECOVERY

Until the last decade, the immediate postoperative interval was a time in which patients who had just had surgery under general anesthesia were carefully monitored. The recovery room was considered a temporary station where patients recovered consciousness and full reflex function before being sent to their hospital room. They would then recover in their room overnight from all the effects of the medications received during surgery. Today, popularization of outpatient surgery makes the immediate postoperative recovery an even more critical aspect of the surgical experience.

Rapid recovery from anesthesia and early ambulation are the major objectives of the immediate postoperative period.[8] One cannot predict that a patient can be safely discharged from the hospital on the sole basis of stable vital signs and return of consciousness. The criteria for discharging a patient may vary from institution to institution. Some require only immediate recovery; others accept partial recovery; and some insist on delaying release until complete recovery is achieved. Each type of anesthesia is associated with a range in recovery period; moreover for any anesthetic modality use of different drug combinations give rise to special effects. Once the in-hospital observation period is over and the patient has been discharged, the laparoscopist resumes his or her role as the primary (or perhaps only) health care resource for the patient. Therefore, it is imperative that the physician be familiar with all aspects of the recovery period subsequent to a laparoscopic procedure.

POSTOPERATIVE PAIN

Following a surgical procedure, pain is accepted by physicians, nurses, and patients as a common effect of the operation. Standard postoperative orders include prescription of medications to help relieve pain as soon as the anesthetic effect has abated. After laparoscopy, patients can expect to experience a certain amount of discomfort. Incisional pain, diffuse abdominal discomfort, and referred shoulder pain are among the most common symptoms reported by patients. Evaluation is difficult because there is a wide range of variation in the pain patterns and quite diverse degrees of pain tolerance from subject to subject. One has to differentiate between average postoperative discomfort and the early signs of some complications. This is an essential component of immediate postoperative care.

The laparoscopist must not rely on the anesthesiologist or recovery room nurses to evaluate the patient's complaints. Instead, he or she should assess each case individually. Nobody is in a better position to identify an unusual pattern of recovery than the surgeon who has performed the operation. The common practice of administering medication for pain relief, other than a mild analgesic, on a standard time schedule is mentioned only to be decried. Although there are many available agents for effective pain relief, the routinized indiscriminate pharmacologic suppression of pain may mask a serious condition. It thus delays the diagnosis and inappropriately postpones corrective measures.

Incisional Pain. The degree of postoperative incisional pain expected varies according to the laparoscopic technique used. Closed laparoscopy, done with small or medium size instruments (5 to 7 mm) used for primary and secondary punctures, is usually associated with minimal discomfort at the puncture sites. The appearance of moderate to severe pain under these circumstances raises the possibility of a subcutaneous or subfascial extravasation of blood with hematoma formation. Palpation of a mass or induration in or near the incision sites during the early postoperative period makes this complication likely. Bleeding from small subcutaneous vessels is often self-limited. As the local tissue pressure builds up at the hematoma site, the lumen of the lacerated vessel is occluded and the bleeding ceases. Subfascial hematomas can also be self-limited, but continued bleeding is a much greater possibility in the subfascial layer than subcutaneously. A longer observation period, with hospitalization if indicated, is required when such a condition is suspected. The treatment of abdominal wall hemorrhage is covered in Chapter 17.

The degree of postoperative incisional pain after open laparoscopy is in direct proportion to the size of the incision and the difficulty experienced by the operator in entering the abdominal cavity. There is still a risk of localized bleeding after these open laparoscopic procedures. Therefore, one has to evaluate each case on its own merits. In some, the usual incisional pain may be aggravated by metal skin clips used to approximate the edges of the incision. It may be necessary to release their tension or remove them altogether to aid in the differential diagnosis.

Abdominal Discomfort. The most common cause of lower abdominal discomfort (other than incisional pain) after laparoscopy is attributable to the instrumental or manual tension used to lift the abdominal wall when the Verres needle or laparoscopic trocar is being inserted. This condition is more likely to occur in patients undergoing laparoscopy under general anesthesia. Greater force (and trauma) is possible under this circumstance because there is no constraining feedback from the patient. In procedures performed with local infiltration anesthesia, excessive manipulation is limited by the patient's pain perception.

If abdominal discomfort occurs following an operative laparoscopic procedure, the patient has to be evaluated thoroughly. As described in Chapter 8, irritation of the visceral peritoneum may produce symptoms. The pain is usually described by the patient as mild generalized discomfort. Early identification and evaluation of cases with more than mild discomfort may disclose an unsuspected complication that had not previously been evident at the time of the procedure. Therefore, whenever a patient experiences an unusual amount of abdominal discomfort, thorough evaluation—sometimes entailing prolonged in-hospital observation—is the indicated course of action. As to operative laparoscopy, a wide range of abdomino-pelvic discomfort can be expected following different types of translaparoscopic sterilization procedures (see Chapters 5 and 22).

Shoulder Pain. It is generally accepted that shoulder pain is almost a universal occurrence after laparoscopy. It is created by irritation of the peritoneum underlying the diaphragm. This results from the subphrenic pneumoperitoneum that remains at the conclusion of the procedure. The pain is referred to the shoulder region because diaphragmatic sensory innervation travels by way of the phrenic nerve. This nerve originates from the fourth cervical nerve trunk; it also receives some fibers from the third and fifth cervical nerves. The fourth and fifth cervical nerves also receive afferent sensory fibers from the brachial plexus which innervates the upper limbs.

Shoulder pain is more common on the right than on the left. This is thought to be due to traction on the falciform hepatic ligament from downward displacement of the liver. While still in the recovery room, the patient usually complains of shoulder pain on sitting or standing. This symptom may be delayed in onset for several hours if perihepatic adhesions are present. Not clearly explained is the initial occurrence of shoulder pain the day after surgery, as is experienced by a few women.

Patients should be given a thorough explanation of the physiopathology of shoulder pain. They must be reassured as to its benign nature. Control of this type of discomfort rarely requires more than a mild analgesic agent (such as acetaminophen). Nevertheless, patients must be informed that, if this particular discomfort continues without abating for more than 48 hours, they should notify the physician. Although intraperitoneal gas may last for up to 7 days, it is not usually accompanied by unremitting pain for that extent of time. The persistence or reappearance of shoulder pain more than 48 hours after the procedure should prompt a full work-up to rule out other more serious complications, such as perforation of a hollow viscus.

RECOVERY FROM NEUROMUSCULAR BLOCKING AGENTS

One of the main advantages of the use of general anesthesia for a laparoscopic procedure is the profound degree of relaxation it can produce. In the past, the relaxation needed to provide an optimal surgical field required the use of high concentrations of anesthetic agents. Such deep anesthesia was far from innocuous. The desired relaxation is now accomplished by the administration of neuromuscular blocking agents.[2] Use of these paralyzing drugs helps reduce the total amount of anesthetic medication that needs to be given. Only the level required to achieve analgesia and unconciousness is required.

Neuromuscular blockers used as adjuncts for general anesthesia can be divided in two groups according to their mode of action. The depolarizing agents (e.g., succinylcholine) combine with acetylcholine receptors to cause depolarization of the end-plate region. The competitive agents combine with acetylcholine receptors to prevent depolarization (e.g., d-tubocurarine).[2] Although a detailed description of the mode of action of these drugs is beyond the scope of this book, their main effect, duration of action, and side effects must be known to the operating surgeon. Such information is necessary because intraoperative use of these agents is a common source of postoperative complaints.

Depolarizing Agents. Depolarizing neuromuscular blockers, of which succinylcholine is the most commonly used, exert the same action as acetylcholine at the neuromuscular junction. By reacting with the end-plate receptors, they lead to depolarization of the chemically excitable membrane. Depolarization spreads to the adjacent electrically excitable membrane, thus causing muscular contraction. This generalized depolarization causes an uncoordinated type of myocontractile response known as fasciculation.

Succinylcholine is not eliminated as rapidly as acetylcholine. Therefore, it depolarizes the end plate for a longer period of time. When it is used as the single agent for muscular relaxation, fasciculations may persist for an extended period of time. Commonly, patients receiving large amounts of depolarizing agents complain of muscle pain postoperatively. The use of intravenous succinylcholine is believed to be the cause. Although there is no correlation between the occurrence of pain and the degree of fasciculation, uncoordinated muscular contractions may be the underlying mechanism. Administration of a competitive agent prior to the injection of a depolarizing drug prevents fasciculations and reduces the incidence of postoperative muscle pain.

Competitive Agents. The most commonly used drugs in this group are d-tubocurarine and pancuronium. Their long duration of action, although easily reversed with anticholinesterase, interdicts their use for short procedures such as laparoscopy. Long acting competitive agents are also associated with cardiovascular changes and histamine release. Competitive agents act synergistically in combination with depolarizing drugs to achieve adequate muscular relaxation and at the same time avert some of the undesirable side effects. Even though d-tubocurarine is used in conjunction with succinylcholine for purposes of reducing fasciculations, postoperative myalgia is not entirely eliminated. Newer short acting competitive-type drugs, such as atracurium and vecuronium, appear to be equally effective in producing muscle relaxation of short duration; yet, they can be given without depolarizing agents altogether.

The duration of side effects resulting from neuromuscular blocking agents may persist for up to 48 hours after laparoscopy. The generalized myalgia may not be readily differentiated from the easy fatigability seen so often postoperatively in patients who have had general anesthetic. Knowledge of these side effects is useful when counseling a patient for laparoscopy. It may influence the patient's choice of anesthesia. As will be described in a later section (see Discharge Instructions, p. 216), patients undergoing outpatient laparoscopy must be made aware of the possibilities of the common after effects. This applies in particular to those related to the use of muscle relaxation agents.

RECOVERY FROM LOCAL ANESTHESIA

Recovery time of the patient who has a laparoscopy under local anesthesia is short. Its duration depends on the amount of adjuvant medication (sedative, hypnotic, or analgesic agent) given to supplement the local infiltration anesthesia. Premedication is generally given in conjunction with local anesthesia to provide amnesia and analgesia.[5] As was shown in Chapter 8, such preoperative drugs do prolong the postoperative sedative period. This makes the practice questionable for outpatient procedures. If parenteral diazepam is to be given as the sole agent for supplementation of local anesthesia, it should be carefully titrated to minimize dosage and effect. Its biphasic action (described in Chapter 8) may prolong the postoperative recovery for as long as 5 to 7 hours.

The appearance of postoperative pain may require parenteral drugs for relief. Dosage and potency of the analgesic agent may also prolong the required period of observation before the patient can be discharged. Morphine and a number of similar narcotic medications have a biphasic effect similar to diazepam. The operating surgeon must be cognizant about the type and quantity of analgesics the patient has received both during and after the laparoscopic procedure.

One of the advantages of local anesthesia is that it does not require highly sophisticated equipment to follow the patient postoperatively. This helps reduce the overall cost of the procedure. Patients are able to ambulate soon after the conclusion of the procedure. Similarly, they are better able to tolerate fluids and solid food so that oral intake can begin much sooner than with other anesthetic techniques.

The duration of the recuperative period and the degree of discomfort after laparoscopy under local anesthesia are inversely related to the patient's knowledge about the procedure and its side effects. Good doctor-patient rapport, coupled with realistic expectations by patients, reduces the amount of systemic pain relief required. In turn, this facilitates more rapid recovery and earlier discharge from the surgical facility. The postoperative course is sometimes characterized by prolongation of discomfort. This applies even when laparoscopy is performed under general anesthesia. Because this may be a problem these women cannot be discharged unless they are accompanied by a responsible adult. They should not be allowed to leave the surgical center alone. It is especially important that they not drive themselves home.

RECOVERY FROM REGIONAL ANESTHESIA

Postoperative recovery from a laparoscopy performed under regional block anesthesia (e.g., spinal and epidural) differs from that after one performed under local or general anesthesia.[4] The observation period is perforce longer than with the other techniques. The criteria of an acceptable end point for discharging the patient remain controversial. It is important for them to be clarified, especially since there is growing demand for undertaking laparoscopy in the outpatient setting. This issue has to be resolved before regional anesthesia can be recommended for laparoscopy.

Care of the laparoscopy patient during her period of immediate postoperative recovery is usually the responsibility of the anesthesiologist who administered the regional anesthesia. It is carried out in a fully equipped recovery room. Although the laparoscopist may not be called upon to deal directly with problems that may arise, he of she must be familiar with the usual events occurring during recovery. Without such information, the laparoscopist would not be able to counsel the patient appropriately. Even though the recovery from spinal anesthesia is similar in many respects to that from epidural, there are enough differences to warrant considering them separately.

Spinal Anesthesia. The rate of recovery following spinal anesthesia depends on the anesthetic drug used and the maximum level of sensory and motor block achieved. The duration of the block is directly related to the concentration of anesthetic agent in the cerebrospinal fluid. Return of motor function to the lower extremities precedes return of sensory perception. The patient's ability to flex and extend the knee and hip joints enables her to sit and walk. The capacity to move the large toe (representing motor function transmitted via L3 and L4) marks one end point of recovery from spinal block.

Sensory deficits usually regress over 6 hours, but they may persist for up to 24 hours. The return of anal sensation may be a useful end point for resolution of low spinal block. Residual block of the parasympathetic system (mediated by way of the reflex arc of S2 to S4) may produce bladder distention with urinary retention. Therefore, after spinal anesthesia the patient must be able to void spontaneously before her discharge from the surgical facility is permitted.

The postoperative assessment of a patient who has received a spinal anesthesia requires monitoring of her circulatory system. The extensive blockade of the autonomic nervous system prediposes to hypotension during and after surgery. Treatment of hypotension includes hydration, proper positioning, and administration of vasopressors, if indicated. Head-down shock position generally proves helpful in these cases. Early recognition of a fall in blood pressure requires that it be measured at regular intervals, specifically no less often than every 15 minutes.

Contrary to previously held concepts, spinal headache is not prevented by keeping the patient supine for 6 to 8 hours. It is current practice to encourage ambulation as soon as the motor and sensory blockade have disappeared. Adequate hydration helps prevent the appearance of postlumbar puncture headache. Treatment of this condition is detailed in Chapter 14.

Epidural Anesthesia. The duration of postoperative recovery after epidural anesthesia for a laparoscopy is somewhat shorter than after spinal block. The addition of vasoconstrictors to the anesthetic agent prolongs both motor and sensory block. When spontaneous movement of the ankle and the big toe is elicited, one can rely on the fact that there is little residual sympathetic blockade.

Although less than with spinal block anesthesia, the risk of hypotension is still present during the postoperative recovery period after epidural anesthesia. In contrast to the clear benefit of head-down position after spinal block, steep Trendelenburg position may actually aggravate circulatory difficulties in the patient with an epidural anesthesia (see Chapter 14). Therefore, it should be avoided. Adequate hydration and, if needed, vasopressor administration medication are usually sufficient to correct neurogenic hypotension.

RECOVERY FROM GENERAL ANESTHESIA

The popularization of outpatient laparoscopy has been accompanied by modifications in the type of general anesthesia patients are given. General anesthesia for procedures of short duration, such as laparoscopy, has to be designed to ensure rapid return to normal function, while minimizing side effects such as nausea and vomiting. The definition of normal function after a general anesthetic is controversial and is still being debated.[1]

In most institutions, anesthetists and highly specialized nurses are in charge of the immediate postoperative care of patients who have had laparoscopy under general anesthesia. Nevertheless, the laparoscopist remains the primary care physician. Therefore, he or she must be familiar with the events the patient can expect to experience during the recovery period. It has to be reemphasized that conveying this information is an integral part of the preoperative counseling. It is necessary in order to ensure one has obtained proper informed consent prior to a laparoscopy. Furthermore, experience has shown that a recently operated patient appreciates the surgeon's participation in the postoperative care activities, and she responds better as a consequence.

In the recovery room, there must be close monitoring of the protective gag and swallowing reflexes, respiratory function, and circulatory status.[3] Prior to complete recovery of reflexes, the patient is at serious risk of aspirating regurgitated gastric contents. The danger of accidental aspiration is present even in the wakened patient in whom the effects of neuromuscular blocking agents have not been adequately reversed.

After general anesthesia it is not unusual for there to be a right-to-left shunt in pulmonary blood flow. If the shunt is large and the patient is breathing room air, this may result in arterial hypoxemia. It can be easily corrected by the administration of 30 to 40 percent oxygen by mask. To allay patient anxiety, it is wise to provide information about this phenomenon preoperatively.

As indices for assessing full recovery, neither stabilization of vital signs nor early return of consciousness are particularly valuable. Moreover, return of the blood pressure to the patient's normal range does not necessarily signify full recovery of the circulatory system. Prolonged depression of myocardial performance has been seen after thiopental was given for induction and/or maintenance of anesthesia. This diminished activity may not be reflected in the arterial blood pressure.

Circulatory disturbances such as severe hypotension or persistent tachycardia during the immediate postlaparoscopy recovery period are uncommon. Their appearance strongly suggests that a vascular injury may have occurred at the time of surgery. Such vessel damage is seldom recognized intraoperatively. Immediate reevaluation by the operating surgeon is indicated.

Similar deficiencies exist in our ability to evaluate the psychologic status of patients recovering from laparoscopy under general anesthesia. Return of consciousness has to be recognized as reflecting mental awareness. It need not be indicative of intellectual efficiency and performance. Simpson et al compared the effects of two drugs commonly used for short anesthesias, namely fentanyl and halothane.[7] They evaluated mental efficiency by testing logical reasoning, addition, and cancellation of letter pairs, at regular intervals. Patients who awakened after fentanyl administration performed 40 percent below their normal level for up to 8 hours. Patients receiving halothane responded significantly better than those in the fentanyl group. They performed better on all three tests.

Korttila et al evaluated psychomotor skills and simulated vehicular driving after a brief period (3.5 minutes) of general inhalational anesthesia.[6] The drugs used were halothane or enflurane, both common general anesthetic agents. They found that psychomotor performance remained significantly worse than that of a control group for up to 5 hours afterward. Impairment of driving skills persisted for 7 hours. Diminished psychomotor performance and driving skills were observed even after the patients considered their abilities to have returned to normal. Therefore, following adequate recovery from general anesthesia, it is critical for patients to be discharged in the care of a competent adult. They should not be allowed to leave by themselves. Furthermore, they should be clearly instructed not to operate a motor vehicle for the next 24 hours.

One must differentiate between the manifestations of immediate recovery (the return of consciousness and even the ability to ambulate) and those of full recovery. The laparoscopist has to be familiar with the current anesthetic techniques in order to be able to counsel a patient properly when a laparoscopy is indicated. The endoscopic surgeon performing a laparoscopy under general anesthesia must also carry out the precautionary measures needed to ensure the patient's safety in conjunction with the anesthetist.

DISCHARGE INSTRUCTIONS

The growing need to discharge patients on the same day of surgery requires that they be instructed and well informed about what they may expect over the following days. Information concerning the postoperative period encompasses matters dealing with recovery from both the laparoscopy and the anesthesia. The term ''discharge instructions'' deserves clarification because it can be misinterpreted. Whereas it literally alludes to advice about activities that are permitted or interdicted, it does not imply that such instructions are to be given shortly before discharge. For a laparoscopic procedure, as for any other operation, details about postoperative recovery events and constraints are integral to the counseling they must receive before they can intelligently decide to undergo the surgery. They are an essential feature of good medical practice. Furthermore, as will be discussed in Chapter 25, the physician has a medicolegal obligation to inform the patient about what she may expect to happen as a consequence of the procedure.

Anesthetic Considerations

Local Anesthesia. For cases in which laparoscopy is done under local block, the anesthesia has little impact after the patient has been discharged. This is because most of the anesthetic agent has been metabolized or excreted by that time. If premedication or supplementary sedation has been administered, the patient must be given the same instructions as if she had received a general anesthesia. The magnitude and duration of psychomotor performance impairment is similar to those experienced by patients receiving these drugs for premedication purposes or in addition to general anesthesia.

Regional Anesthesia. Patients who have been given epidural anesthesia for a laparoscopic procedure must be fully recovered insofar as their sensory and motor functions are concerned. Exceptionally, one may encounter patients who develop paresthetic complications related to the epidural anesthesia; they require longer and more extensive care. All other patients can be instructed in the same manner as those who had the procedure performed under local anesthesia.

Patients in whom the laparoscopic procedure was done under spinal anesthesia should be instructed to report any headache or backache. Readmission to the hospital may be needed in case a severe spinal headache occurs. If a mild headache does not respond to increased fluid intake, bedrest, and mild analgesic medication, any further delay exposes the patient to unnecessary prolongation of discomfort.

General Anesthesia. The most common symptoms reported by patients after general anesthesia are muscle pain, which can last 24 to 48 hours; dizziness, sometimes persisting for up to 72 hours; inability to concentrate, a problem reported by approximately one-third of patients, continuing in some for up to 72 to 96 hours; and headache, nausea, and vomiting, occurring usually within the first 24 hours. Patients may experience a sore throat if endotracheal intubation had been used; this is usually self-limited, subsiding within the first 48 hours.

These side effects may also be encountered in patients who were not subjected to general anesthesia, but have been given a variety of drugs either before or during the laparoscopy. Thus, the same instructions given to patients receiving a general anesthetic for laparoscopy also apply to those receiving premedication or supplementary sedation for local or regional anesthesia. They include the following admonitions:

The patient must be discharged into the care of a competent adult.

She cannot be permitted to drive an automobile or operate complex machinery for at least 24 hours after the procedure.

She should be advised to avoid signing documents or make important decisions for the first 24 hours following surgery.

She must not drink alcoholic beverages for 24 to 48 hours if she has been given intravenous barbiturates or long-acting inhalation anesthetics.

Laparoscopic Considerations

Discharge instructions for patients undergoing a laparoscopic procedure have to take into account the extent of the explorational and operative manipulations. Some side effects are common to all forms of laparoscopy (both diagnostic and operative); others are special to the type. To avoid apprehension and anxiety, patients need explanations and instruction about possible future events resulting from laparoscopy.

Vaginal Bleeding. The use of a single-toothed tenaculum to grasp the cervix may cause vaginal bleeding. Packing the vagina with 3 or 4 medium sized sponges applied firmly against the cervix for 1 to 2 hours is generally sufficient to control this problem. If a uterine mobilizer is used, local damage to the endometrial lining may also contribute to the appearance of blood per vaginam. This may last for up to 24 hours and is generally self-limited. Patients who undergo dilatation and curettage at the time of laparoscopy should expect a certain amount of vaginal staining afterward. This is not different from the bleeding expected after dilatation and curettage done as an isolated procedure. Vaginal bleeding following laparoscopy, unaccompanied by curettage, may produce undue anxiety in a patient who is not aware that it can occur. Unusual or unexpected bleeding should be evaluated at once.

Shoulder Pain. Nearly all patients complain of shoulder pain immediately following the laparoscopy or shortly after they are discharged. They should be warned about it and advised that it is self-limited in duration, rarely lasting more than 24 to 36 hours. A short explanation about the pathophysiological mechanism of shoulder pain (see p. 210) helps reduce the patient's anxiety.

Incisional Pain. Patients should be warned that they will probably experience some incisional pain. At the same time, they benefit from a review of the care of the incision. They should also be told about the type of suture material that was (or will be) employed to approximate the incisional skin edges and how that will be managed. Peri-incisional pain lasting longer than 48 hours should be reported to the physician at once. The appearance of incisional drainage (bleeding or suppuration) requires immediate notification of the operator for evaluation.

Special Instructions. Following a translaparoscopic tubal sterilization procedure, varying degrees of pain may be experienced by patients; these are often dependent on the operative method used. Mechanical occlusive methods (and the Falope ring in particular) give rise to a dull pelvic ache that can persist for up to 72 to 96 hours (see Chapter 22). The symptom appears to be due to the ischemic devascularization of the tubal segment produced by the silastic band. This is not the case with electrocauterization techniques. Patients should be forewarned about it and given a prescription for a mild analgesic agent.

After any type of laparoscopy, patients should be instructed to notify the surgeon immediately if any unexpected symptom appears. This is especially important if electrocautery has been used during the procedure (see Chapter 23). Before the patient leaves the surgical facility, she should be given verbal instruction. In addition, it is advisable to provide her with a written set of guidelines. Those instructions must clearly state what can usually be expected to occur during the interval from the time of discharge until the postoperative visit. They must also include specific information about when and how to contact the physician responsible for the patient's care.

References

1. Arlow SM. Recovery time from general anesthetics: A comparison of techniques. J Reprod Med 1978; 20:341-344.
2. Dripps RD, Eckenhoff JE, Vandam LD. Neuromuscular blocking agents. In, Introduction to Anesthesia: The Principles of Safe Practice. 6th ed. Philadelphia, WB Saunders 1982; 160-179.
3. Epstein BS. Recovery from anesthesia. Anesthesiol 1975; 43:285-288.
4. Farhie SE. Postoperative care after regional anesthesia. Int Anesthesiol Clin 1983; 21:157-171.
5. Kanto J. Benzodiazepines as oral premedicants. Br J Anaesth 1978; 53:1179-1188.
6. Korttila K, Tammisto T, Ertama P, Pfaffli P, Blomgran E, Hahhinen S. Recovery, psychomotor skills, and simulated driving after brief inhalational anesthesia with halothane or enflurane combined with nitrous oxide and oxygen. Anesthesiol 1977; 46:20-27.
7. Simpson JEP, Glynn DJ, Cox AG, Folkar DS. Comparative study of short-term recovery of mental efficiency after anaesthesia. Br Med J 1976; 1:1560-1562.
8. Spence AA. Uses of anaesthesia: Postoperative care. Br Med J 1980; 281:367-368.

12 EQUIPMENT FAILURE

Verres Needle
Trocar and Sleeve
Laparoscope
Light Cord
Accessory Nonelectrical Instruments
Insufflator
Electrogenerator and Circuitry
Electro-instrumentation

No surgical instrument should be employed unless the surgeon knows the proper indications for its use, its potential capabilities, and its limitations. The use of automated insufflation for the production of the pneumoperitoneum, high-power cold light for illumination, and electrical power for electrocauterization requires the special education and training of each member of the surgical team.

Correct usage of equipment is essential to the successful completion of a laparoscopic procedure. Deficiency of one or more instrumental components accounts for most failures to successfully complete a planned operation. Familiarity with the proper functioning of each component of the laparoscopy set is essential in order to identify a flaw in the system. Simple problems, such as tubing that is incompletely attached or a trocar sleeve valve that is improperly assembled, are responsible for an inability to maintain an adequate pneumoperitoneum.

It cannot be emphasized strongly enough that it is the surgeon's responsibility to ensure the proper functioning of every instrument to be used during a laparoscopy. Such equipment checks should be performed prior to the laparoscopic process, if possible. Certainly they should have been conducted to the surgeon's satisfaction before the patient is anesthetized for the procedure.

Each instrument in the laparoscopy set has a particular function. Instruments cannot be interchanged as readily as can cutting or clamping instruments. Little room for improvization exists when one of these components fails to function properly. To facilitate the correction of such problems it is important to recognize the exact location of the breakdown in the system and to know how to test the functional integrity of each instrument in use.

Whereas some equipment malfunctions can be corrected by readjustments and calibration, others require the replacement of particular components. Because of the nature of the procedure, failure to carry out a laparoscopy to conclusion means an inconclusive diagnostic or incomplete therapeutic operation. Incomplete laparoscopy may require major abdominal surgery (laparotomy) to fulfill the original indications. Any institution performing laparoscopy should have the necessary back-up equipment that allows replacement of defective components even when a defect develops after the procedure has begun.

VERRES NEEDLE

Spring-Load Function. It is critical for the spring-loaded inner blunt needle to work properly before the Verres needle enters the peritoneal cavity. If it is fixed in the loaded position, any bluntness impedes sharp penetration of the fascial layer. If the needle is fixed in the open or unloaded position, the outer sharp bevelled casing exposes a cutting edge dangerous to intra-abdominal and retroperitoneal structures.

Improperly functioning spring mechanisms are usually caused by faulty assemblage of the Verres needle components. Disassembling the Verres needle into its individual components, followed by its careful reassemblage, should solve the problem. If this proves unsuccessful, it is probable that the inner blunt insufflating needle is bent. A more thorough check by the manufacturer is required before it can be used again.

Needle Patency. Complete patency of the insufflating channel is essential for several reasons. Any material occupying the lumen of the needle is propelled into the peritoneal cavity by the gas insufflated for creating the pneumoperitoneum. If the instruments are disinfected rather than gas sterilized, the narrow lumen may not receive the full benefit of the disinfecting solution. Introduction of unsterile particles into the peritoneal cavity may cause postoperative infectious or irritative morbidity.

An obstruction of the Verres needle lumen also produces false measurements of the intraperitoneal pressure. The pressure recorded by the insufflating machine manometer is affected by the flow of gas and the resistance offered by the inner diameter of the Verres needle (see Chapter 2). Any obstruction reduces the diameter of the flow channel and results in unusually high entrance and insufflation pressures. The mistaken belief that the needle is improperly placed may lead one to remove and reintroduce the Verres needle unnecessarily. By contrast, low entrance and insufflating pressures are obtained if the connecting rubber tubing is not properly attached to the Verres needle. When creating the pneumoperitoneum, another reason for a lower than usual intra-abdominal pressure reading is the use of a Verres needle with a wider lumen.

The obturator knob on the needle barrel should turn easily so as to allow the surgeon to shut off the insufflation of gas entering the surgical field without the need of ancillary assistance or contamination. In my own experience, I prefer the operator to control the inflow of gas at both the Verres needle and the laparoscopic trocar sleeve.

An unusual complication has been described in a patient who underwent uneventful dilatation and curettage and laparoscopic sterilization by cauterization. Eight months after the procedure, a metallic foreign body was seen on radiographic examination of the abdomen.[4] A repeat laparoscopy identified the metal object as the outer sheath of a Verres needle. This foreign body was removed translaparoscopically. Newer instruments avoid this complication because they are constructed with a flare on the outer sheath of the needle where it is attached to the spring-loaded chamber. This prevents slippage into the abdominal cavity. Thus, care should be exercised if older Verres needles are being used.

TROCAR AND SLEEVE

Regardless of the operator's preference for a conical or pyramidal trocar, the instrument should always be sharp. A dull trocar requires additional force to penetrate the fascial layer. The increment in downward thrust may be difficult to control once the resistance is overcome. Sudden deep penetration increases the likelihood of damaging intra-abdominal and retroperitoneal structures (see Chapter 16).

The primary trocar of the laparoscope should be inspected to assure correct functioning of the spring bolt and the automatic valve so that there will be no loss of pneumoperitoneum. This inspection should take place before the laparoscope is inserted and again when it is removed for cleaning purposes. Because the component parts of these devices are rather simple in design and construction, it is likely that faulty assembly is the cause of any malfunction encountered. Most of the time, only disassembly followed by attentive reassembly is required.

The trocar sleeve should be inspected for any distortion of its contour. At any time, a fiberglass sleeve can be easily damaged during the sterilization process or by rough handling. Distortion of the shape of the sleeve impedes the telescoping motion of an instrument placed within it. It can be distressing to find oneself unable to slide the laparoscope up and down the sleeve with ease in order to obtain a clear view of the pelvis. The same applies to the secondary trocar sleeve. The operating instrument must have complete freedom of motion within the abdominal cavity to prevent uncontrolled and forceful motions which can damage the organs being manipulated.

Different sizes of rubber gaskets should be available to allow exchange during a laparoscopic procedure. The material of which they are composed may break during insertion or removal of the sharp trocar. This makes it impossible to obtain a good hermetic seal. Failure allows insufflated gas to escape.

LAPAROSCOPE

The actual laparoscope is a delicate piece of equipment which is easily damaged and which requires careful handling. The nature of its optical components and its sealed assembly makes this instrument the least amenable to any corrective measures when problems arise. The most common problems attributable to laparoscopic malfunction are (a) fogging of the objective lens; (b) fracture of a lens that makes the tool completely useless for image transmission; (c) appearance of water droplets inside the lens container.

The front lens of the laparoscope has a tendency to fog as it enters the peritoneal cavity. This results from the difference between the relatively cool temperature of the instrument (usually room temperature) and the warmer peritoneal cavity (central body temperature). Special devices to warm the laparoscope are available, but are expensive and impractical when several concomitant procedures have to be done. Antifogging detergents, such as hexachlorophene are effective. However, in some patients they have caused irritation when in contact with peritoneum or other tissues. Equally effective in preventing fogging of the laparoscope's front lens, without the risk of allergic reaction, is immersion of the laparoscope in warm normal saline solution.

A more practical maneuver is to equalize temperature by warming the objective lens by means of contact with intra-abdominal organs, such as uterus, ovaries, or the anterior bladder peritoneum.[3] This maneuver can be repeated as often as required without having to remove the laparoscope from the abdominal cavity. This reduces the risk of contamination.

Fogging of the eyepiece lens is also a common occurrence because it is close to the operator's expired air. The use of antifogging masks or masks that are taped to the bridge of the laparoscopist's nose usually circumvents this problem. If it is necessary to clean the eyepiece intraoperatively, the cleaning should be performed at a distance away from the surgical field since the eyepiece has been contaminated by contact with the operator's face.

Fracture of the objective lens should be identified while inspecting the instrument prior to its use. Broken lenses impede clear visualization of the organs to be inspected because refraction of the light occurs at the fracture line.

Water droplets can be found within the lens compartment. They are formed by the condensation of moisture in the closed chamber between the optic lenses. Water usually enters the lens chamber as a result of autoclaving the laparoscope for sterilization purposes.

The amount of liquid accumulated inside the lens chamber determines the size of the droplets. Multiple tiny droplets appear as a thin fog layer which resists any defogging maneuver previously described. Larger accumulations of water form a well defined drop. This can obstruct the field of vision and/or refract the light, thereby resulting in a distorted laparoscopic image.

Preventive measures to assure the long life of this delicate instrument include the following. (a) A program to educate all personnel who handle the cleaning, storage, disinfection, and sterilization of laparoscopes. Personnel should also be familiar with their delicate nature and exercise caution not to drop or mishandle the instruments. (b) Autoclaving should be avoided because laparoscopes only poorly tolerate the process of autoclaving. Even if no immediate damage is apparent from this type of sterilization process, the overall life expectancy of the instrument is greatly reduced by repeated autoclaving procedures. (c) Sterilization by the ethylene oxide gas technique with adequate follow-up aeration before reuse in a patient is preferred (see Chapter 21).

The most appropriate measure to avoid having to interrupt a laparoscopy is to have a spare instrument always at hand. Institutions performing a fair number of laparoscopies should evaluate cost considerations in relation to impact on patient care. One can save by not having an extra instrument, but lose by being unable to complete a procedure once it is started or by being unable to perform any laparoscopic procedures while a damaged instrument is being repaired.

LIGHT CORD

Lack of sufficient illumination within the peritoneal cavity may be caused by a defective light power source or transmitting fiberoptic cord. The light generator has several connecting outlets to accommodate a variety of manufacturers' fiberoptic cords. Anything short of a perfect fit between the cord and the light generator allows the escape of light around the fiberoptic cord. This decreases the illumination at the distal end of the cord. The degree of illumination generated by the light power source depends on the output range of each generator. Knowledge of the particular unit used in each setting is useful so that one does not expect more from the equipment than the unit is able to provide.

The degree of light arriving at the laparoscope is directly related to the number of intact fiberoptic fibers in the bundle forming the light transmitting cord; this varies inversely with the length of the transmitting cord. Individual broken fibers are difficult to identify, but when a sufficient number of fibers are damaged, small black dots are seen at the output end of the instrument when light is supplied at the proximal end. If the light transmitting cord is tightly folded to fit special containers, damage to the fiberoptic light cords can occur usually during the sterilization process. Intraoperatively, these can also be injured if they are fastened to the surgical drapes by passing them through the finger holes of a clamp. However, encasing the light cord with the surgical drapes and securing the drapes with a clamp can prevent damage to this delicate accessory. Proper care and handling of such a delicate component of the laparoscopy set cannot be sufficiently emphasized. Usually, the fiberoptic light cord is not able to be repaired. In most cases, a damaged cord requires replacement.

Of practical importance is that, over the years, equipment may have been acquired from different manufacturers. Such equipment may not be compatible. It is advisable to obtain all necessary adaptors for each component so as to make all laparoscopic equipment easily interchangeable.

ACCESSORY NONELECTRICAL INSTRUMENTS

Each instrument used in conjunction with the laparoscope is susceptible to inherent malfunction and breakage. In the interest of brevity, only the most common problems will be discussed here; a more detailed review of each instrument is left to the manufacturer's catalog or descriptive literature. Two major categories of instruments will be considered: (a) nonelectrical instruments, such as probes, aspiration cannulas, and grasping forceps, and (b) electrosurgical instruments including unipolar forceps, electrodissectors, and bipolar forceps, among others.

Probes. Probes, usually made of solid metal alloy material, are used for manipulating, measuring, and applying traction to intraperitoneal structures. Preventive measures for avoiding damage when using this instrument include the following: (a) A smooth surface to avoid injuring peritoneum or vessels in or around the structures being handled, and (b) an extra-abdominal handle of the probe that is greater in size than the diameter of the lumen of the accessory puncture sleeve. This prevents introducing the probe entirely into the abdominal cavity. Cases in which the probe inadvertently falls into the abdominal cavity require laparotomy for retrieval.

Aspiration Cannulas. Generally, aspiration devices are constructed to allow electrocoagulation by direct unipolar contact and aspiration of intraperitoneal fluid. The most common problem with this hollow tubular instrument is inadequate cleaning prior to sterilization. As a result, the shut-off valve does not function properly. This makes prolonged and intermittent aspiration difficult because of the constant loss of intraperitoneal gas and subsequent deflation of the pneumoperitoneum.

Grasping Instruments. Because of the delicate nature of the intra-abdominal organs and tissues to be manipulated and held with these instruments, it is essential for the grasping tongs to be perfectly smooth and easily manipulated. In addition to ensuring that the tongs are functioning properly, it is advisable to assess the delicacy of their action by grasping a soft and sensitive area of one's own skin; an ear lobe or a lip can serve this purpose. Any malfunction of these types of instuments can create serious complications lacerating the peritoneum or vessels in the structures to be handled.

Silicone Ring Applicators. The interdependent set of movements required for the successful application of a silicone ring to a fallopian tube or to a lacerated vessel necessitates that the applicator be in perfect working condition. During the inspection of the instrument prior to the surgical procedure, the following points should be checked: (a) The protruding tongs should approximate softly without tearing the tissue grasped between them; the ends of the tongs should not be sharp enough to pierce the material they hold, such as the delicate mesosalpinx. (b) Withdrawal of the grasping tongs into the main lumen of the forceps should be smooth and achieved evenly in a single motion. (c) The final motion of sliding the silicone ring over the grasped tissue should also be easily and smoothly accomplished. If the instrument does not perform well during the preoperative inspection, it should not be used but set aside for repair.

The same principles described for testing silicone ring applicators apply to tubal clip applicators. The latter require additional testing for the maneuvers required to release the clip once it has been applied.

INSUFFLATOR

The inability to produce or maintain an adequate pneumoperitoneum may originate in the apparatus used to insufflate the distending gas or in the connecting tubes. When using an insufflating machine, one must be familiar with the function of each individual component as well as the sum of its parts in order to be able to identify a malfunction.

If the reserve gas tank does not register pressures between 50 and 100 kp per square centimeter, it can be due to absence of gas in the tank or failure to open the shut-off valve. The latter is common and readily corrected. An empty reserve tank should rarely be the reason to abort a laparoscopy in progress because it can be easily replaced during the procedure.

The insufflated volume dial measures the amount of gas used from the smaller internal tank. It measures only the amount of gas that has been delivered by the instrument. This need not be the amount that has been insufflated into the patient's abdomen. When this smaller gas tank is refilled, failure of the needle to return to the zero mark may signify a leak between the large and the small tank.

A more hazardous condition exists if the valve in the gas line to the patient's abdomen has not been shut off. In this case the gas leaving the large tank under pressure does not refill the smaller gas reservoir, but instead goes directly into the peritoneal cavity. This situation is dangerous because the surgeon has no idea of the amount of gas being insufflated. Furthermore, the gas in the large cylinder is compressed under high pressure, well above that considered safe for direct administration to a patient. When an uncontrollable amount of gas at a very high pressure enters the abdominal cavity, the risk of cardiovascular and respiratory complications is greatly increased (see Chapters 9 and 10).

The measurement of intra-abdominal pressure can be erroneously affected at any part of the gas line. As previously discussed, a true measurement of the intraperitoneal pressure is obtained only if one has stopped the flow of the insufflating gas. A very low pressure reading usually indicates a leak in the gas circuit. The most common cause of such a leak is faulty attachment of the gas tubing to the Verres needle or the laparoscopic sleeve. Disassembling and reattaching the connection usually resolves this problem. A normal flowmeter reading with a low pressure reflects a leak in the gas circuit rather than a lack of insufflating pressure. Another common source of low pressure is an empty gas tank in combination with an inadvertently deflated pneumoperitoneum. Refilling the small gas reservoir tank reestablishes proper function.

Pressure readings that are higher than expected obligate the operator to rule out abdominal overdistention. Causes for an abnormally high read out related to the instrument include obstruction of the gas circuit by acute angulation or compression of the rubber tubing, often by the operator or assistant. In addition, obstruction may occur at the Verres needle, as previously discussed.

Failure to insufflate the distending gas at the appropriate rate can be determined by allowing the gas to escape freely into the room atmosphere. The amount delivered from the small gas tank is measured by the volume gauge on the apparatus. The normal flow rate should be 1 L per minute and in fast flow, 3 L per minute. If the insufflating apparatus fails to deliver the appropriate volume of gas, an alternative method for increasing the amount of gas delivered into the peritoneal cavity may be used. A second insufflating machine can be attached to the Verres needle or the laparoscopic trocar by means of a three-way Luer-lock adaptor.

ELECTROGENERATOR AND CIRCUITRY

The laparoscopist should be able to identify a malfunction of the high frequency power generator or a disruption in the electrical circuit. This is if electrocauterization cannot be achieved by touching the tissues with the instrument. It is not sufficient to accept the manufacturer's specifications for their equipment on blind faith. If a low power generator behaves like a high power generator or a bipolar instrument adopts the operational characteristics of a monopolar type, it is prudent for the surgeon to adjust the generator setting or change the equipment altogether.

The margin of safety of the electrogenerator is directly related to its proper functioning.[5] Small deviations from normal performance magnify the risks many times over. For example, the magnitude of current leakage is proportional to the square of the current flowing.[1] In turn, this current is directly proportional to the frequency of the generator. Thus, the current leakage from an electrosurgical generator with a low operating frequency of 2 Mhz produces four times as much undesirable heat as the leakage from a 1 Mhz generator.

Leakage of electrical current from the power generator must be within the standards set by the Joint Commission on Accreditation of Hospitals. A sudden increment in current leakage may be a potential source of fire or explosion (see Chapter 23). Periodic maintenance checks should be mandatory in all operating room facilities.

The generator transforms the low frequency current from the commercial electrical utility supplier at the wall outlet into high frequency current. The voltage output is conditioned on the incoming voltage from the electrical source. Fluctuations of the voltage available at the wall outlet may produce irregular fluctuations in the output of the electrogenerator. Spark-gap generators are particularly dangerous for translaparoscopic use because of their output variability.[2] The output can be further influenced by changes in atmospheric pressure and ambient humidity.

ELECTRO-INSTRUMENTATION

Malfunction of any electrosurgical instrument used translaparoscopically may lead to serious complications. Each of the three types of electrically powered instrument—unipolar, bipolar, and thermal—can malfunction in various ways. The laparoscopist must be capable of identifying all of these before any complications occur.

A problem common to all electrosurgical instruments is the accumulation of carbonized tissue debris on the operating forceps. This causes the cauterized tissue to adhere to the jaws of the instrument; thus, it cannot easily detach at the conclusion of the electrocoagulation. Hasty separation of the attached tissue often lacerates surrounding tissues and vessels. The surgeon should allow the jaws of the forceps to cool. In most cases, this makes it easy to free the tissue from the forceps. If this maneuver fails, the laparoscope can be utilized to push the tissue gently away from the adhered site on the forceps under direct visualization. One should ensure that there is no flow of current at this time.

Unipolar Instruments. The older unipolar instruments were designed to act as an active electrode which delivered a ground-seeking current. After the current left the active electrode, the path of least resistance was used in its return to the unit or to other grounded instruments. If, for example, electrocardiographic electrodes were attached, the current could flow to ground via the electrocardiographic equipment. Newer units are made somewhat safer by use of isolated electrical circuits. With this design, the current delivered is not ground seeking. Current has to return to the electrogenerator by a specific return or dispersive electrode. The safety factor built into this kind of unit prevents the release of current by the active electrode (such as forceps or probe) if the return electrode has not been properly connected. Therefore, failure to achieve an electrosurgical tissue effect with this equipment may be due to an incompletely connected electrical circuit and not to a problem with the instrument itself.

Bipolar Instruments. Designed to prevent inadvertent electrical injury to tissue, a bipolar unit functions by the transfer of electrons between the jaws of the grasping forceps. Early instruments did not always deliver an accurate and preestablished amount of current. This sometimes charred the superficial serosal layer of the grasped tissue without cauterizing the entire thickness of the tissue between the jaws. Laparoscopic sterilizations failed as a consequence (see Chapter 22), and there was bleeding from incompletely coagulated vessels.

Increasing the power that these instruments are able to deliver has partially solved the problem, but it has created a potentially new complication. As the tissue between the jaws is coagulated, its resistance increases; as the resistance increases, the electron flow is reduced. Theoretically the flow of electrons between the electrodes (forceps tongs) should ultimately cease. Increased power allows continuous delivery of electrons from the active electrode, so that current seeking the return electrode may burn adjacent tissues. In such instances, the unit is acting as a type of unipolar device. The lack of a dispersive electrode may cause sparks to jump to more distant tissue surfaces. The surgeon may thus have a false sense of security.

Thermal Cautery. The hot wire device exposes the tissue to be coagulated to a 270 ° wire loop. A smooth spring-loading action can lacerate the tissue and produce unexpected bleeding. Smoke always accumulates during tissue coagulation by this method. If visibility is reduced enough, one may not be able to complete the procedure. Evacuating the existing pneumoperitoneum and then reinsufflating solves the problem. Because reinsufflation of the pneumoperitoneum may have to be repeated several times during the surgical procedure, it is advisable to use a high-flow insufflator to deliver 3 L per minute of gas in order to facilitate rapid reestablishment of the pneumoperitoneum.

References

1. DiNovo JA. Radio frequency leakage current from unipolar laparoscopic electrocoagulators. J Reprod Med 1983; 28:565-575.
2. Hays CV. Making laparoscopy electrically safer: An engineer's approach. J Reprod Med 1979; 23:91-93.
3. Jakubowski A. Permanent intraperitoneal defogging of the optics during laparoscopy. Obstet Gynecol 1977; 49:128.
4. Kent SW. Retention of defective Verres needle sheath in abdominal cavity after laparoscopy. Fertil Steril 1977; 28:499.
5. Neufeld GR. Principles and hazards of electrocautery including laparoscopy. Surg Gynecol Obstet 1978; 147:705-710.

13 PROCEDURAL FAILURE

Inability to complete a laparoscopic procedure due to technical difficulties is a frequent occurrence. Phillips reported that the rate of failed attempts to conclude a laparoscopy is related to the operator's experience.[5] The incidence of failure is highest during the learning process. He noted a sharp decrease in the number of unsuccessful laparoscopic attempts after accumulating a case experience of 250 or more procedures.

Failure to carry out a laparoscopy as planned may be due to equipment malfunction (see Chapter 12) or to technical difficulties. Timely recognition of the cause for the latter is essential if complications are to be avoided. Operator experience plays an important role in overcoming procedural difficulties. This chapter will be limited to a description of the most common problems that preclude the successful completion of a laparoscopy and the corrective measures available. Prevention by adherence to proper technique (see Chapter 2) remains the most important step to ensure against a failed laparoscopy.

PNEUMOPERITONEUM

Techniques to obtain a suitable pneumoperitoneum have been described in Chapter 2. A common difficulty encountered by the operator is the deflation of a previously adequate pneumoperitoneum. The causes of this difficulty range from a simple misconnection between the tubing and the Verres needle or trocar sleeve to the more difficult problem of continuous leakage of gas.

Systematic evaluation for the probable source of pneumoperitoneum loss must precede any corrective attempts. This includes examination of the gas reserve and connecting tubing, determination of the source of gas leakage, and the operation of the automatic insufflation mechanism, as follows:

Gas Reserve. Before a laparoscopy is started, the surgeon must make sure there is sufficient distending gas in the reserve tank. Check to see that the valve between the reserve tank and the insufflator tank is open. Refill the insufflator tank before it empties completely (see Chapter 12).

Connecting Gas Tubing. Misconnection of the gas tubing to the insufflator proximally or to the Verres needle or trocar sheath distally results in gas leakage that precludes formation and maintenance of pneumoperitoneum. Low intraperitoneal pressure is registered by the insufflator's manometer. Simple detachment and reconnection of the tubing solves this problem.

Elevated intraperitoneal pressure may be registered because of excessive insufflation (see Chapter 15), but it may also result from inadvertent compression of the gas tubing. This situation may occur as a consequence of sharp bending of the gas line or collapse of the soft tubing at the site of attachment to the drapes on the operative field. Reevaluation of the entire gas circuit must be carried out before insufflation of the distending gas is continued. Absence of a drop in intraperitoneal pressure following the aforementioned maneuvers requires reevaluation of the position of the Verres needle (see Chapter 15).

Gas Leakage. Leakage of intraperitoneal gas may occur around the shaft of the instrument at the point it pierces the abdominal wall. This can be confirmed by filling the umbilical fossa with normal saline and observing for bubbling around the instrument. An Allis clamp placed around the trocar sheath assists in sealing off the leak.

Leakage of gas around the Hasson cannula during the performance of an open laparoscopy can be troublesome. Repositioning the conical adaptor and reanchoring the fascial stitches to the trocar sheath is usually sufficient to overcome this problem. It is better to attempt to reseal the pneumoperitoneum by the aforementioned maneuvers than to increase the rate of insufflation of distending gas when replacing the escaping gas.

Another source of gas leakage occurs when the rubber gaskets surrounding the laparoscope or the auxiliary instruments are damaged. This happens frequently when sharp pyramidal trocars are used to perforate the abdominal wall. Simple replacement of the rubber gasket ought to solve this difficulty.

Use of Automatic Insufflation. Deflation of an established pneumoperitoneum can occur when the insufflator is switched to its automatic mode. In the automatic control mode of insufflation, the apparatus is meant to compensate for any amount of gas lost during endoscopy. Gas flow is regulated to be delivered at 1 L per minute. The flow stops when the intraperitoneal pressure reaches 14 to 18 mm Hg. The machine is adjusted to resume insufflation whenever the intra-abdominal pressure falls below this level.

Major variations in gas flow can be encountered during insufflation in the automatic mode. The level of intra-abdominal pressure regulates the amount of gas the insufflator delivers per unit of time in this modality. The greater the impedance, the lower the flow of gas.

These variations in gas flow secondary to fluctuation in intra-abdominal pressure are of practical significance during laparoscopy. The combination of intraperitoneal pressure within an established pneumoperitoneum, intermittent elevation in pressure during respiration (inspiration), and increased resistance produced by the flow of gas during automatic flow may exceed the shut-off threshold built into the insufflator. This can result in inappropriate cessation of gas flow which in turn leads to deflation of pneumoperitoneum.

FAILURE TO MOBILIZE PELVIC STRUCTURES

Successful completion of a diagnostic laparoscopy depends to a great degree on the ability to mobilize the pelvic structures (see Chapters 3 and 4). This is usually accomplished by displacement of the uterus in various directions. Inability to move this centrally located organ at will may be due to a variety of causes. Fixation by pelvic adhesions as a result of previous surgery, acute retroflexion, and enlarged uterine cavity are some of these. Some can be circumvented, whereas others cannot.

Pelvic Adhesions

As described in Chapter 3, pelvic adhesions are common in patients undergoing diagnostic laparoscopy because of pelvic pain or infertility. At times, these adhesions preclude visualization of important structures or areas which are in need of evaluation. It is not always possible to divide them translaparoscopically.

More often than not, filmy adhesions do not impede uterine mobilization but act instead as barriers to laparoscopic inspection (Figure 13.1). Entrapment of gas used to produce the pneumoperitoneum can sometimes be seen in newly formed compartments walled off by these adhesions (Figure 13.2). This loculated pneumoperitoneum may simulate gas within the bowel wall (pneumatosis intestinalis). It is advisable to manipulate the adhesions to release the enclosed gas. The extent and quality of the adhesive band determines the approach to be taken.

Filmy avascular adhesions can be incised with accessory scissors. Alternatively, access to view can be accomplished by perforating the adhesions with a secondary sharp trocar under direct vision. The newly created opening permits the passage of the laparoscope to explore the previously occluded area (Figure 13.3).

It is debatable whether the aforementioned maneuver should be undertaken in a patient who requires a subsequent major surgical procedure for reasons of infertility. Nevertheless, it has proven valuable in specific cases. In women

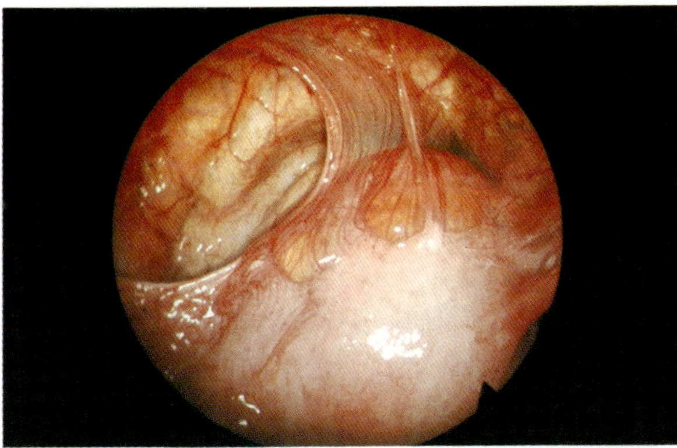

Figure 13.1 Filmy adhesions between the anterior uterine wall and the anterior parietal peritoneum. Complete visualization of the vesicouterine peritoneal reflection is not possible. Vascularization of the adhesions makes electrocoagulation necessary before division is attempted.

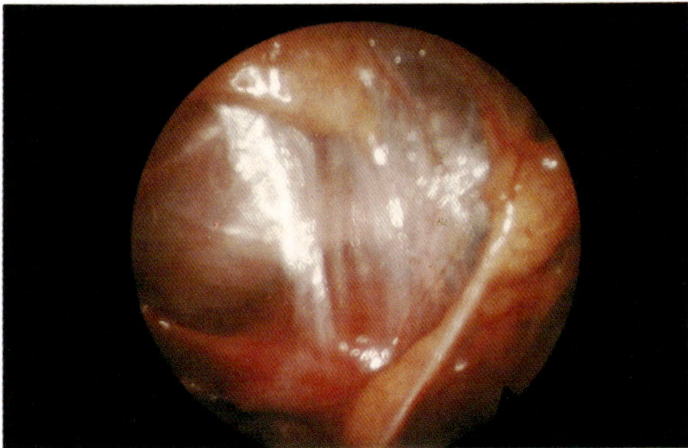

Figure 13.2 Filmy adhesions occluding the vesicouterine peritoneal reflection. Insufflated gas is entrapped behind the adhesions placing them on stretch. Avascularity of the adhesions allows the operator to divide them without prior electrocoagulation and thus visualize the anterior hemipelvis.

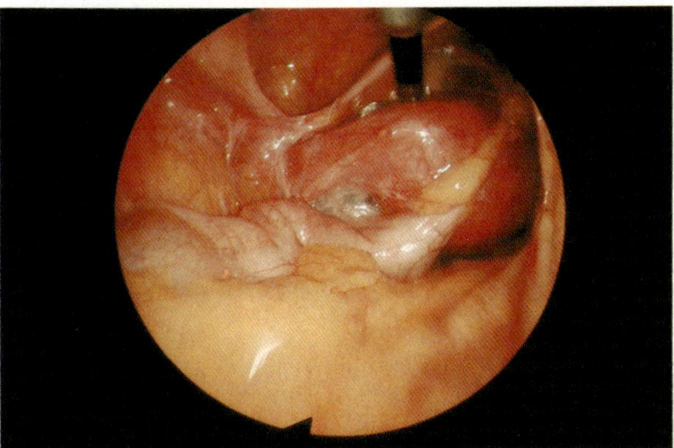

Figure 13.3 Filmy adhesions shown in Figure 13.2 have been divided. Vesicouterine peritoneal reflection can now be inspected.

undergoing a diagnostic laparoscopy to rule out the presence of an ectopic gestation, the ability to explore the entire pelvis may make the difference between a successful evaluation and an inconclusive one (Figure 13.4). Imperfect visualization may require a laparotomy for obtaining a definitive diagnosis. Similarly, successful completion of ovum aspiration may necessitate carrying out this maneuver.

In women undergoing laparoscopy as part of an infertility work up, piercing an adhesion to facilitate visualization with the laparoscope is also useful.

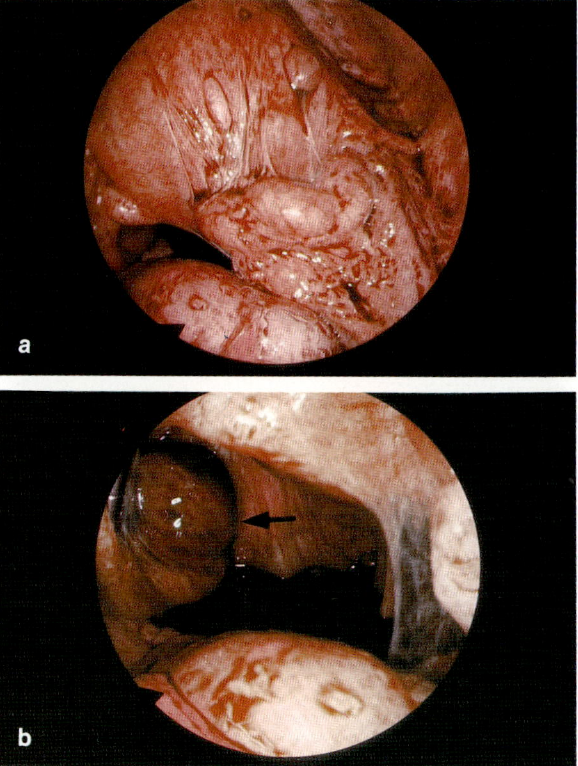

Figure 13.4 Multiple pelvic adhesions encountered during a diagnostic laparoscopy. *a*. Despite right peritubal and periovarian adhesions, the right fallopian tube can be visualized well. However, the left tube cannot be seen. *b*. Lysis of right peritubal adhesions allows mobilization of the right adnexa and exposure of the left adnexa. An ectopic pregnancy is now visualized in the ampullary portion of the left fallopian tube (arrow).

Notwithstanding that future operations will be needed, knowledge about the condition of the hidden fimbria is important. Discussion and counseling regarding future surgery differs from patient to patient according to the findings. Pelvic and peritubal adhesions, which are accompanied by bilateral fimbrial occlusion or tubal distention, have a different prognosis for subsequent pregnancy than when no fimbrial abnormalities are present. Anatomic distortion limited to peritubal adhesive bands has a better fertility prognosis (Figures 13.5 and 13.6).

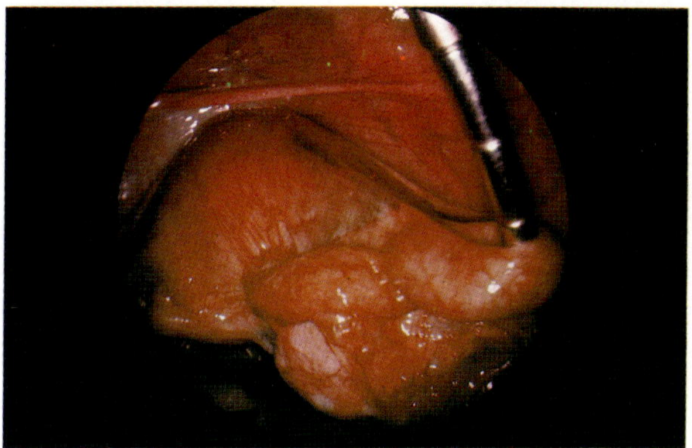

Figure 13.5 Peritubal adhesions. Tubal dilatation suggests the possibility of hydrosalpinx. The diagnosis requires observation of fimbrial obstruction with demonstration of intraluminal accumulation of fluid.

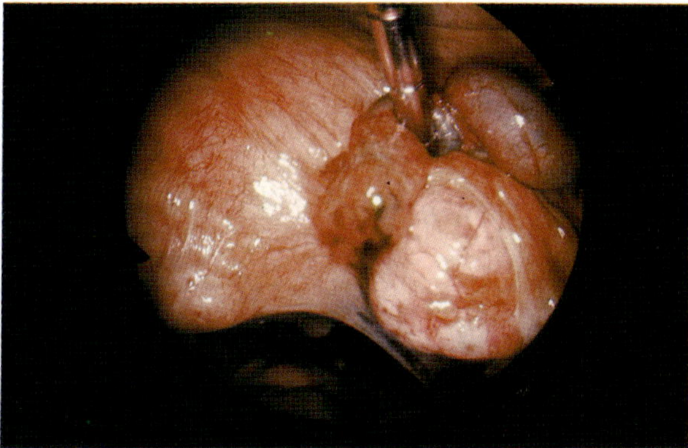

Figure 13.6 Adhesions shown in Figure 13.5 have been lysed. The fimbria have normal configuration. Tubal patency is confirmed by free flow of dye solution. Minor translaparoscopic surgery (lysis of adhesions) enabled the operator to arrive at a correct diagnosis.

Omental adhesions may also impede one's view of the pelvic organs. Displacement with a probe inserted through an accessory puncture enables the surgeon to inspect the pelvis (Figure 13.7). Carefully increasing the distention of the peritoneal cavity—while ensuring that the pneumoperitoneum never exceeds 20 mm Hg—may facilitate visualization by placing the adhesion on stretch. Omental adhesions to the anterior abdominal wall may be moved out of the field of vision by this extra insufflation. Caution should be exercised to avoid tearing a vascular adhesion which may be the source of subsequent intraperitoneal bleeding. Makanji and Elliott reported rupture of the spleen during laparoscopy.[4] They attributed this complication to stretching of perisplenic adhesions during the induction of pneumoperitoneum.

At times, omental adhesions following previous pelvic surgery, especially if they are located in the midline, require that inspection of the pelvis be performed in two stages. One begins by visualizing the hemipelvis accessible upon entrance into the peritoneal cavity (Figure 13.8). A 360° sweeping motion of the laparoscope (clockwise or counterclockwise as the circumstances dictate) relocates the endoscope to the opposite face of the omental adhesion. This maneuver enables the surgeon to visualize the contralateral hemipelvis.

The rotation of the laparoscope has to be carried out under direct observation. In its rotational trajectory, the endoscope traverses the upper abdomen. Therefore, caution is needed so as not to injure the falciform hepatic ligament during this step (Figure 13.9).

The falciform ligament is composed of peritoneal folds. It lies obliquely, coursing from the abdominal surface of the diaphragm to the dorsal surface of the rectus abdominis sheath as far caudad as the umbilicus. The round ligament of the liver (ligamentum teres) is the remnant of the obliterated umbilical vein. It connects the umbilicus to the umbilical notch of the liver and is usually found in the free margin of the falciform ligament.

Before rotation of the laparoscope is attempted, the operator must evaluate the extent of intra-abdominal penetration of the laparoscopic sleeve. Intrusion of this sleeve beyond the depth required to traverse the anterior abdominal wall may itself be the cause of trauma to the suspensory hepatic ligament. Withdrawal of the sleeve as needed, and visual identification of the ligamentum teres must precede rotation of the laparoscope.

The operator may take advantage of the opportunity to explore the upper abdomen under vision while performing this motion. Omental adhesions to the lateral abdominal and pelvic walls can impede the completion of a laparoscopic evaluation. Visual exploration is indicated to evaluate whether the bowel is involved in the adhesion (Figure 13.10). Displacement of the adhesion with a probe must be done gently because bowel serosa can be lacerated. Any disruption of vascular integrity may give rise to small localized hematomas.

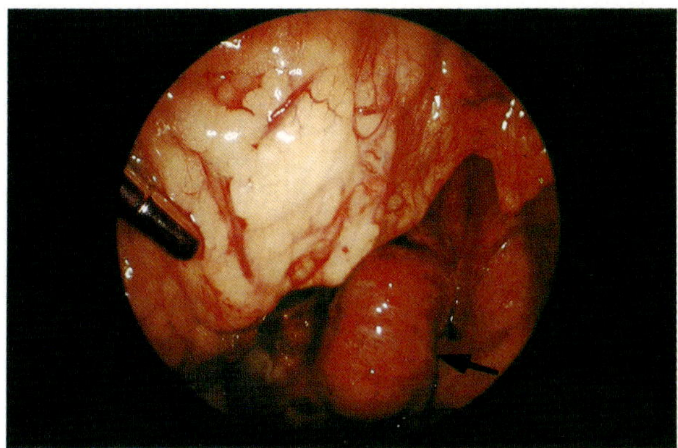

Figure 13.7 Omental adhesion to the uterus. Displacement with a metal probe inserted via a secondary puncture allows exploration of the pelvis. An ectopic pregnancy is thus visualized in the right fallopian tube (arrow).

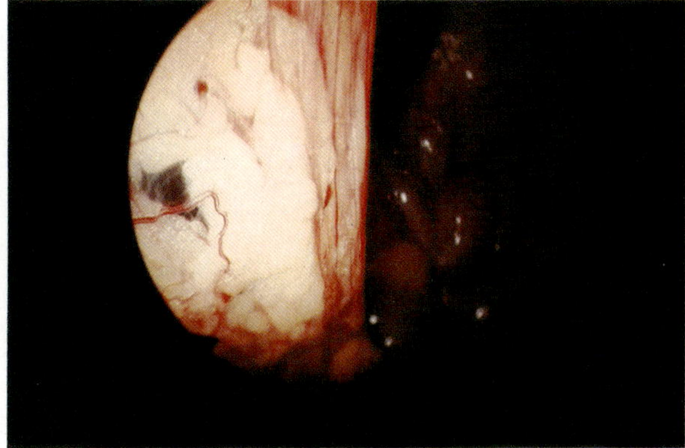

Figure 13.8 Midline omental adhesion. Patient had undergone abdomino-pelvic surgery in the past through a subumbilical vertical incision. Upon insertion of the laparoscope, the right hemipelvis can be seen. Exploration of the left hemipelvis requires a 360° clockwise circular sweeping rotation of the laparoscope and sleeve to bring the laparoscope into the free space on the contralateral side of the adhesion.

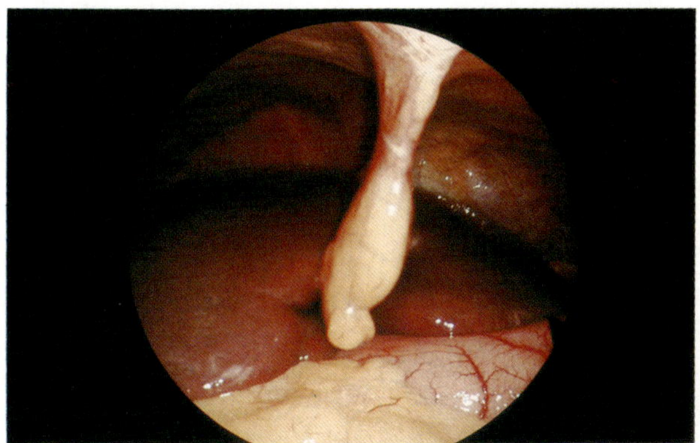

Figure 13.9 Falciform hepatic ligament. Rotation of the laparoscope into the upper abdomen must be performed under direct vizualization. The laparoscopic sleeve should not intrude more than 2 cm. into the peritoneal cavity.

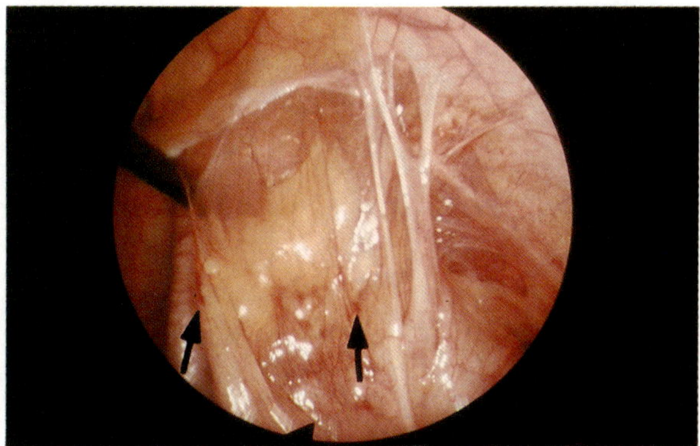

Figure 13.10 Omental adhesions to pelvic wall. Bowel is included within the adhesive bands. Undue stretching of the adhesion produced vascular disruption (arrows).

Uterine Enlargement

The ability to move the abdominopelvic organs freely is essential during diagnostic and operative laparoscopy. Uterine dislocation plays an important role in a laparoscopic procedure since displacing the uterus is usually accompanied by mobilization of the adnexal structures. Uterine fixation may occur as a consequence of adhesions to adjacent structures or a significant enlargement.

Uterine enlargement can be seen with uterine fibroids and pregnancy or following an interruption of pregnancy (Figures 13.11 and 13.12). Expansion of the uterine muscle mass is often accompanied by a concomitant expansion of the endometrial cavity. This makes mobilization of the organ with standard instrumentation difficult if not impossible.

Most uterine mobilizers are designed to be used with a normal sized uterus. The short endocervical-endometrial stem is often inadequate to manipulate a larger organ because of its distended cavity. Use of inapproprate instruments under these suboptimal conditions increases the risk of trauma, such as uterine perforation.

When confronted with this problem, the laparoscopist ought to resort to ancillary maneuvers to mobilize the uterus. These include digital manipulation of the organ, the use of additional accessory punctures, and the transcervical insertion of a large Hegar dilator.

Digital mobilization of the uterus requires the participation of an assistant. Pressing the cervix against the posterior vaginal fornix by fingers inserted vaginally anteverts the uterine corpus. This is possible because the uterus is suspended on a fulcrum at the level of its internal os by the cardinal ligaments. Lateral displacement of the cervix projects the uterine corpus to the contralateral direction and thus facilitates visual exploration of the adnexal structures.

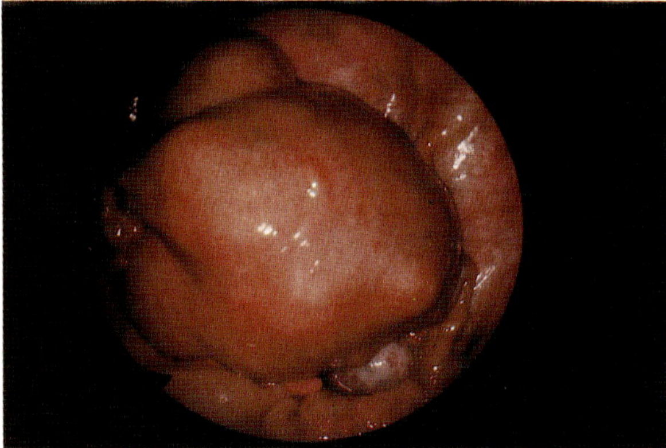

Figure 13.11 Enlarged fibroid uterus. Multiple fibroids distort the normal configuration of the uterus. The large uterine size occludes adequate visualization of the pouch of Douglas and the adnexal structures. Use of the usual uterine manipulators are of little help for mobilizing the uterus.

Manual displacement of the uterus for laparoscopy is not limited to cases in which there is enlargement of this organ. If an intrauterine pregnancy is supected, this maneuver is valuable because the uterine cavity does not have to be invaded. This is particularly beneficial for a patient who may have an ectopic gestation, but who wishes to retain the pregnancy, if it is located within the uterus.

Quite often, the enlarged uterus can be readily dislocated by means of accessory probes. One should not hesitate to insert a third or even a fourth additional probe, if warranted. Diagnostic or operative laparoscopy requiring several accessory punctures is usually preferable to a laparotomy. A more benign postoperative recovery period and a more desirable cosmetic result justify this practice.

The use of a large-bore Hegar dilator (No. 15 or larger) has also proved helpful in mobilizing a larger than normal uterus. Its large diameter and blunt tip reduce the risk of perforating the uterine wall. Dynamically, this technique accomplishes adequate ventrodorsal displacement of the uterus by changing the position of the cervical canal.

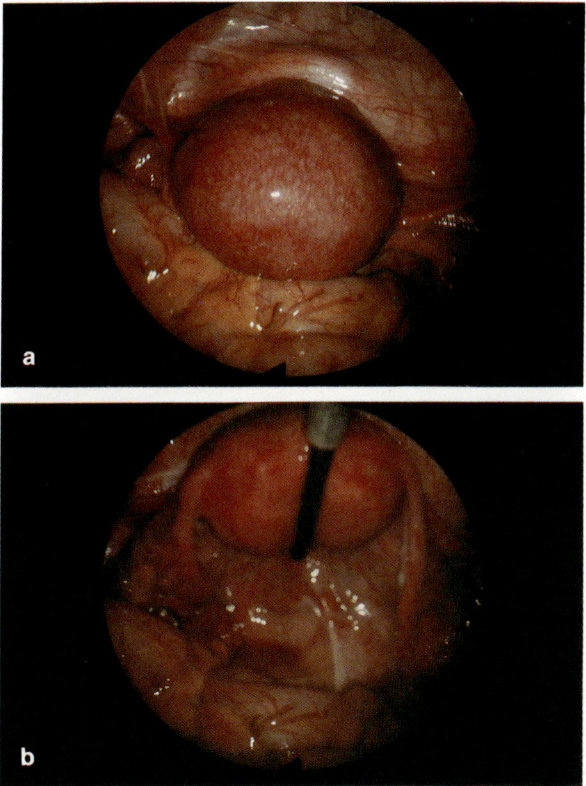

Figure 13.12 Uterine enlargement following pregnancy interruption. *a.* Uterus enlarged to twice its normal size makes displacement difficult. The expanded endometrial cavity makes the average uterine manipulator ineffectual. *b.* Utilization of auxiliary probe displaces the uterus ventrally and allows visualization and access to the adnexal structures.

Adequate cervical dilatation is required for the insertion of a large Hegar dilator into the endometrial cavity. This does not appear to present a problem in a recently pregnant uterus. However, it may present difficulties for a non-pregnant patient in whom dilatation to such large dimensions exposes the cervix to the risk of traumatic laceration.[1]

OBESITY

Obesity confronts the surgeon with a difficult challenge whenever abdomino-pelvic surgery is indicated. Laparoscopy is no exception (Figure 13.13). Frequently cited as the cause of failure to complete a planned laparoscopy, obesity has been classified by some as a relative contraindication for this procedure.[3]

Creation of pneumoperitoneum seems to be the most difficult obstacle to the successful completion of laparoscopy in the obese patient. Attempts to insert the Verres needle through alternative areas other than the infraumbilical site—such as transfundal or through the posterior vaginal fornix—do not seem to overcome all difficulties. Use of a longer Verres needle has been recommended.[3]

Personal experience does not substantiate the need to vary the standard technique described in Chapter 2 for the overweight patient. The umbilical anatomy is essentially unchanged in the obese patient. Skin, fascia, and peritoneum are apposed to each other and form a single tissue layer similar to that found in the patient of average weight.

The Verres needle should be inserted perpendicularly to the fascia layer plane. If the peritoneum has not been pierced after the needle has been inserted to a depth of 5 cm, it should be removed and reinsertion attempted. The

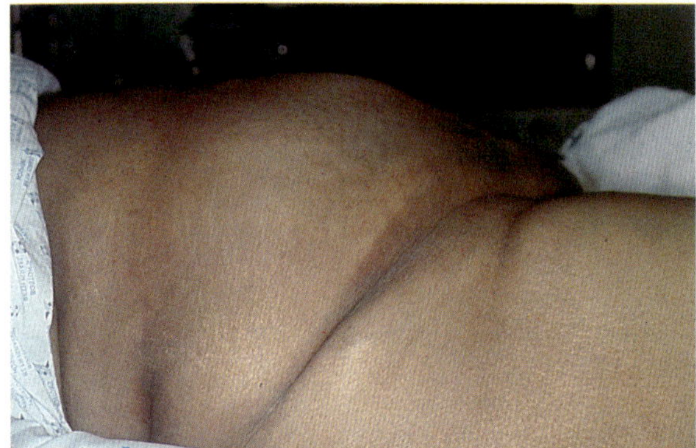

Figure 13.13 Abdominal configuration in an obese patient. Use of standard laparoscopy instrumentation (Verres needle and laparoscopic trocar) is recommended. Proper site and angle of insertion is more relevant than the length of the instruments for a succesful procedure under these circumstances.

saline injection-reaspiration test (see Chapter 2) is essential to confirm the intraperitoneal position of the needle tip. Insufflation of the distending gas should not to be started until the test is successfully performed.

The obese patient with a pendulous abdominal panniculus and/or short stature presents a special problem to the laparoscopist. The reduced subumbilical-suprapubic distance limits the space between the primary and secondary punctures (Figure 13.14). Intra-abdominal collision of instruments and limitation of their motion is a common occurrence. Positioning the patient in the Trendelenburg position and cephalad displacement of the periumbilical abdominal wall by a surgical assistant prior to the insertion of the Verres needle has proved helpful. A similar maneuver must be employed when the laparoscopic trocar is being inserted.

The abdominal capacity is increased in the obese patient. The volume of gas insufflated into the peritoneal cavity offers little guidance to the operator. Repeated measurements of the intraperitoneal pressure, coupled with assessments of diaphragmatic resistance the anesthesiologist must overcome to properly ventilate the patient, are the best guides to the amount of distending gas that can be safely used for pneumoperitoneum. Continuous interaction between the operator and the anesthesiologist is crucial for the performance of laparoscopy in the obese patient.

Schoeffler et al reported the hemodynamic and respiratory changes experienced by obese women undergoing laparoscopy.[6] Decreased cardiac index and increased systemic vascular resistance were observed during peritoneal insufflation. Diminution in venous return was responsible for the decrease in cardiac output. A slight increase in $PaCO_2$ was seen under controlled ventilation. These results did not differ from those obtained with nonobese patients (see Chapters 9 and 10).

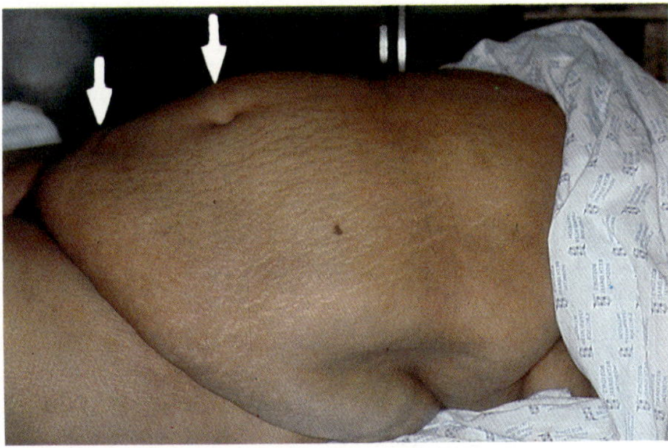

Figure 13.14 Pendulous abdominal panniculus. Distance between pubis and umbilicus is foreshortened (arrows). Perpendicular insertion of instruments is recommended to avoid intra-abdominal collision.

Insertion of the sharp laparoscopic trocar in the obese patient can be more difficult than is usual. Inability to manually elevate the anterior abdominal wall adds to this problem. The use of towel clips to raise the periumbilical area has been suggested.[3] I do not find this maneuver particularly helpful. At times, it may even produce an additional obstacle to the introduction of the sharp trocar by elevating only the skin and superficial subcutaneous tissue. This enlarges the distance that has to be traversed by the trocar before the sleeve enters the peritoneal cavity.

Personal experience has shown that insufflation of somewhat more distending gas than usual offers the operator the necessary abdominal wall resistance to insert the sharp trocar without the need to elevate the abdominal wall. Normally, a maximum pressure of 18 to 20 mm Hg on manual insufflation is sufficient to perform laparoscopy in the nonobese subject. In the overweight patient, intra-abdominal pressures of 20 to 22 mm Hg may be required for trocar insertion. Once the laparoscope is in the peritoneal cavity, the excess pressure can be released. It is mandatory that the laparoscopist inform the anesthetist in advance of his or her intention to create this temporary elevation in intra-abdominal pressure.

INSTRUMENTAL COLLISION

Intra-abdominal collision between the laparoscope and the accessory instruments inserted through the secondary puncture may interfere with a planned laparoscopic procedure. Constraining the full intra-abdominal motion of the instruments precludes their proper intended use. Such limitations can also obstruct visualization through the laparoscope.

Commonly, instruments hinder each other as a result of excessive penetration of their trocar sleeves into the peritoneal cavity. Careful withdrawal of the trocar sleeve is generally sufficient to overcome this difficulty. Caution is recommended to avoid excessive withdrawal of the sleeve or there may be need for reinsertion by trocar puncture.

Reinsertion of the laparoscopic sleeve following accidental removal is facilitated if performed under direct visualization. With the laparoscope pulled back somewhat into its sleeve, the original pathway can be identified (Figure 13.15). Gentle advancement of the sleeve can occasionally regain its intraperitoneal position, thus avoiding the need to create a new perforation.

If the aforementioned maneuver is unsuccessful, reinsertion with the sharp trocar may be required. When this is required after the auxiliary sleeve is in place, it should be performed under visual guidance. Replacing the auxiliary instrument (probe, forceps) with a 5 mm laparoscope enables the operator to select the peritoneal site for the laparoscopic trocar to reenter.

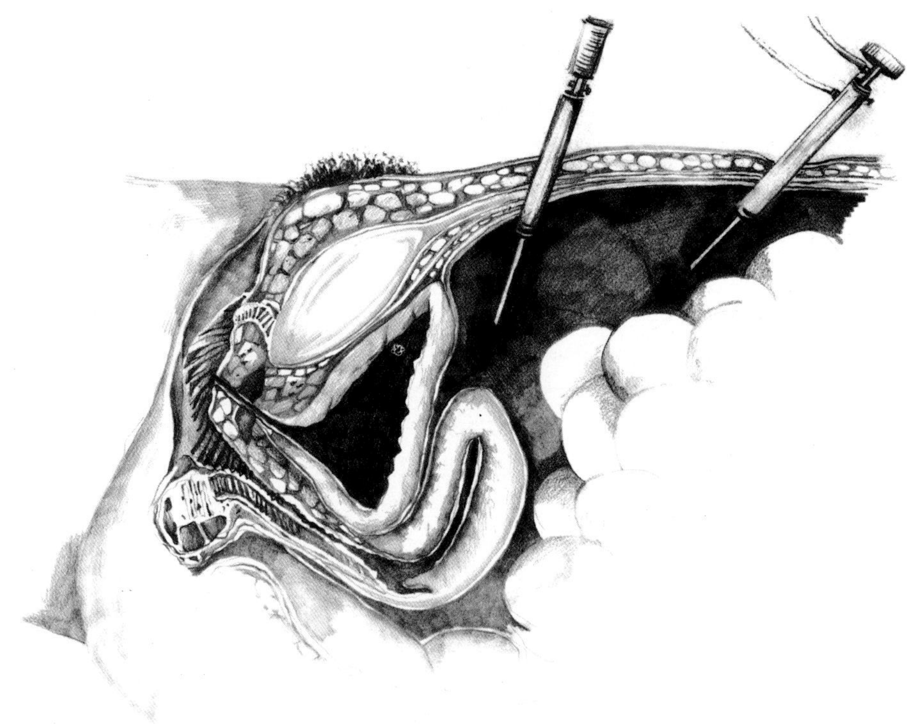

Figure 13.17 Similar subumbilical view as shown in Figure 13.16, but with proper angulation of laparoscope and accessory instrument. Perpendicular insertion of the sleeves maximizes the intraperitoneal entry distance between instruments.

SINGLE PUNCTURE OPERATIVE LAPAROSCOPY

Advantages and shortcomings of the single puncture operative laparoscope have been previously described (see Chapter 1). Advent of translaparoscopic laser surgery aroused a renewed interest in the utilization of this instrument. The skill of individual operators permits some laparoscopic procedures to be successfully completed through a single incision. Nevertheless, the technical difficulties previously described remain unresolved.

Counseling the patient in whom a single puncture operative laparoscope is to be used should include advising her of the probable use of secondary punctures. Consent limitations and/or reluctance by the laparoscopist to make use of additional punctures ought never to be the reason for an incomplete diagnostic laparoscopy.

AUXILIARY PUNCTURES

Notwithstanding the advantages previously described (see Chapter 3), the use of auxiliary punctures during diagnostic laparoscopy remains controversial. Proponents of their use in all laparoscopic procedures point out the need to visualize both sides of the ovary and to facilitate exploration of the entire pelvis. Opponents of the routine use of secondary punctures claim a reduction in complications when insertion of another sharp trocar is avoided (see Chapter 16).

Personal experience supports the use of an auxiliary trocar in all diagnostic and operative laparoscopies. Inability to completely visualize all intraperitoneal aspects of the reproductive organs must be considered aspects of an inconclusive laparoscopy. If laparoscopy is inconclusive as a consequence of the reluctance to use an auxiliary puncture, it must be judged a procedural failure (in reality, the operator's failure) and not a limitation of the technique itself.

Inability to fully evaluate the pelvic region may expose the patient to a life-threatening risk. On cursory exploration, an expanding mass may be diagnosed as a uterine fibroid or hydrosalpinx when instead it actually represents an ectopic pregnancy (Figures 13.18). Not as serious, but nonetheless important, is the identification of hidden peritubal or periovarian adhesions. Without such information, correct and adequate counseling about the need of future surgery is not possible.

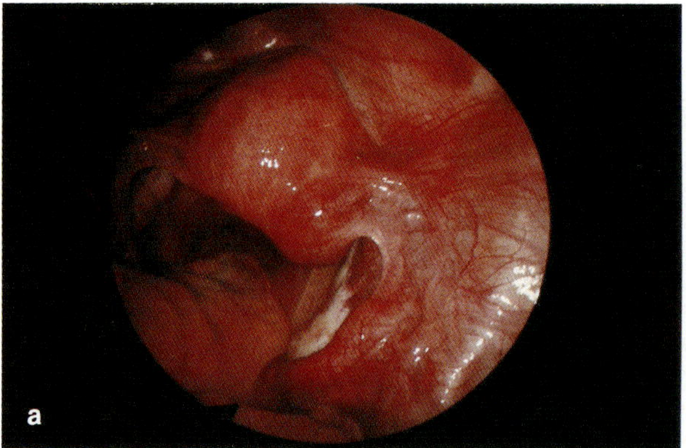

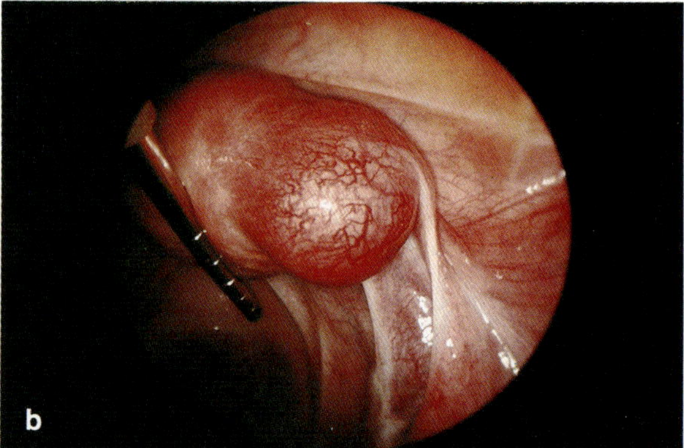

Figure 13.18 Auxiliary trocar benefit demonstrated. *a.* An expanded tumor mass located in the right cornual region. Maximal anteflexion of the uterus allows visualization of the anterior aspect of this mass only. A preliminary diagnosis of cornual fibroid was made. *b.* A solid probe has been inserted through a midline suprapubic auxiliary puncture site to provide additional anterodisplacement of the uterus and reveals the mass to be hypervascular and originating from the interstitial portion of the fallopian tube. The unruptured cornual tubal pregnancy was confirmed at the subsequent laparotomy (same case as Figure 3.17).

References

1. Chi I, Felblum P. Uterine perforation during sterilization by laparoscopy and minilaparotomy. Am J Obstet Gynecol 1981; 139:735-736.
2. Hulka JF, Higgins G. Trauma to the internal cervical os during dilatation for diagnostic curettage. Am J Obstet Gynecol 1961; 82:913-919.
3. Loffer FD, Pent D. Laparoscopy in the obese patient. Am J Obstet Gynecol 1976; 125:104-107.
4. Makanji HH, Elliott HR. Rupture of spleen at laparoscopy: Case report. Br J Obstet Gynaecol 1980; 87:73-74.
5. Phillips JM. Complications in laparoscopy. Int J Gynaecol Obstet 1977; 15:157-162.
6. Schoeffler P, Haberer JP, Manhes H, et al. Circulatory and respiratory effects of celioscopy in the obese. Ann Fr Anesth Reanim 1984; 3:10-15.

14 ANESTHETIC COMPLICATIONS

Anesthetic complications associated with laparoscopy are rare. Their incidence is difficult to establish because only serious morbidity and mortality tend to be reported. Nevertheless, the operator must include proper preoperative anesthetic evaluation as an integral part of the patient's preparation for the procedure.

Selection of the anesthetic technique for laparoscopy varies in accordance with the indication for the procedure, the condition of the patient, the availability of personnel and the operator's preference (see Chapter 8). As previously indicated, advantages and risks are associated with each anesthetic method. The preventable nature of most anesthetic complications during laparoscopy means they can often be avoided by careful assessment. Knowledge of their existence, identification of the predisposing factors, and close collaboration with the anesthetist are essential in this regard.

Exploration of all possible anesthetic complications is beyond the scope of this book. For a description of the techniques of each anesthetic method, the reader is referred to the standard anesthesiology literature. The aim of this chapter is simply to emphasize those complications that are more commonly seen in association with laparoscopy.

Anesthesia for pelvic laparoscopy presents peculiar problems. They include those related to pneumoperitoneum, carbon dioxide insufflation, and the Trendelenburg position (see Chapters 9 and 10). The potential detrimental effects of these factors vary with the type of anesthesia (general versus regional).

GENERAL ANESTHESIA

General anesthesia is used for pelvic laparoscopy around the world. The advantages of this technique were previously described (see Chapter 8). Circulatory and respiratory variations secondary to the laparoscopy itself, which may influence selection of the anesthetic, have also been reviewed (Chapters 9 and 10).

Generally, the aforementioned changes are well compensated for during inhalation anesthesia. Nevertheless, a propensity to serious complications, such as inadvertent endobronchial intubation and regurgitation of gastric contents is increased during general anesthesia for laparoscopy. Awareness of these problems by the primary surgeon will help select and counsel patients appropriately.

Endobronchial Intubation

Inadvertent endobronchial intubation is a serious complication associated with general anesthesia. It results as a consequence of the mislocation of the tip of the endotracheal tube when it is advanced below the carina. Ventilation may then be limited to the ipsilateral lung of the intubated mainstem bronchus.

Trendelenburg position is routinely used for pelvic laparoscopy. The degree of head down tilt in the conscious subject (under local or regional anesthesia) is limited by the discomfort that accompanies this position. Patients experience symptoms due to vascular engorgement of the head and neck. These limitations do not exist under general anesthesia. Thus, the operator's request for a steeper Trendelenburg position are usually accommodated by the anesthetist.

Heinonen et al studied the position of the endotracheal tube in patients placed in the Trendelenburg position.[6] They found an upward displacement of the hilum of the lung when the subject is tilted head down. Inadvertent bronchial intubation may ensue as a consequence. The use of a short endotracheal tube may prevent this from happening.

Regurgitation of Gastric Content

Regurgitation and aspiration of gastric content into the lungs is one of the most serious complications associated with anesthesia.[8] During general gynecologic operations, gastroesophageal regurgitation is not a common problem. Lack of manipulation of the upper abdominal organs keeps this risk at a minimum. This is not the case during laparoscopy.

At the time of pelvic laparoscopy, several factors contribute to the increased risk of gastroesophageal regurgitation. The lithotomy position compounded by a steep head down tilt, exposes the patient to reflux of gastric contents. This augmented risk is counterbalanced by the preventive benefit offered by the Trendelenburg position in the event regurgitation does occur. The refluent material is unable to enter the airway by gravity.

The sequelae of pulmonary aspiration of gastric content relate to the quantity and quality of the inspired material. Solid particles can produce obstruction at any level of the bronchial tree and may cause asphyxiation. Large amounts of fluid can flood the air spaces. The most serious complications resulting from inhalation of regurgitated material are those due to the relative acidity of the gastric reflux.

Severe bronchoconstriction and necrosis of the tracheal mucosa result from aspirating substances with a pH of less than 2.5. Patchy pneumonitis is seen as a white out on chest roentgenogram. Pulmonary edema may occur and the patient develops what is known as adult respiratory distress syndrome or Mendelsohn's syndrome.

Similar to all other surgical complications, prevention is essential. When in doubt, aspiration of gastric contents by nasogastric suction is important prior to anesthesia induction. If needed, suction should be repeated intermittently throughout the entire operation. Endotracheal intubation with immediate inflation of the cuff ought to be standard procedure for all laparoscopies under general anesthesia. This occludes the trachea around the endotracheal tube and prevents aspiration even if regurgitation occurs.

When regurgitation and aspiration of gastric contents is suspected, the pH of the aspirate must be measured. Solid particles must be removed under bronchoscopic visualization. Tracheal lavage with small amounts of physiologic saline solution is followed by suction. The patient must be hospitalized for continuous observation and intensive care.

Duffy evaluated 93 young females undergoing pelvic laparoscopy for evidence of gastric regurgitation into the pharynx.[5] All patients received general halothane anesthesia. The trachea was intubated with a 7.5 mm cuffed tube which was subsequently inflated. All subjects underwent the laparoscopic procedure in the lithotomy position with steep head down tilt. At the end of the procedure, laryngoscopy was performed. Fluid was aspirated with a syringe and analyzed by a pH electrode.

Two of the 93 women studied showed evidence of regurgitation by fluid pooling in the pharynx. In one, 12 ml of fluid with a pH of 2.3 was found. The other patient revealed a bile stained 3 ml pool with a pH of 8.05. None of these patients had a history of peptic ulceration or indigestion.

Carlsson and Islander studied the incidence of gastric regurgitation in 138 women undergoing gynecologic surgery.[2] Subjects were divided into two groups: elective and emergency operations, respectively. At the conclusion of the surgical procedure, the mouth and pharynx were inspected by laryngoscopy and suctioned before extubation.

Suctioning of the pharynx yielded a small amount (less than 2 ml) of fluid in most patients. None of the 56 women who had an elective laparoscopy revealed evidence of gastric regurgitation. The pH of the pharyngeal fluid measured 5.7 ± 0.7. By contrast, 7 of the 35 patients (20 percent) subjected to emergency laparoscopy had pharyngeal contents with pH of 3.0 or less. When compared with other types of operations, emergency laparoscopy was associated with a high risk of silent regurgitation.

Unlike vomiting, which is readily apparent, regurgitation can be slow and silent. During laparoscopy, in addition to the mechanical causes that predispose to regurgitation (Trendelenburg position, increased intra-abdominal pressure), there are pharmacological factors. Patients receiving atropine and hyoscine have diminished lower esophageal sphincter tone. This, in turn, increases the propensity for stress reflux of gastric contents.

Women with a history of incompetent cardiac sphincter are also at a greater risk of gastric reflux. O'Mullane demonstrated that the esophagus in these subjects can retain large volumes of material.[9] Utilization of the Trendelenburg position in combination with muscle relaxant drugs predisposes these patients to regurgitation.

Acute Hypotension

A significant drop in blood pressure (acute hypotension) can occur during gas insufflation to create or maintain the pneumoperitoneum. The acute decline in peripheral blood pressure may lead to a shock-like state. This may even cause cardiac arrest, as reported by Arthure.[1]

Several conditions may produce acute hypotension during laparoscopy. These include: (a) cardiac arrhythmia due to hypercarbia; (b) hypertonic vagal reflex; (c) severe hemorrhage; (d) gas embolism; and (e) compression of the inferior vena cava by excessive intraperitoneal pressure.

Seed et al first reported tachycardia and acute hypotension in a patient whose intra-abdominal pressure rose above 40 mm Hg.[10] They attributed the fall in blood pressure to compression of the inferior vena cava and a decrease in venous return. Recovery was immediate following decompression of the abdomen by evacuation of the insufflated carbon dioxide. As a consequence, they recommended that the intraperitoneal pressure should not be allowed to increase beyond 20 mm Hg.

Patients who present for laparoscopy with decreased blood volume are at increased risk of developing acute hypotension during creation of the pneumoperitoneum. This includes women with established hemoperitoneum or excessive external hemorrhage. In these situations, the operator may have to limit the intraperitoneal pressure to no more than 16 mm Hg.

If acute hypotension occurs, the operator must discontinue the intraperitoneal insufflation of gas at once. Simultaneously, the gas already within the peritoneal cavity must be evacuated. This has to be accomplished irrespective of the amount of gas delivered into the abdominal cavity. The procedure may resume as usual once the blood pressure has returned to normal values.

Lee reported an episode of acute hypotension in a young woman following the insufflation of only 3 L of carbon dioxide.[7] The pressure registered by the insufflator's manometer had reached 40 mm Hg. Blood pressure returned to normal within seconds after evacuation of the intraperitoneal gas. No evidence of bradycardia or cardiac arrhythmia was present, thus making compression of the inferior vena cava the most likely cause of the hypotensive episode.

Acute hypotension secondary to excessive intraperitoneal pressure is a preventable accident. The laparoscopist must keep the intra-abdominal pressure under close surveillance. During the visual exploration of the pelvis, the assistant or nurse should assess the intra-abdominal pressure and report any elevation above 20 mm Hg to the surgeon. The anesthetist should also check the intraperitoneal pressure at regular intervals.

At times, the need to reduce the illumination in the operating room prevents constant visualization of the insufflator. This is dangerous and avoidable. A source of illumination must be maintained at all times during the procedure. This can be accomplished by dimming the lights in the room (instead of turning them off completely) or by turning on an auxiliary light source (such as the roentgenographic light box present in every operating suite). The practice of illuminating the insufflator's dials intermittently with a flash light is only mentioned to be condemned.

Pulmonary Complications

Pulmonary complications associated with laparoscopy are rare. Nevertheless, their sudden unexpected appearance and seriousness deserve description. Prompt diagnosis and treatment may prevent devastating sequelae.

Desai et al reported the appearance of acute pulmonary edema in a young woman undergoing a diagnostic laparoscopy.[3] Following the insufflation of between 1 and 2 L of carbon dioxide to create a pneumoperitoneum, tachycardia and hypotension ensued. This was accompanied by copious amounts of pink frothy secretions recovered through the endotracheal tube. The sudden appearance of acute pulmonary edema shortly after the onset of insufflation of carbon dioxide suggests the possibility of gas embolization (see Chapter 15).

Other factors that are known to be capable of precipitating acute pulmonary edema include: (a) extreme Trendelenburg position; (b) elevated central venous pressure; and (c) narcotics. All of them are commonly encountered during laparoscopy.

The appearance of unilateral or bilateral pneumothorax during laparoscopy has also been reported.[4] In the absence of trauma to the diaphragm, it is presumed that gas enters the pleural space through a congenital diaphragmatic defect. If previously undiagnosed, such malformations become evident as a result of the increased intra-abdominal pressure. The appearance of pneumothorax complicating laparoscopy is not limited to procedures performed under general anesthesia. It may also occur during laparoscopies done with local or regional anesthesia.

REGIONAL ANESTHESIA

Refinements in technique and better patient selection practices have made regional anesthesia increasingly acceptable for laparoscopy. However, these methods are not free of complications. Resulting problems can be divided into those that are intraoperative in nature and those that occur postoperatively.

Intraoperative complications of regional anesthesia include high or total spinal block and adverse reactions to the local anesthetic agent. Both of these conditions appear prior to the initiation of the laparoscopy and usually lead to postponement of the procedure. Postoperative complications of regional anesthesia include headache, backache, bladder dysfunction, and neural complications. These adopt particular significance for the laparoscopist because he or she will be contacted first by the affected patient. Early recognition prompts appropriate therapy or referral as required.

Headache

Headache following a regional anesthesia is the most common complaint expressed by patients. It may appear following a spinal anesthesia or after inadvertent dural puncture during a peridural attempt. Post puncture headache may appear from 6 to 48 hours after the spinal tap.

The incidence of post spinal headache is affected by the diameter of the needle used (the larger the bore, the higher the incidence). Young women and dehydrated patients are more prone to this complication. The headache is usually of a pounding nature. It is characterized by worsening when the patient moves from the supine to the sitting position. Conversely, it diminishes when the patient lies supine in bed.

Conservative treatment during the first 24 to 48 hours is warranted. This includes bed rest, increased fluid intake, analgesics, and tight support of the abdomen. Most post spinal headaches will subside or disappear within the first 24 to 48 hours.

If conservative means are ineffective, the patient should be hospitalized so that more active measures can be undertaken. The latter include saline injection into the epidural space or the use of an autologous blood patch. Both of these therapeutic modalities are carried out in close collaboration with the anesthetist.

Backache

Backache secondary to periosteal or ligamentous trauma from the needle insertion is not uncommon. This entity can be treated symptomatically. It is self limited and diminishes over a period of days.

Bladder Dysfunction

Bladder dysfuntion may complicate recovery from regional anesthesia. Absent the urge to void, the bladder can accumulate large amounts of urine. Bladder distention can cause severe abdominal pain. This is compounded by the increased administration of intravenous solutions for hydration purposes routinely administered before and during regional anesthesia.

Bladder function returns as the regional anesthesia wears off. On occasion, patients may have urinary retention for up to 24 hours following surgery. Intermittent urethral catheterization is indicated until spontaneous voiding occurs. Patients ought not to be discharged from the facility until bladder function is fully recovered.

Neural Complications

Trauma to a nerve root during insertion of a spinal or epidural needle is rare, but it does occur. Mild pain at the time of needle insertion is not uncommon. Severe sharp pain must be interpreted cautiously. Persistent pain postoperatively requires immediate neurologic evaluation.

Another rare but potentially serious complication of regional anesthesia is the formation of an epidural hematoma. Pain radiating to the back or lower limbs results as a consequence of compression of the spinal contents by the hematoma. Persistent weakness of the lower limbs can also be the presenting sign. Early surgical decompression may reduce the incidence of permanent neurologic disability.

LOCAL ANESTHESIA

Selection of local anesthesia for laparoscopy was previously described (see Chapter 8). Although it is generally believed that local anesthesia offers distinct advantages with few limitations, it is not completely free of complications. These may range from minor side effects to life-threatening conditions due to toxicity of the drugs used.

Laparoscopic sterilizations performed under local anesthesia require multiple site instillations. Paracervical block is needed for placing a cervical tenaculum and uterine mobilizer. Infiltration of the abdominal wall may be at a single site for an operative laparoscope or at two if a suprapubic accessory puncture is utilized. Additionally, the anesthetic is usually applied directly to the fallopian tubes. Because local anesthetic drugs are absorbed into the blood stream from all the aforementioned sites, their blood concentration may reach toxic levels.

Side Effects

Lidocaine and bupivacaine are most frequently used as local anesthetics for laparoscopy. Both are amide-type drugs. Bupivacaine is more potent than lidocaine but it is proportionally more toxic. Qualitatively, their side effects are similar.

Adverse reactions are usually associated with excessive plasma levels of these medications. Elevated blood concentration can be due to excessive dosage, rapid absorption, or intravascular injection, the latter being the most common. Accurate determination of the amount of local anesthetic required to cause these side effects has not been established. Instead, manufacturers provide maximum recommended dosages. Such recommendations may be misleading because they are based on tissue infiltration followed by the average absorption rate for a particular medication. They do not take into account inadvertent intravascular administration of part or all of the instilled amount.

For lidocaine used with epinephrine (which purportedly prolongs its effects by delaying its absorption), the maximum recommended dose is 500 mg for an average size individual. It should not exceed 7 mg per kilogram (3.2 mg per pound) in any given patient. When lidocaine is used without epinephrine, the total dose should be kept below 300 mg or not more than 4.5 mg per kilogram (2.0 mg per pound) of body weight.

The rate of absorption of local anesthetics is dependent upon the concentration and total dose of drug administered. Once absorbed, they are evenly distributed. As a result, high concentrations can be found in highly perfused tissues such as brain and myocardium.

Spielman et al recommends the use of 2-chloroprocaine for periumbilical analgesia.[11] Because it is an esther-type anesthetic that is metabolized by pseudocholinesterase, it does not have additive toxic effects with lidocaine or bupivacaine. This allows the use of larger amounts of these drugs for tubal analgesia.

Side effects due to elevated blood concentration of drug can be classified according to their manifestations. Central nervous system reactions include feeling of generalized warmth, chills, nausea, vomiting, dizziness, blurred vision, ringing in the ears, and numbness of the tongue. Evaluation of a patient experiencing these symptoms consists of repeated observations of vital signs (cardiovascular and respiratory) at frequent intervals. If the patient is breathing spontaneously, expectant management is acceptable. Supportive ventilation with oxygen by mask may be beneficial.

Toxic Effects

Toxic effects are the progression of side effects to the point of placing the patient's life in danger. Anxiety, which advances to the stage of restlessness, is worrisome. The appearance of tremors or localized twitching may be premonitory of generalized convulsions. Unconsciousness may ensue.

Treatment varies according to the type and severity of toxic reactions. When anxiety, localized twitching, or tremor are diagnosed, intravenous administration of diazepam 2 mg can be given slowly. Caution must be exercised since respiratory depression is a side effect of excessive diazepam injection. Establishment and maintenance of a patent airway is essential. Assisted or controlled ventilation with 100 percent oxygen may prevent the appearance of convulsions.

Simultaneously, with the administration of first aid, specialized assistance must be summoned. Further aggravation of the patient's condition may necessitate endotracheal intubation and controlled ventilation.

If convulsions have developed, muscle relaxants should be administered. Intravenous succinylcholine (50 to 100 mg) paralyzes the patient without additional central nervous or cardiovascular depression. The administration of intravenous thiopental or additional diazepam will permit controlled ventilation to be instituted.

Elevated blood concentrations of these amide-type anesthetics cause respiratory depression. Progression to respiratory arrest may cause death by asphyxia. Controlled ventilation must be instituted at once.

High intravascular concentrations of local anesthetics produce myocardial depression. Diminished cardiac output, bradycardia, hypotension, and ventricular arrhythmias (including fibrillation) may lead to cardiac arrest. Cardiopulmonary resuscitation has to be instituted immediately. Resuscitative equipment and personnel must be available whenever local anesthesia for laparoscopy is being used. Appropriate anesthesiologic back up is essential to ensure the patient's safety.

References

1. Arthure H. Laparoscopy hazard. Br Med J 1970; 4:492-493.
2. Carlsson C, Islander G. Silent gastrointestinal regurgitation during anesthesia. Anesth Analg 1981; 60:655-657.

3. Desai S, Roaf E, Liu P. Acute pulmonary edema during laparoscopy. Anesth Analg 1982; 61:699-700.
4. Doctor HN, Hussain Z. Bilateral pneumothorax associated with laparoscopy: A case report of a rare hazard and a review of the literature. Anaesthesiology 1973; 28:75-81.
5. Duffy BL. Regurgitation during pelvic laparoscopy. Br J Anaesth 1979; 51:1089-1090.
6. Heinonen J, Takki S, Tammisto T. Effect of the Trendelenburg tilt and other procedures on the position of endotracheal tubes. Lancet 1969; 1:850-853.
7. Lee CM. Acute hypotension during laparoscopy: A case report. Anesth Analg 1975; 54:142-143.
8. Mendelsohn CL. The aspiration of stomach contents into the lungs during obstetrical anesthesia. Am J Obstet Gynecol 1946; 52:191-205.
9. O'Mullane EJ. Vomiting and regurgitation during anesthesia. Lancet 1954; 1:1209-1212.
10. Seed RF, Shakespeare TF, Muldoon MJ. Carbon dioxide homeostasis during anaesthesia for laparoscopy. Anaesthesiology 1970; 25:223-231.
11. Spielman FJ, Hulka JF, Ostheimer GW, Mueller RA. Pharmacokinetics and pharmacodynamics of local analgesia for laparoscopic tubal ligation. Am J Obstet Gynecol 1983; 146:821-824.

15 COMPLICATIONS OF PNEUMOPERITONEUM

Common to all laparoscopic techniques is the production of an adequate pneumoperitoneum. Insufflation of the distending gas into an area other than into the peritoneal cavity not only is a common cause of procedural failure, but also may be the origin of serious morbidity and mortality. To ensure that the inflating gas is injected into the proper location, several safety checks are prescribed. Some are more safe than others, but all are associated with some degree of error. In the case of misapplication, identification and correction of a faulty technique is paramount for preventing more dangerous complications.

On diagnosing any abnormality at this stage of the procedure, the surgeon must discontinue the process and reevaluate the situation. The use of alternative methods to accomplish the original surgical objectives should be entertained. This is necessary even if it entails cancelling the laparoscopic procedure in order to assure safety and to avoid iatrogenic morbidity.

INSUFFLATING NEEDLE COMPLICATIONS

Although any fine trocar or paracentesis needle can be used to insufflate the distending gas for a pneumoperitoneum, the spring-loaded Verres type needle has gained universal acceptance for this purpose. The error that results in the formation of an extraperitoneal gas chamber is almost always due to improper placement of the tip of the Verres needle. Diverse maneuvers and checks have been described to ensure proper positioning of the insufflating device (see Chapter 2). Some are more successful than others, and some can cause unexpected morbidity. Tests utilizing a 360° circular motion and Cohen's suggestion to move the needle back and forth to ensure that the needle is in a free space are both capable of transforming a minimal injury into a serious one[3].

Perforation of the muscular wall of a medium sized artery by a small Verres needle (1.7 mm diameter) need not produce serious hemorrhage. This type of perforation is a common occurrence in transarterial catheterization; it is not generally associated with major complications and can be expected to heal spontaneously. If the tip of the insufflating needle cannot be verified to be intravascular in location, any motion of the needle serves only to enlarge the original perforation site, thereby transforming a simple puncture injury into a traumatic laceration of the vessel wall. The sweeping circular motion safety check may cause laceration of periumbilical adhesions between the bowel or the omentum and the parietal peritoneum periumbilically (Figures 15.1 to 15.3). This has the paradoxical effect of creating a complication while attempting to prevent one.

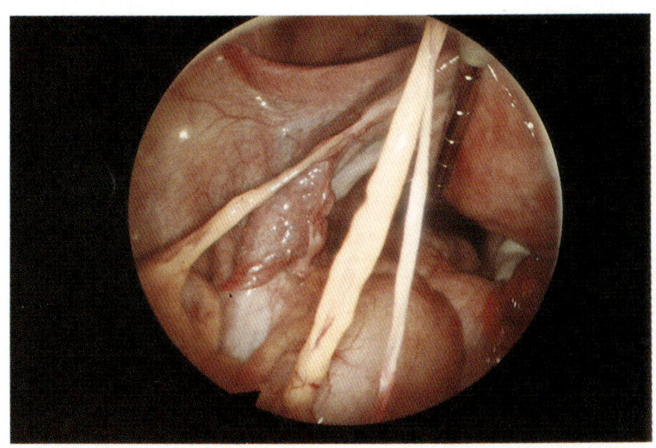

Figure 15.1 Intra-abdominal adhesions. Adhesive bands between bowel and the posterior aspect of the anterior abdominal wall and lateral pelvic wall are depicted. These adhesions are not visible to the operator during the formation of pneumoperitoneum.

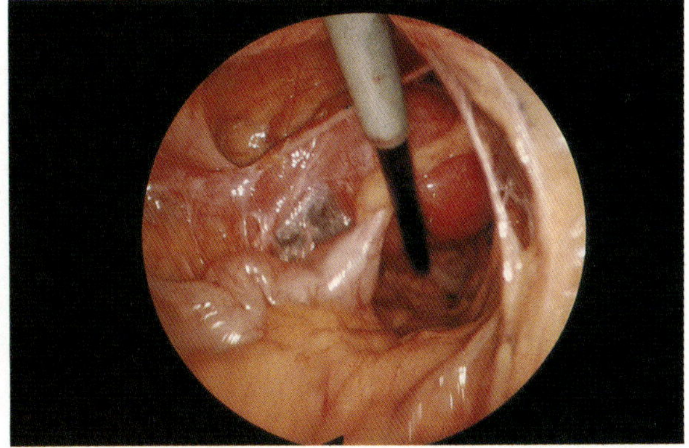

Figure 15.2 Periumbilical adhesions. Insertion of the Verres needle may pierce or narrowly miss the midline adhesion. Circular or sweeping motions of the needle may iatrogenically create trauma.

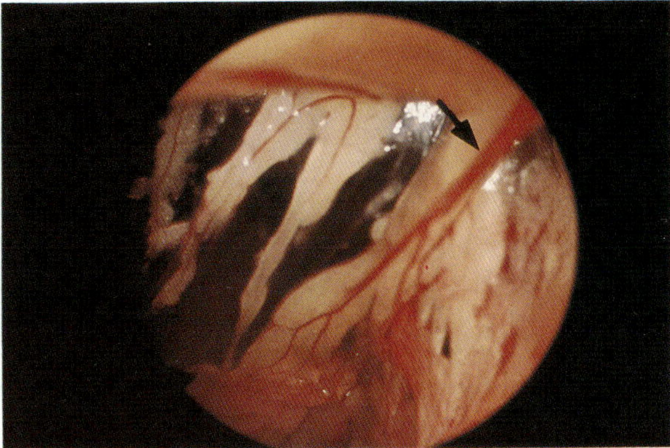

Figure 15.3 Omental adhesion to the parietal peritoneum. Large omental vessel (arrow) is susceptible to trauma during insertion of the Verres needle. When adhesions are found, visual exploration to verify the integrity of the omental vasculature is indicated.

The experienced laparoscopist customarily uses a combination of several methods to ensure the proper location of the Verres needle tip. If an abnormality is encountered in any of the safety checks prompt reevaluation of the entire insufflation process is necessary. In Chapter 2, the usual pneumoperitoneum technique was described. In this section, the safety signs and their derangements are enumerated and discussed.

Insufflating Pressure

As the peritoneal cavity is entered intra-abdominal pressure should be low (less than 6 mm Hg). Gas insufflation is begun at the rate of 1 L per minute. This usually increases the pressure to 10 to 12 mm Hg. Although a low entering pressure does not guarantee intraperitoneal insufflation (bladder and bowel are also low pressure compartments), a pressure greater than 16 to 20 mm Hg is a sure sign that gas has entered a closed space which is not easily distensible. The degree of elasticity of the tissue being expanded is inversely proportional to the pressure elevation.

One should be cautious about interpreting the pressure during insufflation, especially during administration of the first 100 cc of gas. The pressure is often elevated at first until the bowel and the omentum separate from the parietal peritoneum. This occurs because the peritoneal cavity is collapsed as a virtual cavity with all surfaces in close apposition. After the initial 100 cc volume is insufflated, a quick fall in pressure should become apparent.

An additional source of high pressure measurement is the lateral location of the distal opening of the Verres needle. If the aperture of the needle lies against the parietal peritoneum, there is increased resistance to the flow of gas; this is reflected in an elevated pressure reading. Rotating the needle 180° along its own axis dislocates the needle opening away from the adjacent peritoneum and results in an immediate drop in pressure. The Verres needle could be modified to have two lateral apertures to avoid this problem; however, the modification has yet to be implemented.

Periodic fluctuations in intraperitoneal pressure with inspiration and expiration are due to diaphragmatic motion. Once believed to be a sign of correct intraperitoneal insufflation of gas, this interpretation is now known to be erroneous. It is often a misleading index in cases with extraperitoneal injection of gas. On inspiration, the intra-abdominal pressure always increases with the downward movement of the diaphragm. In turn this pressure is uniformly transmitted to contiguous tissues. Thus, one can see quite typical respiratory pressure patterns even if the gas collection is located preperitoneally or even subcutaneously.

Liver Dullness

As gas enters the peritoneal cavity, it diffuses in all directions. It sequesters preferentially in the subphrenic space because of the lower pressure in the subdiaphragmatic area. The accumulation of distending gas under the right hemidiaphragm displaces the liver caudally. This creates a pocket of gas which has a tympanitic characteristic to percussion (see Chapter 2). If dullness to liver percussion fails to disappear, one should be alerted. Absence of tympany is the most accurate sign that the insufflating gas is not intraperitoneal in location.

Aspiration of Injected Saline

By far the most important safety check involves the recovery of fluid injected intraperitoneally. A medium sized syringe with approximately 5 to 10 cc normal saline solution is attached to the Luer-Lok connector at the proximal end of the Verres needle. The fluid is injected into the peritoneal cavity (see Chapter 2). While injecting, one should evaluate subjectively the necessary pressure. After the saline has been injected, an attempt is made to reaspirate the fluid. This may result in the retrieval of (a) no fluid, (b) a small amount of saline, (c) blood, (d) bowel content, or (e) urine.

No Fluid. When the tip of the Verres needle is in the peritoneal cavity, the injected saline may become dispersed between loops of bowel. If one is unable to recover any saline, proper positioning of the insufflating needle is suggested. Gentle aspiration avoids injuring any organ that may be sucked in against the sharp end of the Verres needle.

Small Amount of Saline. Recovery of any amount of saline confirms that the fluid has been injected into a closed space or a newly created space (namely, a fluid collection) within the confines of the abdominal wall. The appropriate corrective measures to undertake at this point are removal and reinsertion of the Verres needle. The saline solution injection-aspiration test should be repeated whenever the tip of the Verres needle is moved to a new position.

Blood. If blood is retrieved through the Verres needle, it indicates either that there is free blood in the peritoneal cavity or that the tip of the needle has entered the lumen of a blood vessel. Under no circumstances should gas be insufflated before a correct diagnosis is made. In the case of hemoperitoneum, it may be appropriate, depending on its degree, to bypass the laparoscopic procedure completely and proceed directly with a laparotomy to deal with the underlying disorder. In the case of a vascular injury, corrective measures must be undertaken immediately (see Chapter 17).

Bowel Content. Aspiration of intestinal fluid suggests injury to the intestinal tract (Figure 15.4). If an accidental puncture of the small or large intestine occurs with the Verres needle, the needle is removed. A new Verres needle is then reinserted and the laparoscopy is carried out in the usual manner. Upon entering the peritoneal cavity, one should attempt to identify and evaluate the site of the injury. If such identification is not possible, close observation for 24 hours is indicated in order to watch for and rule out the development of peritonitis. In most cases, simple puncture of the intestinal tract heals spontaneously without complications.

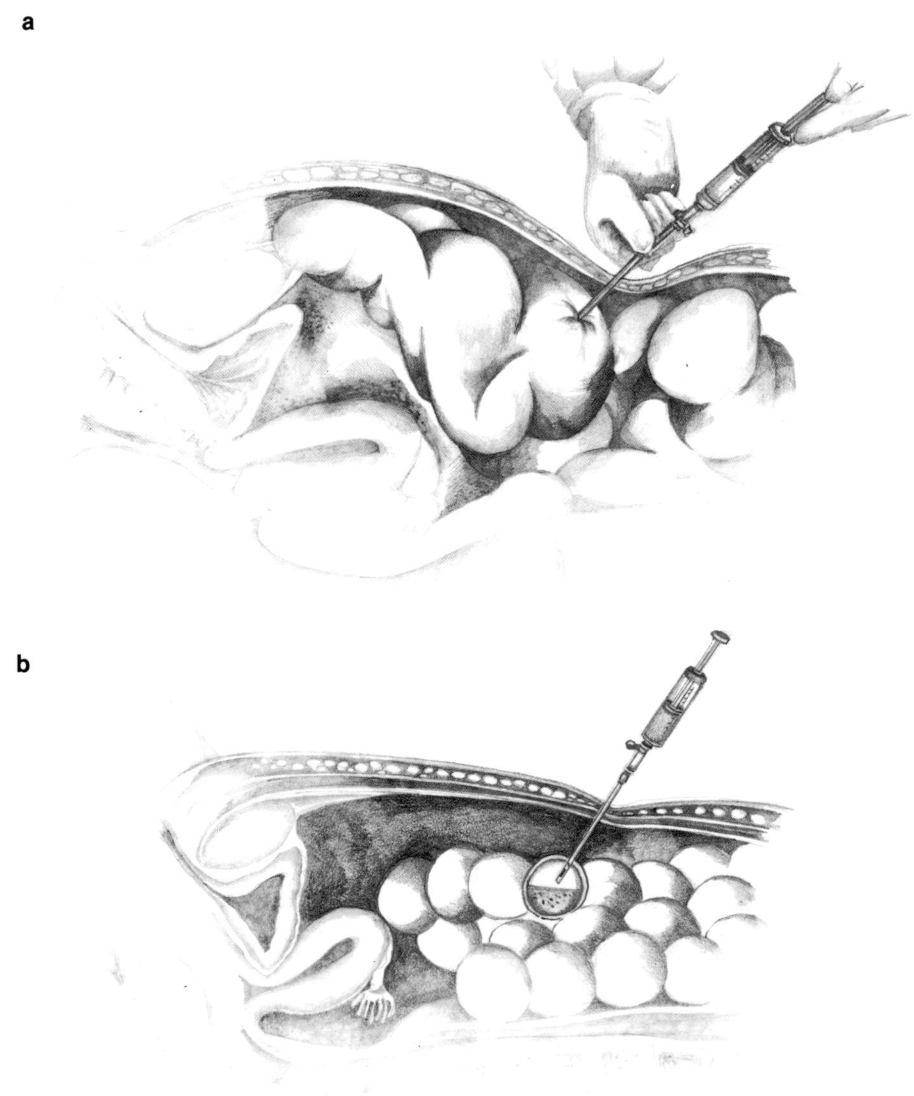

Figure 15.4 Bowel perforation with Verres needle. *a*. Saline aspiration test may yield intestinal fluid. *b*. Aspiration may retrieve gas with a foul smelling odor. Under normal conditions no gas or fluid can be aspirated into the syringe.

Urine. When urine is aspirated through the Verres needle, the needle is usually withdrawn and reinserted. Puncture of the bladder wall is generally well tolerated, and ordinarily heals spontaneously. The laparoscopy then proceeds in the normal fashion. If urinary leakage into tissues is believed to be a possible result of bladder injury, constant bladder drainage for 48 to 72 hours may help prevent major complications.

It has been suggested that the needle be left in place in the case of bowel or bladder perforation. The site is thereby marked for clear identification and later assessment. A second site is chosen for an accessory needle. However, this approach may not be advantageous. The manipulations required to proceed with the laparoscopy while the primary perforating needle is in place may further complicate the case by transforming a simple puncture into a laceration.

Dingfelder felt one could reduce the incidence of complications associated with needle-induced pneumoperitoneum by omitting this step prior to inserting the laparoscopic trocar.[5] He claimed a reduced risk from trocar insertion by avoiding a tense, overdistended abdomen. Injury to retroperitoneal vessels was much less likely to occur if the trocar were advanced through a relaxed abdominal wall because it was so much easier to elevate. Copeland et al evaluated this technique and found it to be useful in most cases.[4] Exceptions included (1) patients who had had previous abdominal surgery, (2) thin athletic nulliparous women, and (3) those in whom direct entry failed after one or two attempts.

In our institution, establishing a pneumoperitoneum prior to sharp trocar insertion is regarded as an integral aspect of a successful laparoscopic procedure. Strict adherence to proper technique reduces the frequency of complications and minimizes their seriousness. However, one cannot eliminate all complications arising from this part of the technique.

TENSION PNEUMOPERITONEUM

A common preventable complication of a laparoscopy is creation of a tension pneumoperitoneum. The inordinate rise in intraperitoneal pressure is the result of excessive insufflation of gas used to distend the peritoneal cavity. In extremely obese patients, the degree of pneumoperitoneum may be masked by the thick adipose layer. A much more common cause of increased intraperitoneal pressure is brought about by continuing to insufflate the distending gas beyond that which is reasonably necessary to carry out the procedure. As described in Chapters 9 and 10, adverse circulatory and respiratory effects are rare if the intraperitoneal pressure is maintained below 20 mm Hg.

In tension pneumoperitoneum the abdomen is ballooned out, barrel-shaped, and tympanitic in all areas. Subjective evaluation of the intra-abdominal tension reveals a hard abdominal wall that is not easily indentable. If the patient is awake, she experiences a gradually increasing difficulty in breathing. This occurs from limitation of the diaphragmatic excursion. The rapid distention and stretching of the peritoneal surface causes pain which further aggravates the respiratory embarrassment created by the increased subdiaphragmatic pressure.

In patients undergoing a laparoscopic procedure under general anesthesia, the diagnosis of tension pneumoperitoneum is technical rather than clinical. Initially, the anesthesiologist notices increased resistance to inspiratory effort on the manual or automatic ventilator. The degree of pressure required to expand the lungs is directly related to the limitation of diaphragmatic excursion created by the rise in intraperitoneal pressure. The increased pressure required to maintain an adequate ventilatory volume is by far the most sensitive index of excessive peritoneal gas insufflation.

Normally, the insufflator dispenses 1 L per minute of the distending gas. The rate can be assessed by a flowmeter with a floating ball which signals the rate of gas flow. An increase in intraperitoneal pressure enhances the resistance in the gas line and results in reduced gas flow. The decrease in the flow of gas lowers the level of the floating ball in the flowmeter.

An additional factor to be considered is the total amount of gas insufflated as measured by the insufflator. Albeit important, it is not as reliable a marker of increased intraperitoneal pressure as is the measurement of intraperitoneal pressure. It provides a measurement of the volume of gas dispensed, but any gas leakage along the gas line gives a false impression of the total amount actually insufflated.

Measurement of a large elevation in the intra-abdominal pressure has to be evaluated carefully. As previously described, the flow of gas should be discontinued when obtaining the intraperitoneal pressure. This is necessary in order to eliminate the flow component of the equation, $P = F \times R$, where P is pressure, F is flow, and R is resistance. The size of the laparoscopic trocar is a factor in this regard. Removal of the laparoscope while evaluating the intraperitoneal pressure also affects the accuracy of the measurement. Whereas intra-abdominal pressure recording is not completely accurate, any abnormality must be thoroughly evaluated before the procedure is continued.

To avoid high intraperitoneal pressure, one should switch from constant insufflation of the distending gas at 1 liter per minute (manual control setting) to replacement insufflation (automatic control) after an adequate pneumoperitoneum has been established. By using the automatic feature, with which most mechanical insufflators are equipped, the surgeon sets a level of intra-abdominal pressure to be maintained (usually 14 to 18 mm Hg). Thereafter, only sufficient gas to replace that lost is insufflated. Newer insufflators have a safety valve that cuts off the flow of gas when a preset pressure is reached. When utilizing an insufflator, which does not possess this safety feature, the surgeon, anesthesiologist, and circulating nurse must check the intra-abdominal pressure readings at regular intervals. The surgeon concentrating on the endoscopy in a darkened room with the insufflator dials out of his view may not realize that the pressure is excessive. Therefore, it is essential for the whole operating team to be aware of the need for frequent checks. Thus, the surgeon can be alerted of any undesirable rise in intraperitoneal pressure.

SUBCUTANEOUS EMPHYSEMA

Extraperitoneal insufflation of the distending gas (carbon dioxide or nitrous oxide) can occur at any depth in the anterior abdominal wall as well as retroperitoneally. These sites of gas collection create both undesirable morbidity and technical problems. These may force the procedure to be terminated without accomplishing any of its original goals. Each abnormal location at which the gas could be insufflated has its own particular set of potentially complicating factors. In this section, the mechanism by which subcutaneous emphysema is created will be detailed along with discussions about its dispersion, prevention, and management.

Failure of the insufflating needle to penetrate the rectus fascia results in a prefascial gas collection known as subcutaneous emphysema (Figure 15.5). Early recognition of the abnormal location of the insufflating tip is enhanced by the maneuvers discussed earlier in this chapter and in Chapter 2. A distinctive sign of subcutaneous accumulation of gas is the sensation of crepitation obtained by palpating the abdominal wall. In extreme situations when the amount of gas is excessive, the distending medium extends along paths of least resistance, thereby dissecting its way in all directions within the subcutaneous adipose tissue layer. The continuity of the subcutaneous suprafascial adipose tissue layer allows the gas to extend downward into the vulvar area, thus creating emphysematous distention of the mons veneris or upward to reach as high as the loose areolar tissue of the neck.

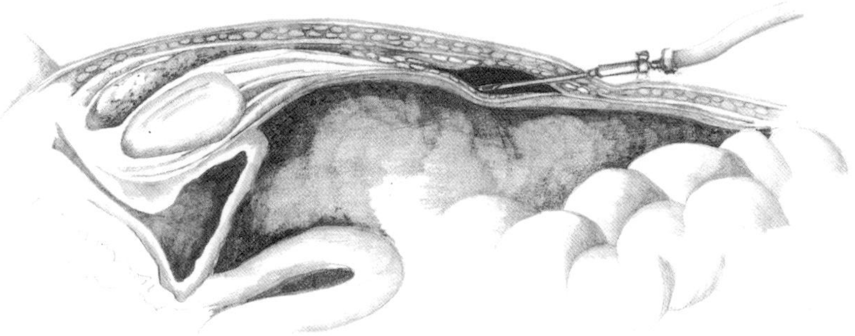

Figure 15.5 Subcutaneous emphysema. Verres needle failed to traverse the fascial layer. Rapid increase in insufflation pressure and crepitation on palpation of the abdominal wall are distinctive signs.

Although the subcutaneous areolar tissue is usually loosely constituted, one always finds a mild to moderate elevation of the insufflating pressure when it is distended by gas. Failure to obtain tympanitic percussion in the right subcostal area (the expected loss of liver dullness to percussion) is strong evidence that the insufflating gas is extraperitoneal in location. If one recognizes that the needle tip is in an improper site, after a small amount of distending gas is injected into the prefascial subcutaneous layer, one can remove and reinsert the needle, perhaps changing the angle of introduction. The gas already insufflated is rapidly reabsorbed without interfering with the operation.

If the error is not identified until a large volume of gas has been introduced subcutaneously, disconnection of the gas tubing from the needle, without moving it, permits most of the gas to escape. The procedure can then be restarted. A similar maneuver can be performed if the diagnosis is made visually through the laparoscope. Disconnecting the insufflating tube and withdrawing the laparoscope from its trocar sheath allows exsufflation of the accumulated gas.

Despite the rapid reabsorptive properties of carbon dioxide, every attempt should be made to aspirate the misplaced gas. Reduction of a major subcutaneous emphysema diminishes the degree of discomfort the patient experiences during the postoperative period. Strict adherence to the aforementioned safety checks ensures the intraperitoneal location of the insufflating needle and averts subcutaneous emphysema. Early identification of the developing gas collection limits its extent in the event the preventive maneuvers fail.

EXTRAPERITONEAL INSUFFLATION

Insufflation of gas outside the peritoneal cavity, but below the rectus fascia layer can create preperitoneal emphysema (Figure 15.6). Unlike subcutaneous emphysema, this condition is less likely to be identified prior to the insertion of the laparoscopic trocar. Preperitoneal emphysema creates greater technical problems that are more difficult to overcome and that are not easily managed once they occur.[1]

The extraperitoneal location of the Verres needle tip is thought to be produced by the following mechanism: as the sharp outer trocar perforates the fascia, the blunt inner needle pops up to protrude ahead of the sharp point of the outer sheath. The blunt inner needle tip then pushes the peritoneum away instead of piercing it. Another factor abetting misplacement of the Verres needle is the practice of using skin clamps (of the towel clip type) to elevate the abdominal wall during needle insertion. When one elevates the skin and subcutaneous tissue by this technique, the peritoneum is not elevated in similar fashion. One actually elongates the path that the needle has to traverse, thus increasing the risk of improper preperitoneal needle placement. The only means for identifying the erroneous placement of the needle tip is recovery of injected saline (discussed earlier in this chapter).

High insufflating pressures are not seen because the resistance encountered by the dissecting gas is not much different from that of the peritoneal cavity. Moreover, a tympanitic response to transabdominal percussion can often be obtained over the newly formed gas chamber. If the full volume of gas (equivalent to that for pneumoperitoneum) is insufflated preperitoneally, the peritoneum is merely displaced (Figure 15.7).

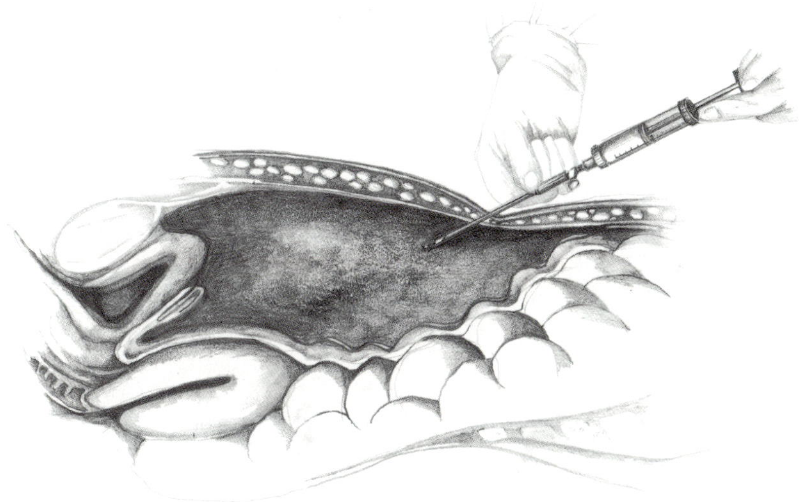

Figure 15.6 Preperitoneal emphysema. Failure to pierce the anterior parietal peritoneum by the blunt inner component of the Verres needle is thought to be the cause. Insufflation pressure may remain within normal levels.

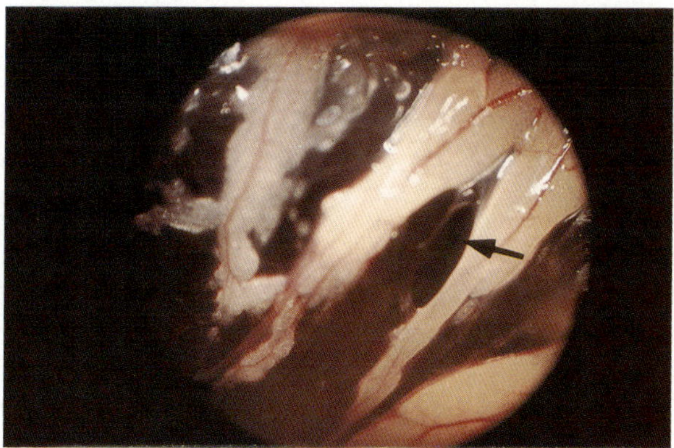

Figure 15.7 Laparoscopic view of preperitoneal emphysema. Bright reflection of the light by the peritoneum is characteristic. Perforation created by the sharp outer sleeve of the Verres needle can sometimes be identified (arrow).

The diagnosis of preperitoneal emphysema is usually made through the laparoscope (Figures 15.8 to 15.10). Once diagnosed, a secondary transcutaneous sharp aspirating needle should be inserted (an 18-gauge spinal needle is adequate) at a nearby location (Figures 5.11 and 5.12). Deflation is performed under direct vision. No attempt should be made to pierce the peritoneal layer because of the increased risk of damaging intraperitoneal structures lying beneath it. The operator should also refrain from pressing on the abdominal wall to accelerate the escape of gas. This maneuver results in further lateral and even posterior retroperitoneal extension of the emphysematous collection of gas.

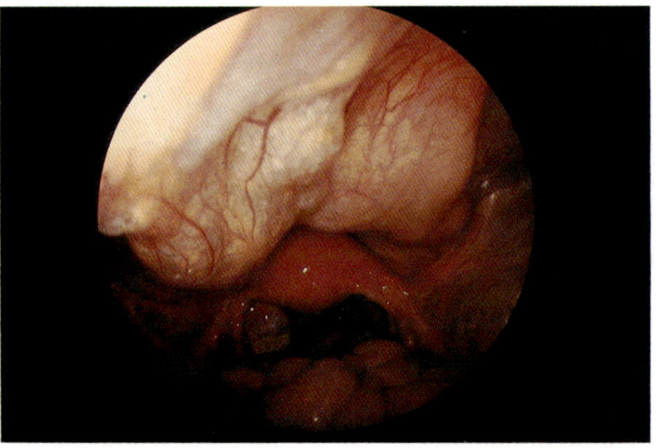

Figure 15.8 Preperitoneal emphysema. Bulging of the detached anterior parietal peritoneum obstructs visualization of the anterior hemipelvis. Uterus is seen at the center of the photograph.

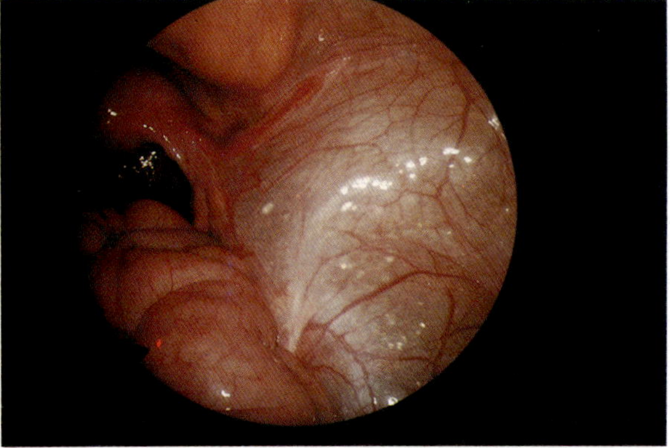

Figure 15.9 Right lateral extension of preperitoneal emphysema. Bullous appearance of gas insufflated into the extraperitoneal subfascial tissue as seen transperitoneally. Separation of the parietal peritoneum is facilitated by its lax preperitoneal areolar tissue attachment.

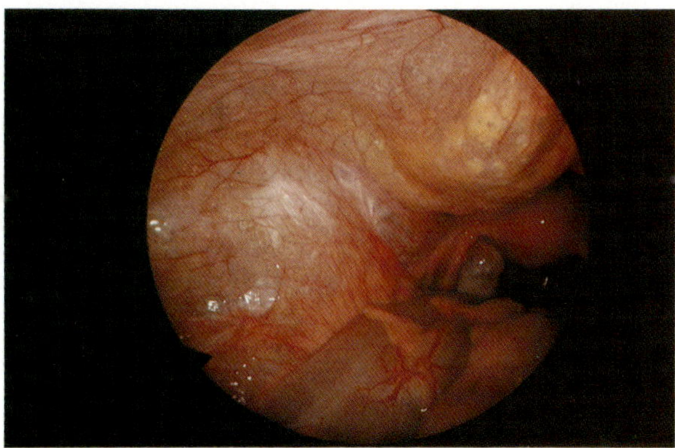

Figure 15.10 Left lateral extension of preperitoneal emphysema. Sigmoid colon is displaced medially by the gaseous dissection of the left posterolateral parietal peritoneum.

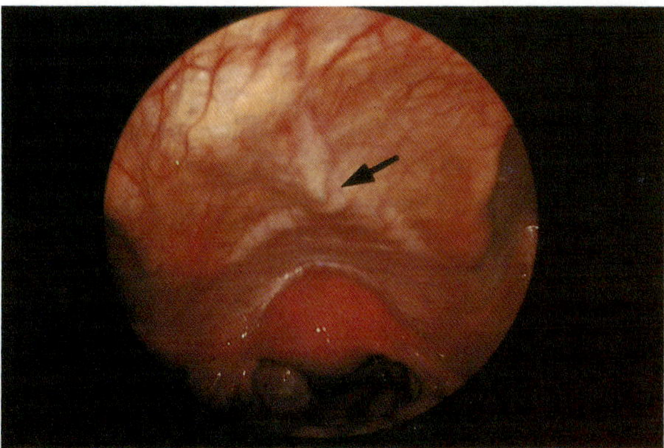

Figure 15.11 Deflation of preperitoneal emphysema. Transcutaneous insertion of a sharp aspirating needle into the gas collection. Needle is left in place extraperitoneally (arrow) during intraperitoneal insufflation.

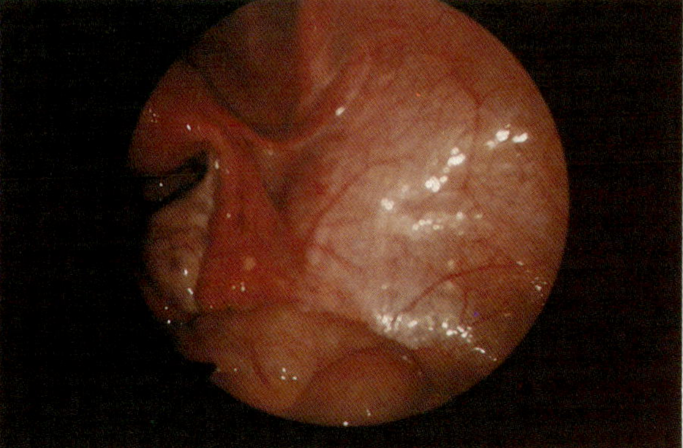

Figure 15.12 Deflated preperitoneal emphysema. Right lateral pelvic wall following escape of preperitoneal accumulation of gas (same case as Figure 15.9). Round and infundibulopelvic ligaments have regained their normal appearance. External iliac vessels can be seen beneath the posterior parietal peritoneum.

Alternative routes can be used to create a pneumoperitoneum in these cases (e.g., by way of the pouch of Douglas or transfundally). Even if a pneumoperitoneum is successfully established, every effort should be made to evacuate the previously created preperitoneal emphysema. This can be accomplished by leaving the laparoscopic trocar sheath in place and by allowing the gradually increasing intraperitoneal pressure to slowly squeeze out the gas.

Caution should be exercised when translaparoscopic surgery is performed in the presence of preperitoneal emphysema. The posterolateral extension of the gas may have advanced the ureters medially (Figure 15.13). This occurs because they are adherent to the posterior parietal peritoneum. When dislocated in this way, the ureters are at increased risk of injury.

Direct retroperitoneal insufflation can occur as a result of inserting the Verres needle too deeply in a thin, low-weight patient (Figure 15.14). This complication is also more likely to occur if insufflation is done by way of a needle inserted through the posterior vaginal fornix. As with other accumulations, if there is only a small gas collection, it is best left undisturbed. Resolution can be expected to occur by spontaneous reabsorption. A large volume of distending gas should be aspirated under direct laparoscopic vision with a sharp 18-gauge aspirating needle.

GAS REABSORPTION, DURATION OF PNEUMOPERITONEUM

Ordinarily, the spontaneous appearance of free gas in the peritoneal cavity is evidence that a hollow viscus has been perforated; prompt operative intervention is indicated. It is common to identify the presence of intraperitoneal air by radiologic study following an abdominal surgical procedure; this includes paracentesis. Its incidence may be as high as 75 to 80 percent. It presents a diagnostic dilemma in cases where postoperative abdominal symptoms require evaluation. Improved diagnostic roentgenography can identify intraperitoneal free air in amounts as small as 1 cc.[2,11]

Because the observation has such obvious clinical relevance, it is important to know how long it takes for any introduced gas to disappear from the peritoneal cavity. The time it persists is proportional to the amount of gas or air left in the abdominal cavity at the conclusion of the procedure. Amounts less than 500 cc are completely reabsorbed by the end of 7 days; volumes up to 1,000 cc may still be detectable for 10 to 12 days. Thin patients tend to retain more air than obese patients after a laparotomy.

Based on extrapolation from the experience reported by urologists who injected carbon dioxide retroperitoneally to delineate the kidney and perirenal structures, postlaparoscopy pneumoperitoneum was once believed to last just a few hours. Gases usually used for gynecologic laparoscopy (specifically carbon dioxide and nitrous oxide) have higher blood solubility indices; this characteristic was thought to enhance clearance from the peritoneal cavity.

Sequential radiographic studies by Lemay et al after laparoscopy showed the volume of residual gas in the abdominal cavity to vary from 25 to 500 ml.[6] The degree and duration of postlaparoscopy discomfort was in direct proportion to the amount of gas remaining in the abdominal cavity at the conclusion of the procedure. Contrary to general belief, almost no reabsorption of gas was seen during the first 24 hours following the operation; 80 percent was absorbed in the second 24-hour period; after 72 hours, no free gas was found in 80 percent of the patients. Some of them still had residual gas as late as the ninth day following the laparoscopy; Lemay et al conjectured this might be room air that entered the abominal cavity during the laparoscopic procedure.

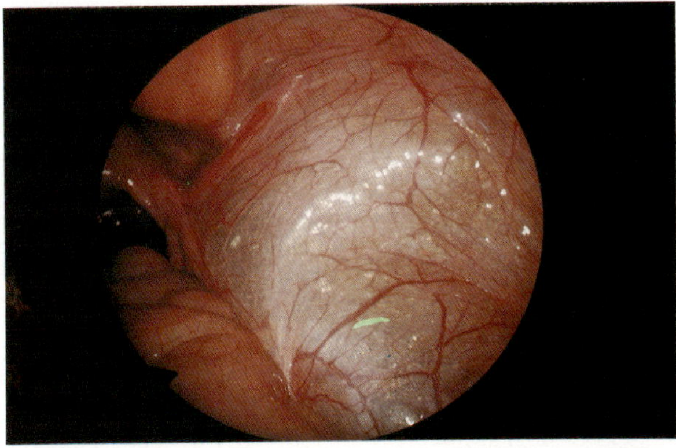

Figure 15.13 Posterolateral extension of preperitoneal emphysema. Apposition of the ureters to the posterior parietal peritoneum advances them medially. Relocation places the ureters at increased risk of inadvertent injury.

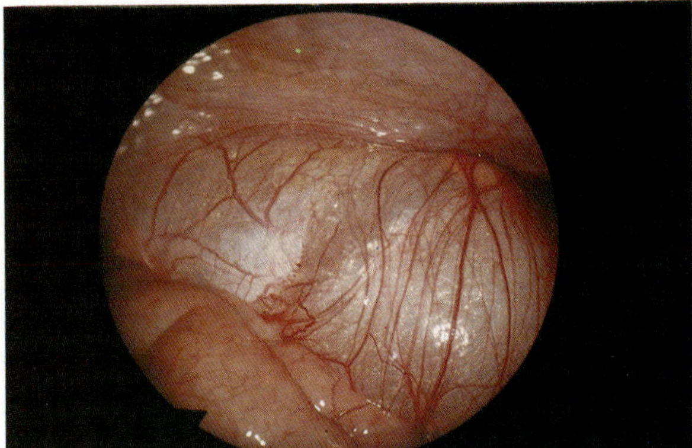

Figure 15.14 Cephalad extension of preperitoneal emphysema. Diminished resistance offered by the preperitoneal areolar tissue facilitates upward dissemination of the insufflated gas. Tympanism heard on percussion of the abdominal wall may mislead the operator.

It seems probable that carbon dioxide is rapidly reabsorbed and cleared from the peritoneal cavity. However, there is always the possibility that some room air has been introduced during insufflation or while other maneuvers are performed. This makes the identification of persistent pneumoperitoneum following laparoscopy an unreliable marker of intra-abdominal disease for at least 4 to 7 days after the procedure. This should not be interpreted to signify that this sign should be ignored, but rather that it has to be taken into account as part of the entire clinical evaluation. As an isolated incidental finding, a persistent pneumoperitoneum does not have the same importance in the postlaparoscopy patient as it would have in other patients after other procedures.

An open laparoscopic type of procedure (using the Hasson cannula, for example) should be considered the same as a laparotomy with respect to the duration of the pneumoperitoneum. Although carbon dioxide or nitrous oxide are used for the insufflation in this method, air enters in large quantities at the time of entering and closing the abdomen. Air is not resorbed at a rate as fast as the gas used to distend the cavity.

GAS EMBOLISM

Gas embolism is a rare but potentially lethal complication of laparoscopy.[14] Its incidence is unknown, but it is likely to be more common than suspected. Minor amounts of gas entering the circulatory system are absorbed and excreted without ever being recognized. Cardiovascular collapse (see p. 257) can develop by diverse mechanisms from a variety of factors including gas embolism. The only absolute criterion to confirm a diagnosis of gas embolism is the identification of intravascular gas bubbles at surgery (by venous catheterization) or at postmortem. With this in mind, the accepted incidence of diagnosed gas embolism as a direct consequence of a laparoscopic operation is approximately 1 in 65,000 procedures.

Many mechanisms have been implicated in the pathophysiology of this complication. Intravascular injection of gas may result from direct vascular injury or indirectly from insufflation of gas into the substance of an organ (e.g., the wall of the uterus). It has been suggested that carbon dioxide accumulated under tension in the peritoneal cavity may enter the circulation by way of minor vessels traumatized during peritoneal stretching.[7] This hypothesis has been advanced as an explanation for gas embolism in some cases.

Insufflation by direct needle access into a large vessel seems the most likely underlying cause of gas embolism. Aspiration by syringe through the Verres needle is essential prior to insufflating any amount of gas (see Chapter 17). This simple precaution ought to eliminate this risk completely. Direct injection of gas into the uterine or urinary bladder wall should be avoided by prompt identification of any error of needle placement.

The outcome of gas embolization is influenced by early recognition and by the type of gas used as the distending medium. Early diagnosis depends on the appearance of cardiac arrhythmias, fall in blood pressure, and characteristic electrocardiographic changes, as well as auscultatory changes of the heart sounds (metallic clicking and gurgling). The most sensitive method for detecting embolized gas is by precordial Doppler ultrasound monitoring.[8] Rapid astute recognition limits the amount of gas reaching the vital organs (particularly heart and brain) and facilitates correcting the homeostatic derangement with prompt return to normality.

The physicochemical properties of the gas insufflated to produce the pneumoperitoneum influences the extent and duration of the morbidity associated with its intravascular injection. Carbon dioxide is highly soluble in blood and is rapidly eliminated from the blood stream by hyperventilation. In angiocardiographic studies, it has been well tolerated in single intravenous doses up to 7.5 ml per kilogram. Only negligible electrocardiographic changes are seen with amounts as high as 400 to 500 cc injected intravascularly. Nitrous oxide is less soluble in blood than is carbon dioxide and it is not eliminated as quickly. Smaller amounts can produce comparable symptoms that may persist for a long time relative to larger amounts of carbon dioxide.

Although no longer used in the United States, air insufflation for the pneumoperitoneum is still used in technologically less well-developed countries. The exact amount of intravenous air which can cause death in humans is not known. The rate at which it enters the circulation is perhaps as important as the total volume. As little as 20 cc per minute have produced toxic effects (including specifically gurgling heart sounds) and transient quadriplegia.[13] Neurological sequelae and deaths have been described with small volumes of air embolism associated with the insertion of central venous catheters. Given that the amount of gas required to distend the abdominal cavity is measured in liters, it becomes clear that room air should not be used in laparoscopy for creating a pneumoperitoneum.

If gas embolization is suspected or diagnosed, an intravenous catheter is advanced to the level of the superior vena cava or right atrium. This facilitates aspiration of the gas from the heart. The practice is based on experience gained with this condition during neurosurgical procedures. If has been shown effective in reducing morbidity and mortality. If carbon dioxide is the gas used, mechanically controlled hyperventilation should enhance its elimination and reduce the duration of the condition.

Verification that the Verres needle is intra-abdominal in location does not rule out the possibility of the distending gas accumulating in an undesirable location (Figure 15.15). Omental emphysema, resulting from insufflation of gas into the omentum, may not be immediately recognized. Because the adipose tissue in this area is elastic, one may not encounter any increment in resistance or measurable pressure. This complication prevents adequate visualization of the abdomino-pelvic structures. If the degree of omental distention is great, the best course of action may be to interrupt the laparoscopic procedure and await spontaneous reabsorption. One may then repeat the operation 1 to 2 weeks later.

Root et al reported a fatal gas embolism one hour after the completion of a diagnostic laparoscopy.[12] Postmortem roentgenographic studies revealed large volumes of gas in the portal system, heart, and brain. They postulated the trapping of gas in the portal circulation with delayed release of the gas into the systemic circulation. Experiments in dogs performed by the same authors confirmed their hypothesis.

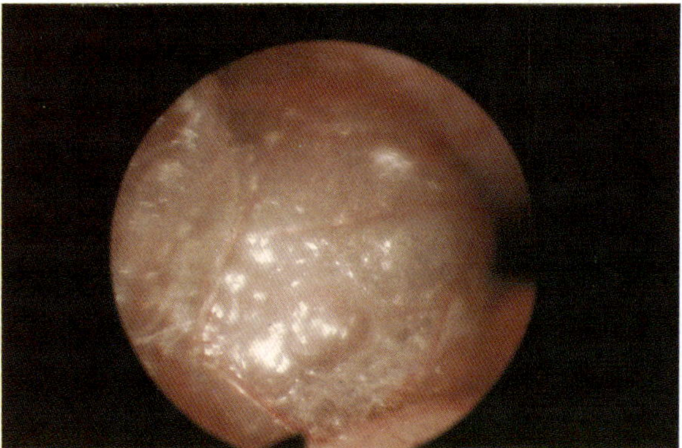

Figure 15.15 Omental emphysema. Low pressure is registered when the omentum is being distended by the insufflated gas. Minimal omental emphysema is of little consequence. Large accumulation of gas in the omentum may preclude successful completion of laparoscopy.

ALTERNATIVE METHODS FOR PRODUCING A PNEUMOPERITONEUM

Occasional failure to create an adequate pneumoperitoneum by inserting the Verres needle in the umbilical or periumbilical area stimulated investigation of new puncture sites. Alternative transabdominal sites have been explored, such as the McBurney point, midline subumbilical point (4 cm below the umbilicus in midline), and the left upper quadrant, an area often used by internists for celioscopy. It is difficult to envision any advantages of any of these over the periumbilical insertion site now commonly used by most gynecologists. It is alleged that some traumatic complications may be preventable by way of these locations, but this is yet to be confirmed.

Two additional approaches recommended for creating pneumoperitoneum are gaining support at the present time. They are the posterior vaginal fornix and the transfundal routes. The posterior vaginal fornix site was once popular for inducing pneumoperitoneum preceding a culdoscopy. Experience showed this method of peritoneal insufflation was not free of complications, as is currently claimed.[10] Morbidity ranged from minor complications, such as bleeding from the vaginal puncture site, to more serious ones that included perforation of the rectum, the sigmoid, or the small bowel adherent to the pouch of Douglas. Extraperitoneal insufflation (usually retroperitoneal) is not unusual. Perirenal and mediastinal emphysema has been reported, especially if the error in regard to the location of the insufflating needle is not promptly recognized.

The posterior fornix site for insufflation of the distending gas is being advanced by gynecologists experienced with culdoscopy.[10] For a culdoscopy, the knee-chest position is used. This allows the uterus and adnexa, as well as other freely mobile intraperitoneal organs located in the pelvis, to move in a cephalad direction. It frees the posterior cul-de-sac. For laparoscopic procedures, the lithotomy or semilithotomy position is utilized. These positions do not ensure that the pouch of Douglas will be empty, even in the absence of pelvic adhesions.

The transfundal puncture method recommended by Morgan has been used successfully for creating a pneumoperitoneum.[9] Before this technique can be adopted widely, more experience with it is required. Complications ranging from extraperitoneal insufflation to carbon dioxide gas embolism have been reported. To prevent such mishaps, the same safety checks used for the transabdominal insufflation route are applicable. Although this technique may prove useful under some unusual circumstances, its routine application cannot yet be recommended. The presence of uterine fundal fibroids may preempt successful entrance into the peritoneal cavity. Deviations of the uterus from its usual midline position may lead to puncture of the vascular broad ligament or adjacent pelvic structures. Transfundal insufflation for pneumoperitoneum is clearly not recommended in patients undergoing a diagnostic laparoscopy for infertility evaluation because it may damage the uterine serosa and lead to the formation of peritoneal adhesions.

If periumbilical intraperitoneal adhesions are strongly suspected, it is advisable to proceed with an open laparoscopy (using the Hasson cannula) rather than to seek alternative modes for producing the pneumoperitoneum. Although insertion of the Verres needle periumbilically is recognized to be a source of significant complications, alternative routes do not eliminate those risks in patients with intra-abdominal adhesions.

References

1. Ahn YW, Leach JA. A comparison of subcutaneous and preperitoneal emphysema arising from gynecologic laparoscopic procedures. J Reprod Med 1976; 17:335-337.
2. Chandler JG, Berk RN, Golden GT. Misleading pneumoperitoneum. Surg Obstet Gynecol 1977; 144:163-174.
3. Cohen MR. Laparoscopy, culdoscopy and gynecography: Technique and atlas. Philadelphia: WB Saunders 1970; 27-32.
4. Copeland C, Win R, Hulka JF. Direct trocar insertion at laparoscopy: An evaluation. Obstet Gynecol 1983; 62:655-659.
5. Dingfelder JR. Direct laparoscope insertion without prior pneumoperitoneum. J Reprod Med 1978; 21:45-47.
6. Lemay M, Lafortune M, Fugere P. Post-laparoscopy pneumoperitoneum. Clin Investig Med 1978; 1:211-212.
7. McKenzie R. Laparoscopy. NZ Med J 1971; 74:87-91.
8. Michenfelder JD, Miller RH, Gronert GA. Evaluation of an ultrasonic device (Doppler) for the diagnosis of venous air embolism. Anesthesiology 1972; 36:164-167.
9. Morgan HR. Laparoscopy: Induction of pneumoperitoneum via transfundal puncture. Obstet Gynecol 1979; 54:260-261.
10. Neely MR, McWilliams R, Makhlouf HA. Laparoscopy: Routine pneumoperitoneum via the posterior fornix. Obstet Gynecol 1975; 45:459-460.
11. Paster SB, Brogdon BG. Roentgenographic diagnosis of pneumoperitoneum. JAMA 1976; 235:1264-1267.
12. Root B, Levy MN, Pollack S, et al. Gas embolism death after laparoscopy delayed by "trapping" in portal circulation. Anesth Analg 1978; 57:232-237.
13. Tunnicliffe RW, Stebbing GF. Intravenous injection of oxygen gas as therapeutic measure. Lancet 1916; 2:321-323.
14. Yacoub OF, Cardona I, Coveler LA, Dodson MG. Carbon dioxide embolism during laparoscopy. Anesthesiology 1982; 57:533-535.

16 COMPLICATIONS OF TROCAR INSERTION

Traumatic injury to intra-abdominal structures during sharp trocar insertion is a rare complication of laparoscopy. Mintz reported only 51 cases in which damage could be ascribed to the trocar in over 99,000 procedures (1 per 1,940).[4] Nevertheless, the serious morbidity resulting from this type of accident requires detailed description.

Injury to particular systems is discussed in subsequent chapters; these include vascular (Chapter 17), gastrointestinal (Chapter 18), and urologic complications (Chapter 19). Just the technical difficulties associated with insertion of trocars will be described here. Because most of these complications are preventable by adhering strictly to prescribed technique, it is imperative to review the details presented in Chapter 2.

LAPAROSCOPIC TROCAR

With the exception of the open technique of laparoscopy (see Chapter 2), insertion of the laparoscopic trocar is a blind procedure. The risk of trocar injury to an intraperitoneal structure is greatest during this step of the procedure because ordinarily the presence of bowel or omentum adherent to the parietal peritoneum of the anterior abdominal wall cannot be known by the operator in advance.

Accidents created during insertion of the sharp trocar are not limited to patients with intra-abdominal adhesions. Injury can occur even in women who are entirely free of them. Experience shows that most trocar complications are the result of technical shortcuts or shortcomings. Inadequate skin incision, extraperitoneal location of the trocar, and use of faulty instruments can be avoided; thus, damage caused by these factors can be prevented.

Inordinate Resistance

Controlled insertion of the primary and/or the secondary trocar is essential. The operator must be able to discern the position of the sharp point of the trocar at all times during the course of its introduction. He or she should be alert to any increased resistance to trocar placement. If resistance is encountered, a consideration of whether it is due to the instrument itself (dull trocar) or to some problem in or on the abdominal wall is mandatory.

As detailed in Chapter 1, trocars used for laparoscopy can have conical or pyramidal tips. Some laparoscopists prefer the conical trocar point because it traverses the fascia without interruption in a single, smooth motion. Technically, others find the pyramidal point more desirable. Regardless of preference, the trocar must be sharp to avoid increase of the thrusting force needed to accomplish perforation of the abdominal wall.

Use of an unsharpened instrument increases the risk of complications. The greater the force required to traverse the abdominal wall, the greater the risk of injury to an intra-abdominal organ. Large forceps translate to poor control of the depth of the penetration. The sudden loss of resistance that occurs as the fascial layer is perforated under these conditions risks deep intra-abdominal penetration and consequent damage.

Structural abnormalities of the abdominal wall may require added force for inserting the laparoscopic or auxiliary trocar. Scars, for example, are sources of difficulty. The wound site of a previous subumbilical operation can be avoided by selecting a paramedian entry point for the laparoscopy (see Chapter 2). Although for cosmetic reasons it is customary to incise the skin over an old scar, it is advisable to avoid traversing the fascia at the old suture line whenever possible. Fibrotic scar tissue offers increased resistance, thus diminishing the thrust control exercised by the operator.

An incision that is too small to accommodate the trocar sleeve can also produce increased resistance. This can usually be prevented by ensuring that the incision is adequate. Using a sharp scalpel, the incision should be made at least 1 to 2 mm larger than the outside diameter of the trocar. This is particularly important for entering in the umbilical fossa where the skin and fascia are in close proximity.

Extraperitoneal Location of the Trocar Sleeve

If the trocar sleeve does not perforate the peritoneum, the procedure cannot proceed. Should the deep end of the sleeve be covered by the elastic peritoneal layer, the laparoscope cannot enter the abdominal cavity. This is at times difficult to diagnose and correct. Misinterpretation of findings may result.

The peritoneal layer generally offers little resistance to perforation by the sharp laparoscopic trocar. Because there is no distinctive feeling detectable as the peritoneum is pierced, failure to puncture it may not be apparent. Noting the escape of carbon dioxide when the trocar is withdrawn from its sleeve is not a fail-safe method to ensure that the sleeve is intraperitoneal in location. Sometimes the trocar may actually perforate the peritoneum, but not to a sufficient depth to enable the sleeve to enter the abdominal cavity.

One should introduce the laparoscope into its sleeve under direct visualization. If the end of the sleeve is below the fascia, but not yet within the peritoneal cavity, preperitoneal adipose tissue is easily identifiable (Figure 16.1). This layer of fat appears bright yellow and readily reflects the fiberoptic light. By contrast, an adequately formed pneumoperitoneum offers a dark background, making the peritoneum translucent and bluish-gray in appearance.

Attempts to perforate the peritoneum with the front end of the laparoscope can occasionally succeed. However, the lens may be smeared by contact with the adipose tissue. This obscures visibility. Removal of the laparoscope and reinsertion of the sharp trocar is preferable. The peritoneal layer should then be readily pierced.

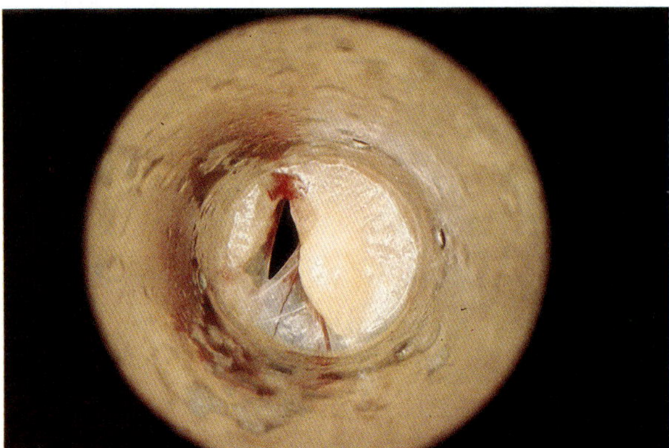

Figure 16.1 Extraperitoneal position of the laparoscopic sleeve. Preperitoneal adipose tissue (yellow) is seen to the right. Translucent peritoneum with its vessels can be identified nearby. The triangular black area represents the site at which the peritoneum was perforated by the sharp pyramidal trocar point. This opening allows intraperitoneal gas to escape when the sleeve is tested for patency.

Intra-abdominal Adhesions

Intra-abdominal adhesions arising as a consequence of previous abdominal surgery or infectious process are predisposing factors to injury of intra-abdominal organs during trocar insertion. If a loop of bowel is fixed to the parietal peritoneum underlying the infraumbilical area, it is not likely to be atraumatically displaced by the sharp point of the trocar at the time of insertion. A similar situation occurs when loops of bowel are adherent to each other; the large mass thus formed is not easily displaced by the perforating instrument without damage.

Careful exploration is essential when the peritoneal cavity is entered. Failure to identify an injury to a segment of bowel can lead to serious morbidity (see Chapter 18). Lacerations produced by the sharp trocar always require evaluation. If indicated, they require immediate surgical repair.

Suspected intra-abdominal adhesions are a relative contraindication for laparoscopy (see Chapter 6). Chi et al evaluated the relative risks of surgical difficulties, immediate complications, and early follow-up complications in women with and without previous abdominal surgery.[1] They found that although the rate of surgical difficulties was significantly higher in women who had had previous abdominal surgery, those obstacles could be overcome without increased complications.

A smaller endoscope (such as a needle laparoscope) may be used to inspect the intra-abdominal periumbilical area and thus to rule out the presence of adhesions prior to insertion of the laparoscopic trocar.[2] The rationale for this recommendation is that unavoidable injury to a loop of bowel adherent subumbilically will cause a negligible laceration (1.7 to 2.2 mm). However, one inherent risk of this approach is the possibility of a through-and-through perforation of a loop of fixed bowel that goes unrecognized by the operator. Personal experience suggests that if a mini-endoscope is used to determine the presence or absence of periumbilical adhesions, it should be inserted in an area unlikely to have underlying adhesions. The left upper abdominal quadrant (commonly used for celioscopy of the upper abdomen) is a preferred site.

Culdoscopic evaluation with a mini-endoscope has also been suggested.[5] This technique itself is not entirely innocuous. I have found obstruction of the pouch of Douglas by abdomino-pelvic adhesions to be much more common than bowel or omentum adherent to the parietal peritoneum of the anterior abdominal wall. Damage is thus likely to occur by using this route.

Attempts to exclude intra-abdominal adhesions preoperatively have met with limited success. The culdoscopic approach requires the mastery of an additional procedure. Moreover, it prolongs the planned surgery. It is more expeditious to consider alternative methods, such as open laparoscopy (see Chapter 2) for cases in which abdomino-pelvic adhesions are strongly suspected.

Depth of Penetration

Injury to intra-abdominal structures by the laparoscopic trocar can occur even in the absence of abdominopelvic adhesions. Traumatic damage can also be created any time the sharp trocar is thrust deeply into the abdomen. The cause of this type of accident is usually technical in nature and, therefore, should be prevented.

Excessive penetration of the laparoscopic trocar generally results from uncontrolled motion during its insertion. This may occur as a consequence of diminished resistance by the abdominal wall (from diastasis of the rectus abdominis muscles, or from inadequate pneumoperitoneum, for example) or as a result of inadequate depth control. Rectus diastasis, a frequent predisposing factor, is common in multiparous patients. The thickness of the midline subumbilical anterior abdominal wall is reduced to that of the linea alba and its covering skin. Thus, diminished resistance to trocar penetration can be expected.

Evaluation of the thickness of the anterior abdominal wall must precede insertion of the laparoscopic trocar. A good practice is to place one's extended index finger over the trocar stem to mark the planned depth of maximum penetration (see Chapter 2). The trocar should not be introduced beyond this point.

Physicians in training frequently neglect to delimit the point of maximal penetration in this way. The most common reason offered is that their fingers are too short. This does not justify compromising the safety of the technique. The problem is solved by shortening the length of the trocar and sleeve accordingly. As discussed in Chapter 2, the thickness of the abdominal wall at the umbilical area is usually no greater than 1 to 2 cm. Thus, a shortened instrument satisfactorily traverses the anterior abdominal wall for laparoscopic purposes.

Adjusting the force of trocar insertion according to the resistance offered by the anterior abdominal wall is important. In addition to the opposition offered by the distention of the anterior abdominal wall by the pneumoperitoneum, some mechanical support is required. This is provided by the operator manually elevating the anterior abdominal wall subumbilically. The elevation is preferably carried out by the surgeon without assistance. Poor distribution of resistance caused by uneven elevation of the abdominal wall is thus prevented.

The resistance due to distention of the anterior abdominal wall by the pneumoperitoneum remains important. Inadequate abdominal distention permits indentation of the wall during trocar insertion. Risk of damage to the retroperitoneal structures is thereby increased (see Chapter 17).

The value of an adequate pneumoperitoneum should not be underestimated. Copeland et al questioned the need to establish a pneumoperitoneum before trocar insertion.[3] They advocated direct trocar insertion without prior pneumoperitoneum. Three bowel perforations with peritonitis complicated this technique in some 2,000 cases performed in this manner.

Faulty Instruments

That the responsibility to inspect all instruments prior to beginning a laparoscopy lies with the operator is a concept often put forward, but not always applied. To encounter faulty instruments in the midst of the procedure is not only frustrating and time consuming, but it may add risk to the procedure and may prevent it from being successfully completed.

The operator must ensure that the sharp trocar slides easily within the sleeve in both directions. Damaged sleeves can prevent the sharp trocar tip from protruding as designed. If this occurs, the opening in the fascia created by the trocar may be too small to accommodate the sleeve. A similar condition is seen when the trocar and sleeve are of different diameters.

It is necessary to be able to withdraw the trocar smoothly from its investing sleeve. If excessive force is needed for this purpose, removal is difficult to accomplish once the instrument is in place in the patient. After insertion, both trocar and sleeve may come out together. Reinsertion of a new trocar and sleeve is then required.

The laparoscopist must check to ensure correct functioning of the laparoscopic valve. The central lumen of the trumpet valve must match the diameter of the trocar and the laparoscope. The pneumoperitoneum leaks if the opening is too big. If too small, the laparoscope is unable to enter the peritoneal cavity.

The surgeon who routinely utilizes a 5 mm laparoscope for the procedure should try to employ interchangeable trocars and sleeves. This makes it possible to insert the laparoscope through the auxiliary sleeve to explore the periumbilical region. Similarly, laparoscopic visualization through the secondary puncture allows one to introduce a metal probe through the umbilical sleeve. This obviates the need for a tertiary puncture to mobilize upper abdominal organs (such as liver and spleen). Procedures of this kind carried out through sleeves of unequal size are hampered by continuous leakage of the distending gas.

AUXILIARY TROCAR

Insertion of the auxiliary trocar carries a smaller risk of injury to intra-abdominal structures because it is performed under laparoscopic guidance. Selecting an entry site free of underlying adhesions helps prevent injuries. Nonetheless, introduction of secondary or tertiary trocars is not altogether free of complications.

The causes of accidents occurring during insertion of the auxiliary trocar range from those that are technical to those that are traumatic in nature. Technical problems, such as extraperitoneal location of the sleeve, can usually be resolved without increased morbidity. Trauma to blood vessels (see Chapter 17) or to bladder (see Chapter 19) requires additional therapeutic maneuvers. Management principles are the same here as for damage resulting from the primary laparoscopic trocar.

Peritoneal Indentation

Failure to pierce the peritoneum can also be seen during the insertion of auxiliary trocars. This occurs as a consequence of the inherent elasticity of the peritoneal layer. The loose areolar attachment of the preperitoneal adipose tissue plays an important role because it facilitates detachment and indentation of the peritoneum.

Several factors are associated with peritoneal indentation by the sharp trocar and sleeve. These include obesity, a perforation site away from the midline, and an inadequate pneumoperitoneum.

In the obese patient, the amount of preperitoneal adipose tissue is markedly increased. As a result, the peritoneum is loosely attached and is thus easily separated from its preperitoneal attachments by the pressure applied to it by the trocar.

Perforation of the peritoneal layer away from the midline also increases the risk of identation. In the midline, the peritoneum is closely adherent to the linea alba; this is not the case paramedially. The absence of the posterior fascial sheath below the semilunar line of Douglas leaves a layer of fat between the peritoneum and the overlying muscles. Peritoneal indentation is more likely to occur in this region.

Creation of an adequate pneumoperitoneum is guided by the level of intraperitoneal pressure (see Chapter 2). To avoid complications associated with excessive intra-abdominal pressure (see Chapter 15), laparoscopy is sometimes attempted with small amounts of insufflated gas. As a result of the low intraperitoneal pressure this produces, the peritoneum offers little resistance to the perforating trocar and shows a propensity to indent.

Insertion of the suprapubic auxiliary trocar is usually carried out under direct laparoscopic visualization. The operator experiences a characteristic sensation when the sharp trocar perforates the fascia. Frequently, the trocar and sleeve enter the peritoneal cavity during the initial thrust.

Occasionally, following perforation of the fascia, the sharp trocar pushes the peritoneum free from its preperitoneal attachments. Under these circumstances, the laparoscopist is sometimes able to see the protruding sharp point of the trocar (Figure 16.2). Nonetheless, the sleeve may remain entirely extraperitoneal. Continued downward pressure only effects a more pronounced indentation of the peritoneal layer (Figure 16.3).

Early withdrawal of the sharp trocar before its sleeve has entered the peritoneal cavity is inappropriate. The elastic peritoneum retracts over the sleeve and obstructs its opening (Figure 16.4). This makes it impossible to insert any instrument into the abdominal cavity through the lumen of the sleeve.

Several corrective maneuvers have proved helpful in assisting the trocar and its sleeve to perforate the peritoneum properly when indentation occurs. They include insufflating additional distending gas, changing the direction of thrust of the perforating trocar, and supporting the indented peritoneum with the laparoscope.

Additional insufflation of distending gas increases the intraperitoneal pressure. The elevated pressure is transmitted equally in all directions. The increment in resistance thus offered to the perforating instrument often makes peritoneal perforation possible. This maneuver has proved particularly helpful in obese individuals.

Once peritoneal indentation has occurred, additional downward pressure by the trocar may separate the peritoneum further from its overlying attach-

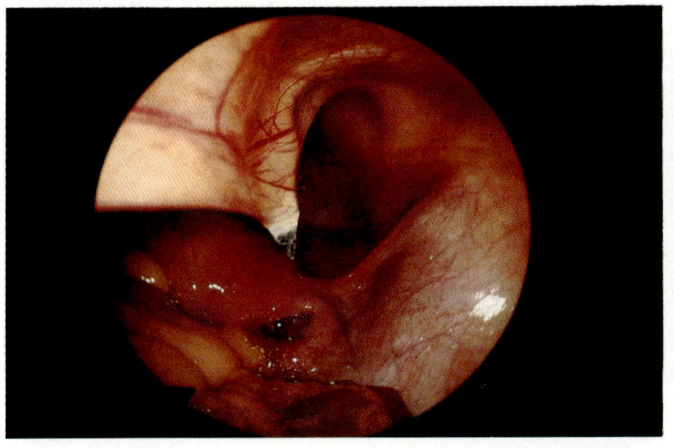

Figure 16.2 Peritoneal indentation as seen from the intraperitoneal vantage. The point of the sharp trocar has incompletely pierced the peritoneum, but its sleeve remains extraperitoneal.

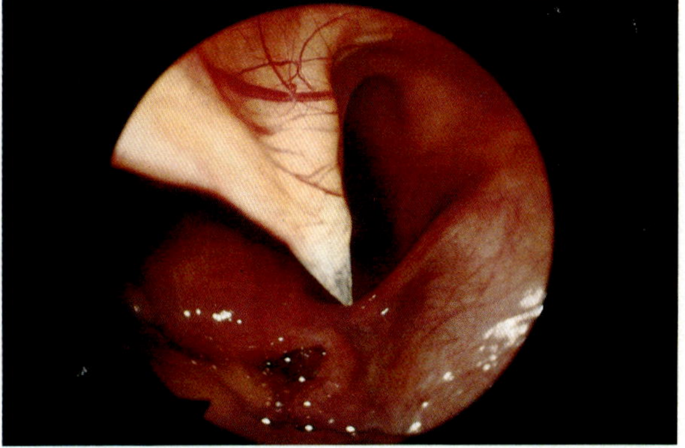

Figure 16.3 Peritoneal detachment, intraperitoneal view (same case as Figure 16.2). Continued downward pressure may further separate the peritoneal layer from its tenuous preperitoneal attachments. Pronounced rotation of the trocar on its longitudinal axis may help the sleeve gain access into the peritoneal cavity.

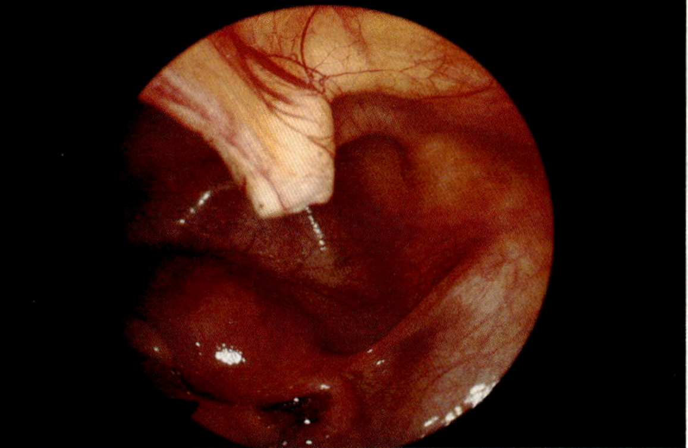

Figure 16.4 Extraperitoneal location of auxiliary trocar sleeve (same case as Figures 16.2 and 16.3). Premature removal of the sharp trocar will occlude the sleeve opening with a peritoneal covering. Reinsertion of the trocar is now required to perforate the peritoneum.

ment. Pronounced rotation on its longitudinal axis may help the sleeve enter the peritoneal cavity. Acute angulation of the trocar can sometimes remedy the situation. Because the direction of thrust is changed, the maneuver must be carried out under laparoscopic visualization to avoid inadvertant intra-abdominal injury.

When all of the aforementioned maneuvers fail to accomplish penetration into the peritoneal cavity, I have utilized the front end of the laparoscope to push the peritoneum over the outer walls of the trocar sleeve. Whereas this may at times smear the front lens, removal, cleansing, and reinsertion of the laparoscope can be accomplished easily.

Traumatic Injury

Traumatic injury arising from insertion of the auxiliary trocar is usually due to technical failures and is thus preventable. Misdirection of the trocar during its introduction and inability to control the depth of insertion account for most of them. Because serious damage can similarly occur during insertion of the secondary trocar, proper technique is no less important during this step of the operation.

Students of laparoscopy are routinely taught that in order to avoid complications during insertion of the primary laparoscopic trocar, their most dextrous hand should be used. Inexplicably, they adhere to an inherited custom of inserting the auxiliary suprapubic trocar with the opposite hand, which is less adroit in most instances. This practice is illogical. Use of the operator's most skillful hand to insert the secondary puncture may require him or her to change from one side of the operating table to the other. This seems a small inconvenience for the counterbalancing benefit of increasing the safety of the procedure.

Direction of trocar insertion is also important. The tendency to aim the auxiliary trocar towards the hollow of the sacrum (Figure 16.5) is inappropriate. This places it in direct line with the retroperitoneal structures. Inability to control the thrust of the instrument risks injury to these structures. Insertion of the auxiliary trocar aiming at an imaginary point on the uterine fundus (Figure 16.6) offers the instrument the largest volume of pneumoperitoneum and space free of any intra-abdominal organs. Failure to control the depth of insertion by this approach could at worst cause injury to the uterus or bladder. Both are less vital organs when compared with the retroperitoneal structures; if damaged, the resulting trauma constitutes much less of a hazard to the patient and is far more readily correctable.

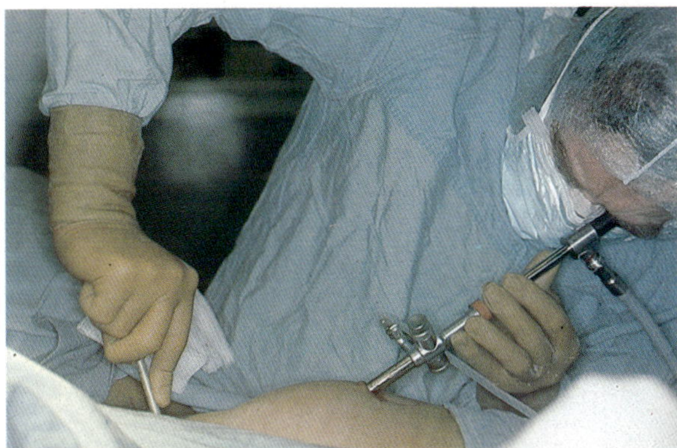

Figure 16.5 Misdirection of auxiliary trocar during insertion. Trocar is pointing toward the hollow of the sacrum. Risk of injury to retroperitoneal structures is increased.

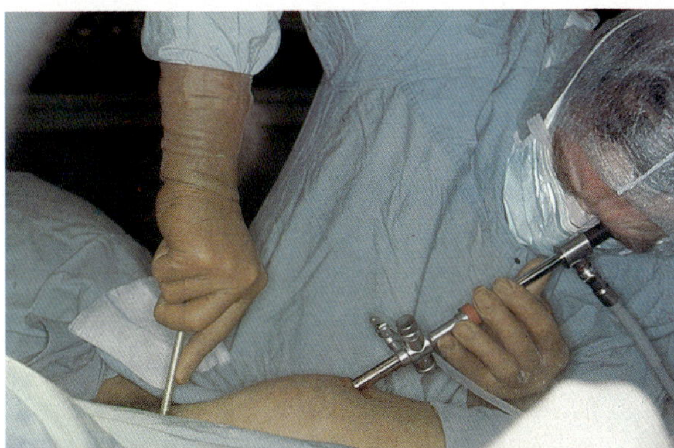

Figure 16.6 Correct direction for auxiliary trocar insertion. Trocar is pointed at the uterine fundus.

References

1. Chi IC, Feldblum PJ, Balogh SA. Previous abdominal surgery as a risk factor in interval laparoscopic sterilization. Am J Obstet Gynecol 1983; 145:841-846.
2. Cook WA. Needle laparoscopy in patients with suspected bowel adhesions. Obstet Gynecol 1977; 49:105-106.
3. Copeland C, Wing R, Hulka JF. Direct trocar insertion at laparoscopy: An evaluation. Obstet Gynecol 1983; 62:655-659.
4. Mintz M. Risks and prophylaxis in laparoscopy: A survey of 100,000 cases. J Reprod Med 1977; 18:269-272.
5. Van Lith DAF, Van Schie KJ, Beekhuizen W. Diagnostic miniculdoscopy preceding laparoscopy when bowel adhesions are suspected. J Reprod Med 1979; 23:87-90.

17 VASCULAR INJURIES

Bleeding problems resulting from laparoscopic procedures account for almost half of all the complications. Injuries to blood vessels range from minor bleeding from superficial vessels at or near the incision site to massive hemorrhage from lacerations of the major retroperitoneal vessels. The nature of the laparoscopic technique, particularly as regards percutaneous insertion of the Verres needle and the laparoscopic trocar, offers neither palpation nor visualization to guide the surgeon. Choice of site and direction rely primarily on knowledge of the usual anatomic landmarks. Such blind instrumentation risks vascular injury. Prompt identification of such injury is indispensable in the prevention of more serious complications, such as intravascular gas embolization (see Chapter 15) or hemorrhagic shock from a concealed retroperitoneal hemorrhage. Some of the minor tegumentary injuries are unavoidable owing to anatomical variations of the abdominal wall vasculature. This does not apply to damage to the major abdominal vascular structures. These latter injuries usually involve technical errors or inappropriate selection of patients for the procedure.

Surveys of large series of laparoscopies indicate that the major vessels are injured in approximately 3 per 10,000 procedures.[10] Vascular injuries may occur from the laparoscopy itself or as a consequence of a surgical procedure performed translaparoscopically. Among accidents resulting from the laparoscopic technique, two thirds are related to the Verres needle used to produce the pneumoperitoneum; the others are caused by the sharp laparoscopic trocar. Bleeding injuries complicating a translaparoscopic surgical procedure are usually related to the operator's technical skills. Just as with any other surgical procedure, it is the surgeon's responsibility to ensure good hemostasis before the procedure is concluded. As an accepted surgical principle, it is the failure to identify these complications rather than the inadvertent injury itself that is responsible for the sequelae.

VESSELS OF THE ABDOMINAL WALL

Trauma to the vasculature of the abdominal wall is common during a laparoscopic procedure. Injury to a large vessel becomes evident intraoperatively when blood is seen dripping down into the peritoneal cavity around the trocar sleeve. Smaller vessels may be traumatized and give rise to late hematoma formation. Hematomas in turn may cause postoperative pain.

Variations in the anatomical configuration and development of the abdominal wall are accompanied by changes in the blood supply to the area. Nevertheless, one must be cognizant of the usual anatomy of the vasculature. This helps one select the site for abdominal entry and thus avoid injury. Several tissue planes are traversed, each with its own vascular supply, as one penetrates from skin to anterior parietal peritoneum. It is important to be familiar with these structures.

Skin

The skin is supplied by capillary vessels running through the subcuticular layer. Damage to these small vessels is usually contained by the pressure produced by the instrument inserted through the tissue. If bleeding continues at the conclusion of the procedure, satisfactory hemostasis can generally be achieved by closure of the skin incision with metal clips or subcuticular sutures.

Subcutaneous Tissue

The subcutaneous adipose layer contains vessels of diverse caliber. Arterioles and venules supply the areas under the skin, and vessels of larger diameter are encountered closer to the fascial layer. Injury to the smaller superficial vessels can be corrected by deep skin sutures (mattress type) or by the application of metal clips (Michel clips).

The operator ought to be aware that the periumbilical venous plexus can be lacerated when the periumbilical incision is extended for the insertion of the laparoscopic trocar (Figure 17.1). It can also be damaged during the initial incision for open laparoscopy. These vessels must be identified, clamped, and ligated to ensure hemostasis. A more common problem is unrecognized trauma produced by the excessive pressure applied by the operator to lift the abdominal wall. This results in ecchymosis or hematoma (Figure 17.2). Gentle handling of tissues is emphasized for all surgical procedures. Rough treatment may cause postoperative pain and poor cosmetic outcome.

Larger hematomas are produced when the deeper subcutaneous vessels are traumatized. The superficial epigastric artery (a branch of the femoral artery) ascends between the two layers of the subcutaneous abdominal wall fascia to reach the periumbilical area (Figure 17.3). It anastomoses with branches of the inferior epigastric artery and the contralateral superficial epigastric artery. It is at greatest risk of being injured during the insertion of the secondary accessory trocar. Transillumination of the abdominal wall with the intraperitoneal laparoscopic light source is helpful for delineating its pathway. Identification of this large vessel facilitates selection of an alternative avascular site for inserting the secondary puncture.

Injury to the deep subcutaneous vessels can sometimes be managed by application of external pressure with a dressing. Alternatively, a small incision can be made for purposes of clamping and ligating the bleeding vessel. If conservative pressure is selected, the patient should be admitted to the hospital for observation because large volumes of blood can be concealed in the subcutaneous layer before it is clinically recognized.

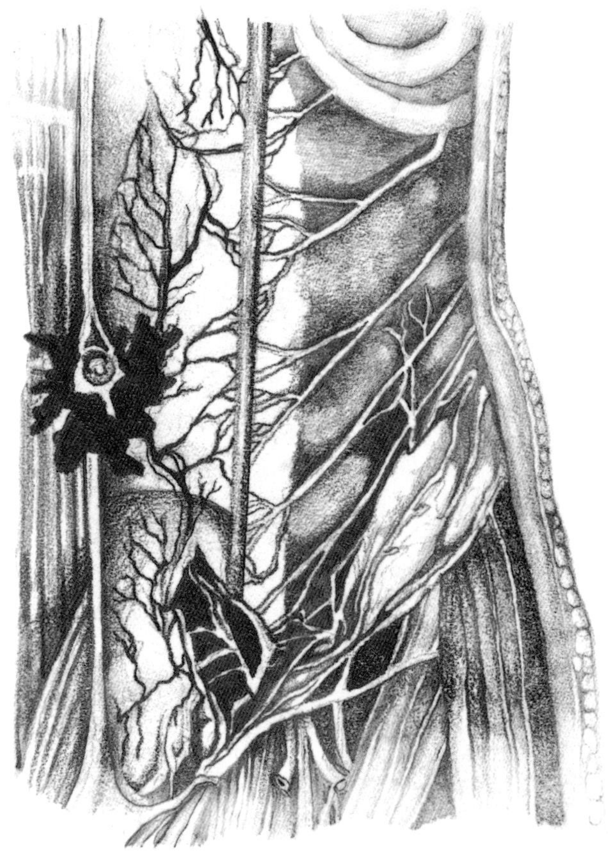

Figure 17.1 Periumbilical bleeding. Incisional bleeding is the result of damage to the periumbilical venous plexus. Individual vessels must be identified and ligated to ensure hemostasis.

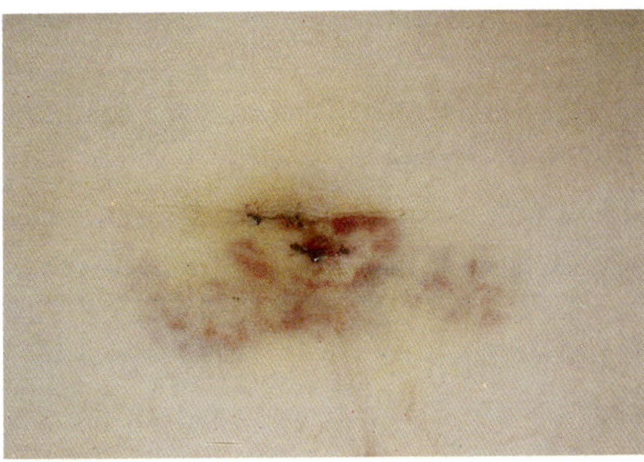

Figure 17.2 Periumbilical hematoma. Seen during the postoperative period, they vary in size and can be very painful. They appear as a consequence of sharp trauma to the periumbilical venous plexus in combination with excessive pressure applied to lift the abdominal wall.

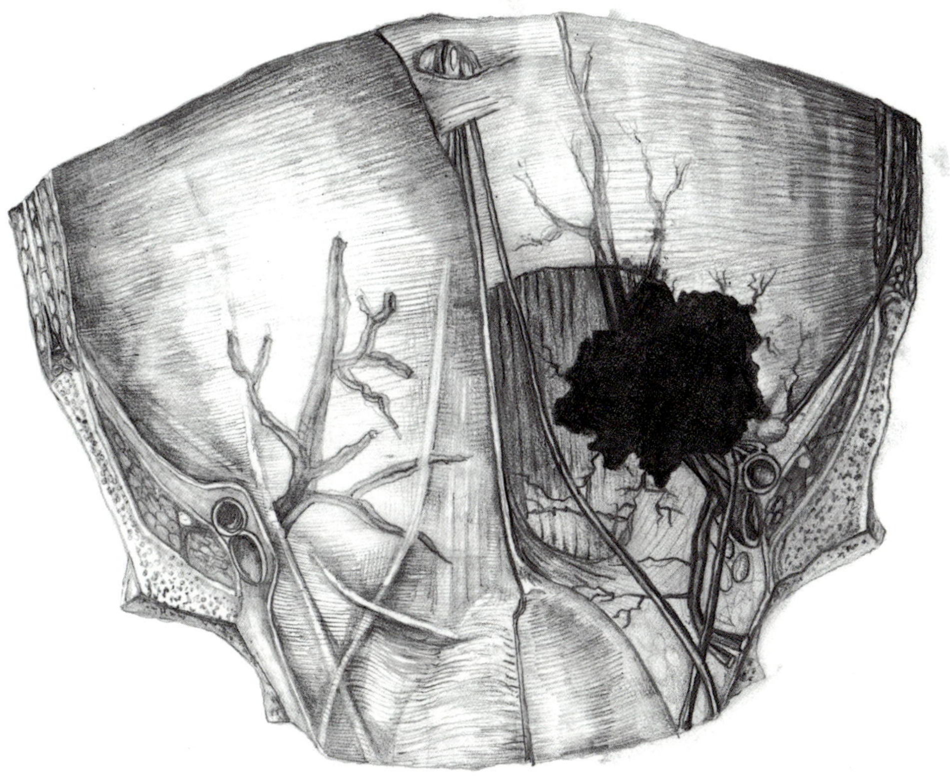

Figure 17.3 Laceration of the superficial epigastric artery. This vessel is at risk of injury during insertion of the secondary accessory trocar. Transillumination of the abdominal wall by means of the laparoscopic light may assist in delineating the vessel's path. Intact contralateral vascularization is shown on the patient's right.

Subfascial Preperitoneal Area

There is abundant vasculature in the anterior abdominal wall except at the midline (linea alba). The rectus muscles, located subfascially, are supplied by moderately large vessels. They arise from the superior epigastric artery (the terminal branch of the internal mammary artery) from above and the inferior epigastric artery (a branch of the external iliac artery) from below (Figure 17.3). Since gynecological laparoscopy is limited to the infraumbilical region, it is mainly concerned with the threat to the inferior epigastric artery. This vessel arises from the external iliac artery immediately above the inguinal ligament (Poupart's ligament) (Figure 17.4). It passes ventrally to the linea semicircularis and continues between the rectus abdominis muscle and its posterior fascial sheath. Above the level of the umbilicus, it anastomoses with the superior epigastric artery and the lower intercostal arteries. Its subumbilical pathway runs parallel to the lateral margin of the rectus muscle, usually in close apposition to the posterior aspect of the muscle.

Translaparoscopic identification of the location of the inferior epigastric vessels is difficult, if not altogether impossible. Light refraction and transmission indices of the rectus muscle (reflecting those of myoglobin) and of the adjacent vessels (mirroring the indices of hemoglobin) are similar. Clear delineation of the path of the vessels by transillumination with the intraperitoneal laparoscopic light source is thus uncertain and problematic.

Laceration of the inferior epigastric artery is not always obvious at the time of laparoscopy. Incisional pain that is excessive for the small auxiliary trocar wound should alert the laparoscopist to this potential complication. Because there is so little resistance to the accumulation of blood by the anterior parietal peritoneum, a large preperitoneal hematoma can form. Its extraperitoneal location means that the signs of peritoneal irritation, usually seen with intraperitoneal bleeding (hemoperitoneum), do not develop. Lateral extraperitoneal propagation further compounds the difficulty of making a correct diagnosis. The large retroperitoneal space can accumulate a considerable amount of blood silently. Injury to the inferior epigastric artery may cause a substantial fall in hematocrit, unaccompanied by any clinical evidence of intraperitoneal bleeding or acute surgical abdomen. Palpation of a unilateral paramedian mass on the anterior abdominal wall is highly suggestive of this complication. Soft tissue roentgenography and sonography are helpful diagnostic aids (Figure 17.5).

Laceration of a retrofascial blood vessel is usually preventable by choosing an avascular area as the site for entering the peritoneal cavity. The midline linea alba is safest for trocar insertion because it is not vascularized. If a paramedian site for the secondary trocar puncture is preferred, Pring suggested that the point of entry be chosen lateral to the external edge of the rectus muscle.[13]

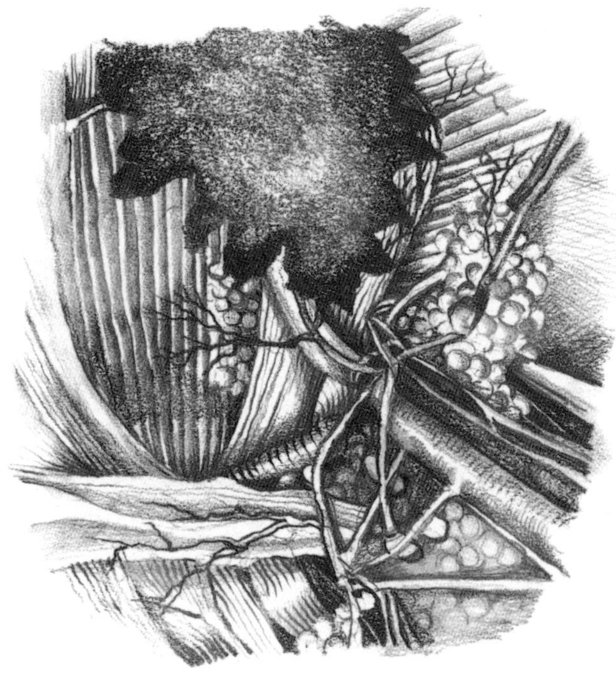

Figure 17.4 Laceration of inferior epigastric artery. A subsidiary of the external iliac artery, it is located between the posterior wall of the rectus abdominus muscle and its posterior fascial sheath. Abdominal transillumination is not helpful for identification.

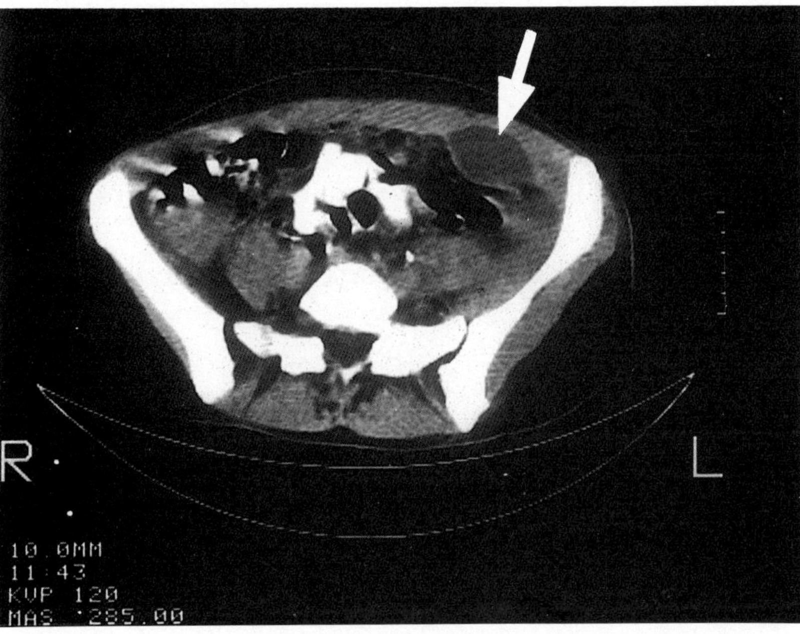

Figure 17.5 Computed tomogram demonstrating rectus muscle hematoma (arrow). The extraperitoneal space can accommodate a large amount of blood silently. A unilateral paramedian mass may be palpable on the anterior abdominal wall.

After one identifies the injured vessel, therapy should consist of exploration of the wound, drainage of the accumulated extravasated blood, and ligation of the lacerated artery or vein. The rich anastomosis of the vascular network in this area requires double ligation (proximally and distally) of the traumatized vessel. If intraoperative inferior epigastric artery injury is diagnosed, full-thickness abdominal wall sutures placed above and below the trocar insertion site may obviate the need for laparotomy. These sutures should be applied under direct laparoscopic visualization to avoid injury to an intraperitoneal organ.

MAJOR RETROPERITONEAL VESSELS

Aside from anesthetic complications, injury to a major retroperitoneal vessel with massive hemorrhage is the most common cause of death associated with laparoscopy. Although the prevalence of this complication is low, the catastrophic outcome makes it one of the most feared iatrogenic complications of the procedure.[12] Thus, it is indispensible for the surgeon to have a thorough knowledge of the abdomino-pelvic anatomy, including the retroperitoneal structures, before he or she undertakes any surgical procedure in the region. Prevention, identification, and management of this complication must be part of the training of every laparoscopist.

The abdominal aorta descends on the anterior surface of the vertebral column slightly to the left of the midline. Below the origin of the renal arteries (between the first and second lumbar vertebra) immediately caudal to the superior mesenteric artery, the ovarian arteries arise from the ventral surface of the aorta. At the level of the third lumbar vertebra, the inferior mesenteric artery originates to supply the left half of the tranverse colon, the entire descending and sigmoid colon, and most of the rectum. There are no other anterior aortic branches.

The aorta terminates in the two common iliac arteries at the level of the fourth lumbar vertebra approximately 3 to 4 cm below the origin of the inferior mesenteric artery. The common iliac arteries diverge for 5 cm in a laterocaudal direction and then divide into the external and internal iliac arteries. This division takes place at the level of the intervertebral fibrocartilage located between the fifth lumbar vertebra and the sacrum. The right common iliac artery is longer than the left, crossing more obliquely over the body of the last lumbar vertebra. Interposed between the common iliac arteries and the vertebral bodies are the common iliac veins and the lowermost aspect of the inferior vena cava.

The external iliac artery continues anteriorly along the psoas muscle and the internal iliac artery dips posteriorly into the pelvis. Both vessels remain ventral to their respective veins, thereby making them susceptible to penetrating trauma during laparoscopy. In the midline, anteriorly to the fourth and fifth lumbar vertebral bodies, runs a small artery which arises from the dorsal aspect of the aorta. This is the middle sacral artery which continues its descent over the sacral promontory, the anterior face of the sacrum, and the coccyx to anastomose with the lumbar branch of the iliolumbar artery.

Topographically, the umbilicus is located directly over the lower end of the aorta in the supine patient. In the Trendelenburg position, the terminal portion of the aorta rotates upward, bringing the common iliac arteries and their subdivisions closer to the horizontal plane. Consequently, the distance between the umbilicus and the aorta is reduced. As will be discussed later, failure to make the necessary technical adjustments for these positional changes increases the risk of injury to the retroperitoneal vessels.

Most penetrating injuries to the retroperitoneal vessels occur at the time of insertion of either the Verres needle or the primary and secondary sharp trocars.[6,7,14] An additional cause of aortic injury is penetration by the sharp scalpel used to incise the abdominal wall prior to the insertion of the Verres needle. This is a special risk in very thin women. It is important to consider some additional factors that predipose patients to this type of injury, such as the patient's habitus, anatomical relationships, and intraperitoneal pressure. These must be recognized in order to reduce the risk.

Patient Size

In very thin patients, the anterior abdominal wall may be as close as 2 to 3 cm from the aorta. It is not unusual to see aortic pulsations transmitted through the abdominal surface in the supine position. In the very obese patient, moreover, relaxation of the flanks, coupled with excessive weight of the anterior abdominal wall, may bring the dorsal aspect of the anterior abdominal wall close to the aorta. It is worth repeating that regardless of the size of the adipose panniculus the abdominal wall is rarely more than 1.0 to 1.5 cm thick in the umbilical region.

Anatomical Relationships

If the patient is placed in the Trendelenburg position prior to the insertion of the Verres needle, the direction of entry has to be adjusted accordingly. In the head-down tilt, the aorta becomes more caudal in location and thus closer to the umbilicus. Lifting the anterior abdominal wall also changes the direction of the underlying parietal peritoneum. Taking these changes into account, one must direct the Verres needle away from the sacral promontory towards the hollow of the sacrum. Aiming at an imaginary target point on the uterine fundus should help in finding a safe pathway for the insufflating needle.

Intraperitoneal Pressure

Creation of an adequate pneumoperitoneum facilitates visualization of the intraperitoneal structures. Additionally, elevation of the intraperitoneal pressure increases the tension on the anterior abdominal wall; this reduces the possibility of the peritoneum tenting downward during insertion of the primary and secondary sharp trocars. Lifting the abdominal wall and the controlled thrusting of the trocar are the most important factors in preventing injury to the abdominal organs. Nevertheless, the increased resistance to penetration due to the elevated intraperitoneal pressure helps keep the anterior abdominal wall away from the retroperitoneal area.

If a major retroperitoneal vessel injury is identified at the time it occurs, adequate surgical repair can usually be accomplished without sequelae. Delayed diagnosis has played a prominent role in all deaths thus far reported from injuries to major abdomino-pelvic vessels.[9] The simple technique of injection of saline and aspiration through the Verres needle shows if it is intravascular in location (Figures 17.6 and 17.7). Blood is characteristically drawn back. When a diagnosis of vessel injury is made, the Verres needle should be left in place. It acts

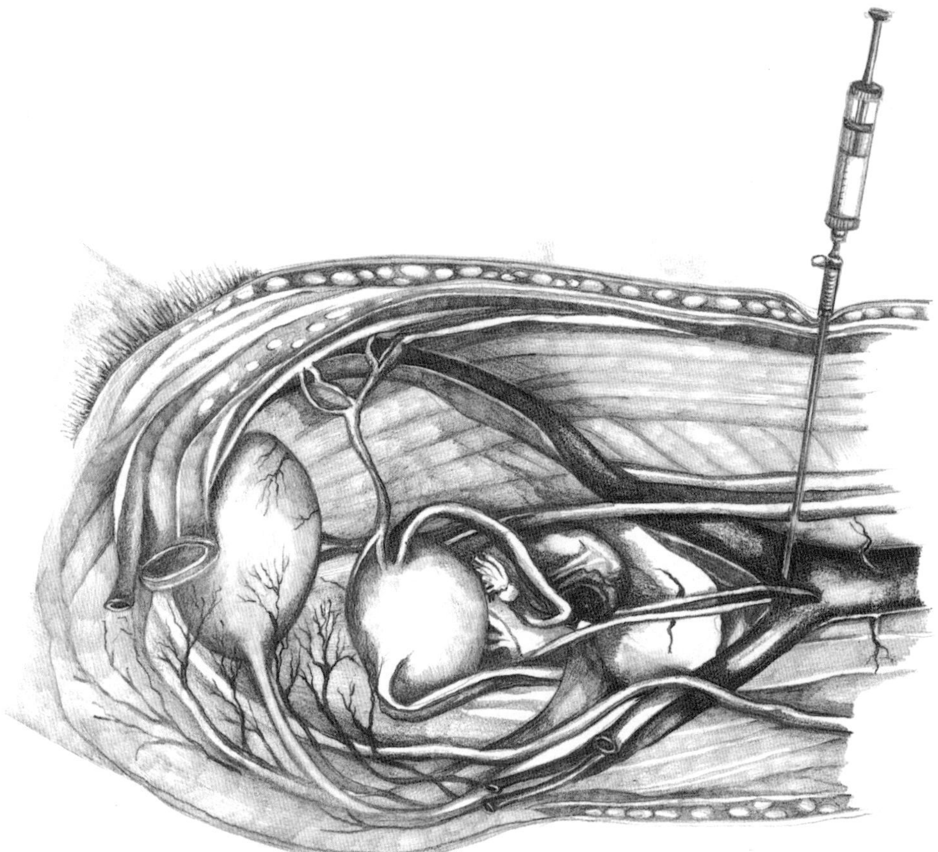

Figure 17.6 Verres needle injury to the aorta. Aspiration of blood through the Verres needle suggests it is intravascular in location. The needle should be left in place to guide the surgeon to the exact location of the vascular laceration.

to obstruct outflow of blood somewhat and it serves to guide the vascular surgeon to the site of the injury. Lesions of the anterior aortic wall tend to bleed freely. This is contrary to what happens when the posterior wall of the aorta is perforated in the course of a translumbar aortography; in this case extravasated blood acts as a tamponade to block the perforation. The posterior parietal peritoneum offers little resistance to pooling of blood, thereby allowing the accumulation of up to 4 L often without clinical evidence of intraperitoneal bleeding.

Vascular injuries created by the sharp laparoscope or auxiliary trocars are larger than those caused by the Verres needle. These give rise to early hypovolemic signs and symptoms. These occur most commonly as a result of lack of adherence to proper technique. If a trocar is not sharp enough, it requires increased force to penetrate the abdominal wall layers and consequently there is less control of the downward thrust.

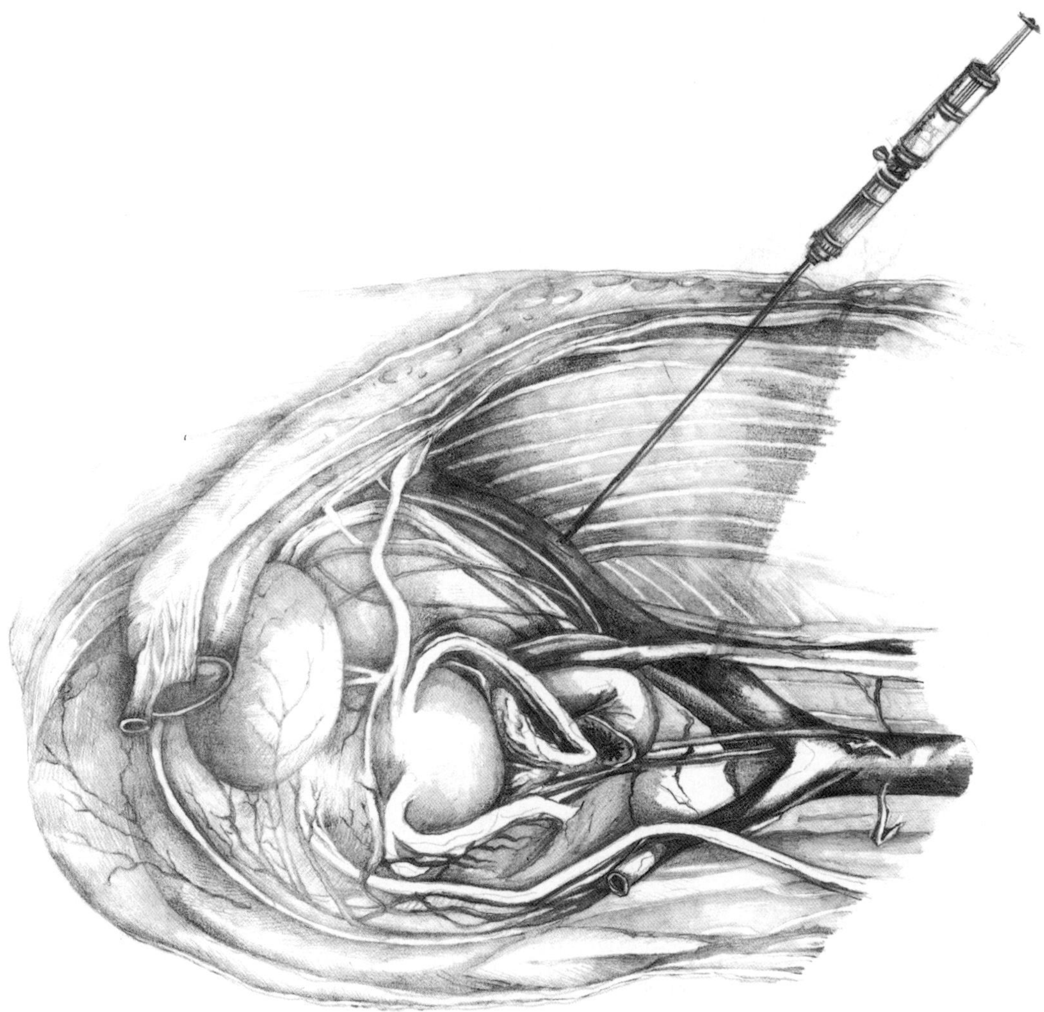

Figure 17.7 Verres needle injury to the external iliac vessels. Deviation from the midline is frequently caused by distortion due to uneven lifting of the abdominal wall at the time the needle is being inserted. Aspiration of blood is a sign of injury to a major vessel.

The auxiliary puncture trocar may produce iliac vessel injury to the common, to the external, and rarely to the internal iliac arteries). Deviation of the instrument from the midline at the time of insertion rather than uncontrolled thrust is thought to be the cause (Figure 17.8). It is advisable for another member of the laparoscopy team to observe the direction of the secondary trocar during insertion to ensure that it is properly introduced.

Whenever a vascular injury is suspected, immediate laparotomy should be undertaken. Exploration of the abdominal cavity and retroperitoneal space should not be delayed until frank shock appears. Concurrently, sufficient amounts of compatible blood should be prepared immediately, if required. Systemic signs (specifically, blood pressure and pulse) are not good indices of the amount of blood loss. Young, healthy patients with normal blood volume and cardiovascular reserve can be expected to maintain normal blood pressure and normal or minimally elevated pulse despite the loss of a large amount of blood.

Upon entering the abdomen, one should exert aortic compression below the level of the renal arteries. This practice effectively and expeditiously reduces or stops the hemorrhage and allows the patient to be stabilized and a vascular team to be assembled. Repairing the laceration with interrupted sutures of Prolene is usually sufficient to correct the problem.

Although nothing can substitute for proper surgical technique, knowledge about this possible complication is needed for early diagnosis. Currently, physicians in outpatient facilities and free-standing surgical centers are performing an increased number of laparoscopies. Appropriate facilities for immediate exploratory laparotomy are essential if these serious complications are to be dealt with expeditiously. In these circumstances long or delayed transfers may make the difference between life and death.

CERVICAL LACERATION

Most uterine manipulators utilized to mobilize the uterus during laparoscopy require attachment to a single-toothed tenaculum applied to the cervix. Bleeding from the tenaculum site is common after the instrument is removed (Figure 17.9). It is necessary to release the tenaculum under direct visualization at the conclusion of the procedure to avoid trauma. Factors that increase the incidence of cervical laceration are superficial application, excessive pull or lateral manipulation, and pregnancy. The last relates to the hypervascularity of the cervix associated with pregnancy.

The exocervical area most commonly used for the tenaculum application, the anterior cervical lip, derives its vascular supply mainly from the descending cervical branches of the uterine artery. They arise at the level of the cardinal ligaments and descend laterally to the cervix. Their terminal branches anastomose

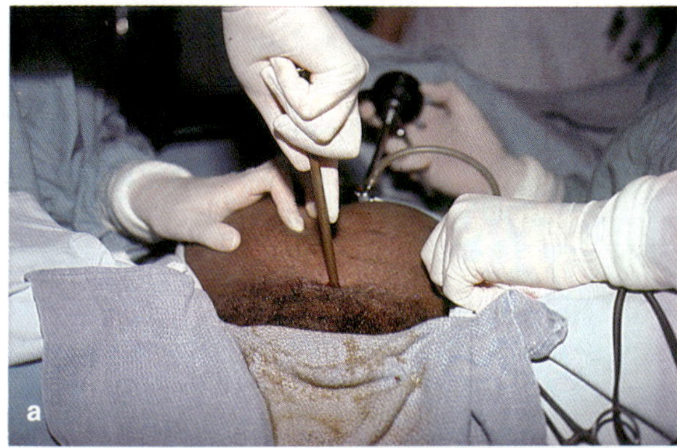

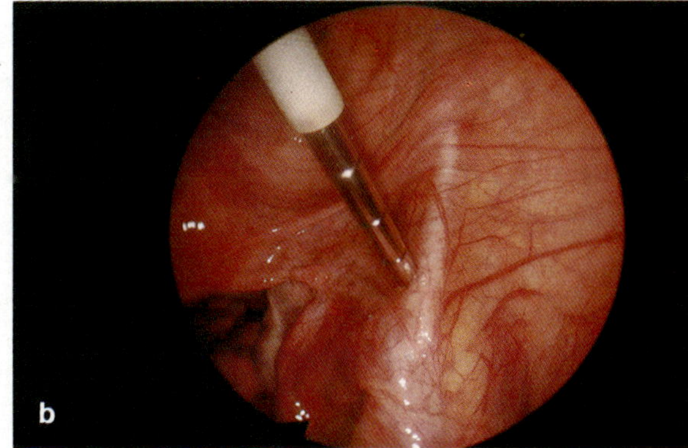

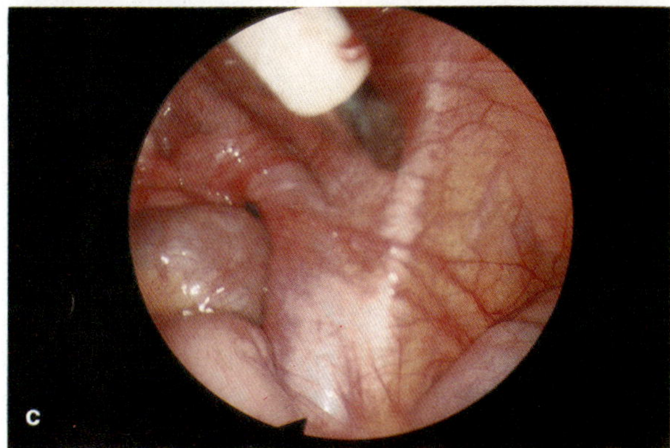

Figure 17.8 Misdirection of the auxiliary puncture trocar risks puncturing iliac vessels. *a*. Deviation from the midline aims the trocar toward the lateral pelvic wall. Use of the operator's more dextrous hand assists in controlling the thrust of the trocar insertion. *b*. Distance between auxiliary trocar sleeve and iliac vessels is generally no more than 4 cm. *c*. Indentation of the abdominal wall during auxiliary trocar insertion brings the sharp trocar in close proximity with the retroperitoneal vessels.

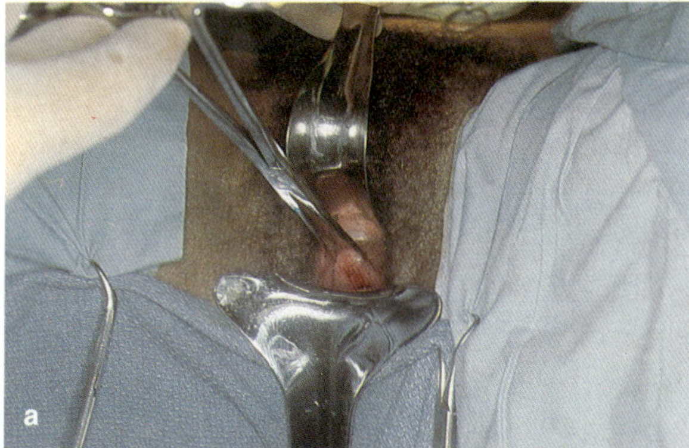

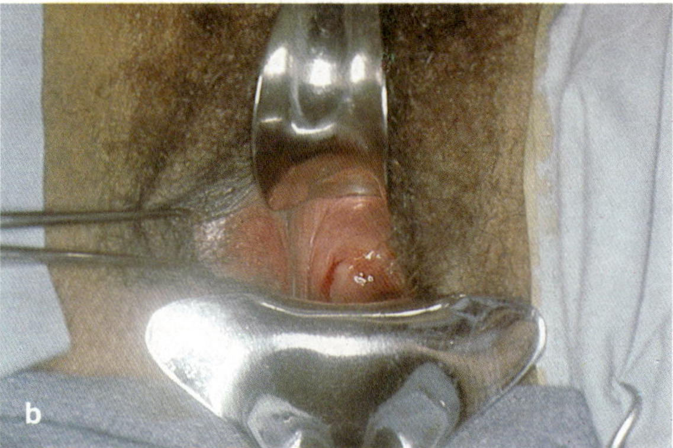

Figure 17.9 Single-toothed tenaculum injury to cervix. *a*. Tenaculum in place prior to its attachment to the uterine manipulator. *b*. Removal of tenaculum at the conclusion of the laparoscopy reveals bleeding from the application site. Packing the vagina with gauze sponges for up to one hour is usually effective in achieving hemostasis. More extensive trauma requires operative repair.

with the azygous vaginal artery to form an arterial circle around the cervix known as the coronary artery of the cervix. The venous drainage of the cervix parallels its arterial supply. The cervical venous network also communicates with a similar venous network draining the neck of the urinary bladder. These profusely distributed vessels are the usual source of bleeding resulting from tenaculum trauma.

If cervical vessel injury is diagnosed while the patient is still under anesthesia, the bleeding source can be easily identified and brought under control. Application of a single suture of absorbable material (4–0 chromic catgut, polyglycolic acid) is the method most commonly used. In patients with a short cervix (such as occurs in women exposed to diethylstilbestrol in utero), caution should be exercised when placing sutures for hemostasis. The close proximity of the base of the bladder and bladder neck to the cervix increases the risk of bladder injury from injudicious suturing.

Owing to the small caliber of vessels from which the bleeding originates, pressure may also be effective for achieving hemostasis. The prolonged application of hemostatic clamps (such as Kelly clamps or sponge forceps) is inadvisable since they may produce ischemic necrosis. Experience shows that packing the vagina with 3 or 4 gauze sponges (4 by 4 inches) closely apposed to the cervix for about one hour is equally effective and far less traumatic. Removal of the vaginal packing can usually be accomplished with minimal discomfort before the patient leaves the recovery room.

UTERINE PERFORATION

Uterine perforation complicating a laparoscopic procedure is not unusual. In patients undergoing laparoscopic sterilization, White et al reported an overall perforation rate of 30.4 per 1,000 procedures.[15] In their study factors ascribed as more likely to predispose to this complication were age 34 years or older, parity of four or more, and obesity of more than 20 percent above the ideal body weight for height. Chi and Feldblum reviewed over 20,000 sterilizations (16,379 laparoscopic sterilizations and 4,378 minilaparotomy sterilizations) and found similar rates of uterine perforation.[3] The perforating instrument is either the uterine sound used for evaluating the cervical axis and depth of the uterus or the uterine mobilizer used to manipulate the uterine corpus and facilitate endoscopic visualization of the pelvis.

Perforation of the uterine wall with a thin blunt instrument is not a serious complication unless it involves simultaneous injury of a major artery or vein. Analogous to a uterine perforation occurring at the time of an endometrial curettage, such a perforation can only be visualized translaparoscopically. Anterior and posterior uterine wall and fundal perforations tend not to bleed excessively. Translaparoscopic electrocoagulation of the bleeding site with unipolar or bipolar instruments is often sufficient to obtain adequate hemostasis. Alternatively, one may try application of microfibrillar collagen.[2]

Perforation at either cornual angle is usually accompanied by greater hemorrhage (Figure 17.10). In patients desiring to preserve fertility, the use of electrocoagulation in this area is contraindicated because extensive tubal destruction may occur. It is difficult to preserve tubal integrity under these circumstances. Failure to achieve hemostasis by the application of microcrystalline collagen means that a laparotomy is needed to identify the source and control the bleeding by application of sutures.

Perforation of the lateral wall of the uterus between the layers of the broad ligament cannot generally be seen translaparoscopically. It only becomes evident when accumulated blood separates the anterior and posterior leaves of the peritoneal reflection, thereby allowing the bluish hematoma to be identified visually. In contrast to the less vascularized thick fundal musculature, the lateral uterus is richly supplied by the ascending branch of the uterine artery. If a broad ligament hematoma is identified, a laparotomy is indicated with careful dissection of the region. The close proximity of the ureter to the uterine vessels mandates proper identification before hemostasis is attempted (Figure 17.11)

If a uterine perforation is identified in a recently pregnant uterus (that is, in a patient in whom a combined abortion-sterilization procedure is being done), the use of uterotonic agents may achieve adequate hemostasis by stimulating a sustained uterine contraction. Intramuscular or intramyometrial prostaglandin $F_{2\alpha}$ analogue has proved successful in this regard. Care should be taken when attempting to electrocauterize such an injury because it may increase the damage and further complicate the problem. Microfibrillar collagen can also help control bleeding from a perforation of a recently pregnant uterus.[2]

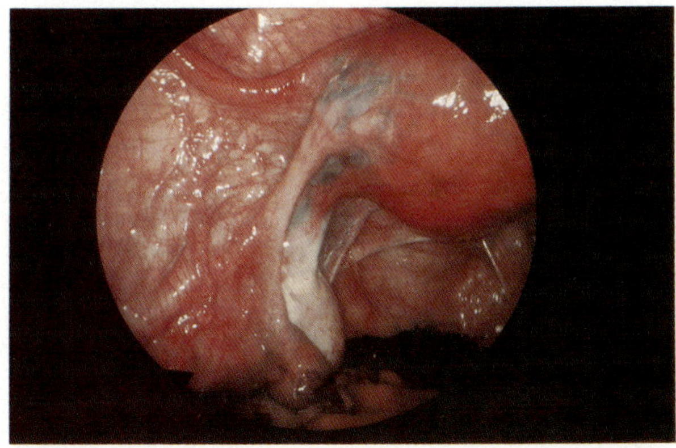

Figure 17.10 Vasculature of left uterine cornual area. Absorbed dilute methylene blue injected in the uterine cavity delineates the vascularity of the region. Perforation here could lead to intensive hemorrhage.

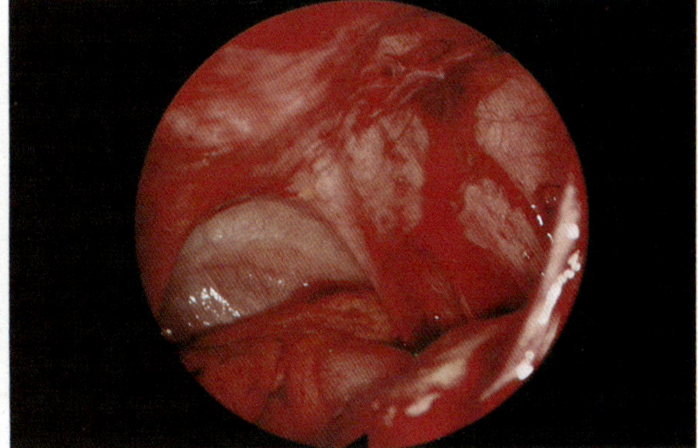

Figure 17.11 Lateral uterine perforation. Laceration of uterine vessels is the source of bleeding. Close proximity of the ureter requires laparotomy for careful identification of the lacerated vessel and dissection of the ureter before hemostasis is attempted.

Steps to prevent uterine perforation during a laparoscopic procedure include the careful sounding of the uterine cavity and the avoidance of excessive force when mobilizing the uterus. The uterus normally pivots on its anchoring ligaments (cardinal ligaments) in both anteroposterior and lateral planes. Attempts to mobilize the uterus in a cephalad direction by applying excessive force to the uterine manipulator predispose to uterine perforation by the cannula. A similar problem is seen when the uterine cavity is large (that is, immediately post abortion or in a fibroid uterus).

The risk of perforating the uterine wall with the uterine manipulator is increased with a small uterus. The standard length of the olive tip attached to the uterine cannula precludes adjustment for different size cavities. The Cohen patency cannula should not be used in patients with a hypoplastic postmenopausal uterus or a very small uterus resulting from prenatal exposure to diethylstilbestrol. In these patients, a negative pressure (suction device) attachment for the uterine manipulator is useful.

MESOSALPINGEAL TEARS

Mesosalpingeal hemorrhage is the most common complication associated with laparoscopic sterilizations. Its incidence, diagnosis, and causes will be discussed in greater detail in Chapter 22. In this section, the vascularization of the mesosalpingeal area will be described along with the different methods for achieving hemostasis in this region.

The arterial blood supply to the fallopian tubes derives from two main sources: the ascending branch of the uterine artery and the ovarian artery. Both of these arteries subdivide into tubal and ovarian branches which anastomose with each other. The tubal artery runs in the mesosalpinx parallel to the lower border of the fallopian tube, thereby supplying the distal portion of the tube (isthmus, ampulla, and fimbria). The ascending branch of the uterine artery gives origin to a cornual branch just prior to its final subdivision; this cornual branch provides the blood supply to the uterine cornu and the interstitial portion of the fallopian tube. Anastomotic arterial channels interconnect the tubal and ovarian vessels; these vary widely in number, but are almost always present. The venous drainage vessels replicate the arteries and run in close apposition. The surgeon must be knowledgeable about this intricate vascular network to enable him or her to secure hemostasis when needed.

Injury to the mesosalpingeal blood vessels may occur as a consequence of direct trauma by the Verres needle or the sharp puncture trocar, but it is most often the result of a laceration or transection at the time of tubal surgery. Translaparoscopic methods available to control hemorrhage in this region include the following: electrocoagulation (unipolar, bipolar), silicone band ligature (Falope ring), microfibrillar collagen topical application (Avitene), and clip application (Hulka clip).

Identification of the bleeding source is important for these methods to be effective. The use of an additional puncture site (secondary or tertiary) may be required in order to aspirate blood pooled from around the bleeding site. Bipolar-type forceps provide pressure occlusion by clamping the source of bleeding, thereby giving the surgeon additional time to attempt hemostasis by other methods. Failure to achieve hemostasis by any one of these techniques or any combination of them requires a laparotomy to accomplish the task.

Bleeding from the cornual region is not amenable to silicone band or clip ligature. Attempts to form an hemostatic loop for banding or pressure occlusion with a spring-loaded clip may lead to increased hemorrhage. Electrode (contact) or application of microfibrillar collagen is preferable. Electrocoagulation of the utero-ovarian ligament should be avoided whenever possible to prevent compromising ovarian circulation. Newer instrumentation, which allows translaparoscopic placement of fine-needle suture ligatures, enhances the operator's ability to control bleeding from this area.

Hemorrhage that originates at the isthmic and ampullary portion of the tube is amenable to a variety of hemostatic procedures. Effective measures can be directed at occluding the point of the vascular laceration or at interrupting the blood flow to the area. The dual origin of the arterial supply to this area must be kept in mind. Electrocoagulation of both tubal branches at their origin from uterine and ovarian arteries is usually sufficient to control the bleeding. Similar occlusion can be achieved by clips or silicone band rings. One should not attempt to electrocoagulate or band the ovarian vessels at the level of the infundibulopelvic ligament because they are too large in this structure. One risks producing more severe hemorrhage. As mentioned previously, every effort should be applied to avoid compromising the ovarian circulation. This may lead to impairment of its function (see Chapter 22).

BIOPSY SITE HEMORRHAGE

As experience is accumulated with diagnostic laparoscopy, the laparoscopist gains increasing confidence in his or her ability to perform translaparoscopic surgery in lieu of a laparotomy procedure. The capacity to biopsy a suspicious lesion enhances the diagnostic value of the laparoscope. Historically, hemostasis by electrocoagulation was once routinely done before any tissue was resected. Today, a biopsy can be free of any artifact or distortion created by such hemostatic measures. Indeed, it should be. However, resection of even a small amount of tissue can be complicated by hemorrhage.

It is of obvious importance for the surgeon to have detailed knowledge of the anatomy of the vascular supply to the organ to be sampled before undertaking a translaparoscopic biopsy. First, it guides the operator to select a biopsy site away from any major vessels in the region, if this is possible. Second, it permits identification of the bleeding artery or vein and its pathway so as to facilitate corrective hemostatic measures. Most critical is recognition of the proximity of large vascular pedicles to the area to be sampled; this perhaps contraindicates the biopsy.

Electrocoagulation of the bleeding biopsy site is the method most commonly used for hemostatic purposes. Although appropriate for mesosalpingeal tears occurring during a tubal sterilization procedure, it possesses some shortcomings when indiscriminately used. This method causes tissue coagulation and subsequent vascular thrombosis. The resulting necrosis and ischemia extends beyond the margins of the original biopsy so that considerably more tissue is destroyed.

Borten and Friedman reported the translaparoscopic use of microfibrillar collagen (Avitene) to achieve contact hemostasis at the site of uterine perforation.[2] This technique has since been successfully used in cases of mesosalpingeal and ovarian bleeding. It involves the application of microfibrillar collagen with an ovarian basket forceps; the material is held in place by a metal probe. If the bleeding is active, it may be necessary to perform a third puncture for purposes of aspirating the accumulated blood while applying the microcrystalline collagen. Microfibrillar collagen should be used judiciously because extensive intraperitoneal proliferative granulomatous response has been reported.[11] Nevertheless, its potential adverse aspects are counterbalanced by its demonstrated ability to provide effective hemostasis, thereby preventing unplanned laparotomy. It may thus shorten postoperative recovery time and reduce hospitalization.

OTHER VASCULAR INJURIES

Vascular injuries are not limited to abdominal wall and retroperitoneal vessels. Any intraperitoneal organ may be traumatized with resulting injury to its blood vessels.[1] Karam and Hajj reported the perforation of a mesenteric vessel by the Verres needle with rapid formation of a large hemoperitoneum.[5] Diagnosis of this complication was delayed until significant hypotension and tachycardia became evident after the laparoscopy was concluded. Failure to identify bleeding intraoperatively was thought to be due to pooling of blood in the upper abdomen while the patient was in the Trendelenburg position. Esposito reported a hematoma of the sigmoid colon produced at the time the Verres needle was inserted.[4] Prolonged visual surveillance through the laparoscope proved sufficient; the hematoma did not continue to enlarge. The patient did well.

Perforation of an omental vessel can also be the source of a large hemoperitoneum. Excessive bleeding from a lacerated omental vein may not occur until the procedure is completed and the pneumoperitoneum is deflated. The elevated intraperitoneal pressure may collapse the vessel walls, thereby acting as a tourniquet. Identification of this type of injury is usually made by direct visualization of the lacerated vessel.

It is not difficult to conjecture that any intraperitoneal structure can be inadvertantly injured during the execution of a blind procedure such as insertion of the Verres needle or the laparoscopic trocar (Figures 17.12 and 17.13). Serious complications may result from failure to identify the accident. Recognition of these unexpected complications is facilitated by panoramically inspecting the entire peritoneal cavity before concluding the laparoscopic procedure.

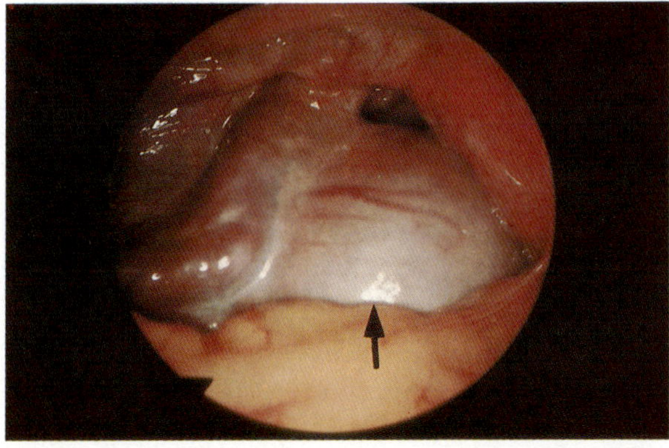

Figure 17.12 Ovarian vessel varicosity. Downward pressure by the left ovarian cyst (arrow) produces venous stasis. Injury to this dilated vein can occur during Verres needle insertion.

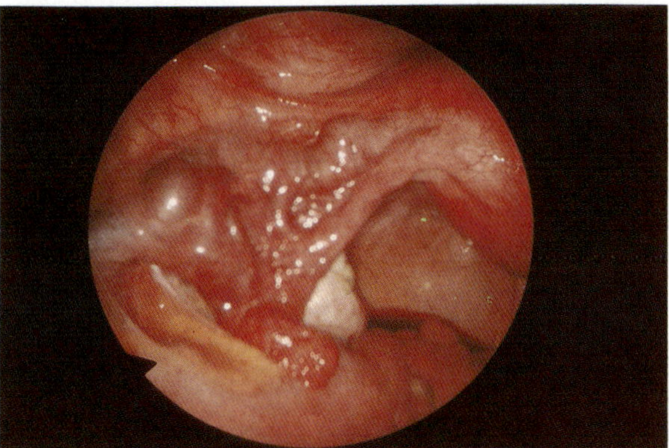

Figure 17.13 Pelvic venous engorgement. Vessels supplying and draining the left ovary fallopian tube appear greatly enlarged. Large vasculature is more susceptible to traumatic injury.

This should be done in all cases. Furthermore, we recommend repositioning the patient from Trendelenburg to supine position at the conclusion of the operation with the laparoscope still in place. This allows the operator to identify any accumulation of free intraperitoneal blood previously hidden in the pouch of Douglas or upper abdomen. It is mandatory to identify the source of any bleeding before the laparoscopy is terminated. Failure to do so exposes the patient to the risk of more severe and even life-threatening complications.

References

1. Bartsich EG, Dillon TF. Injury of superior mesenteric vein: Laparoscopic procedure with unusual complication. NY State J Med 1981; 81:932.
2. Borten M, Friedman EA. Translaparoscopic hemostasis with microfibrillar collagen in lieu of laparotomy. J Reprod Med 1983; 28:804-806.
3. Chi IC, Feldblum P. Uterine perforation during sterilization by laparoscopy and minilaparotomy. Am J Obstet Gynecol 1981; 139:735-736.
4. Esposito JM. Hematoma of the sigmoid colon as a complication of laparoscopy. Am J Obstet Gynecol 1973; 117:581-582.
5. Karam KS, Hajj SM. Mesenteric hematoma: Meckel's diverticulum: A rare laparoscopic complication. Fertil Steril 1977; 28:1003-1005.
6. Katz M, Beck P, Tancer ML. Major vessel injury during laparoscopy: Anatomy of two cases. Am J Obstet Gynecol 1979; 135:544-545.
7. Lynn SC, Katz AR, Ross PJ. Aortic perforation sustained at laparoscopy. J Reprod Med 1982; 27:217-219.
8. Makanji HH, Elliott HR. Rupture of spleen at laparoscopy: Case report. Br J Obstet Gynaecol 1980; 87:73-74.
9. McDonald PT, Rich NM, Collins GJ, et al. Vascular trauma secondary to diagnostic and therapeutic procedures: laparoscopy. Am J Surg 1978; 135:651-655.
10. Mintz M. Risks and prophylaxis in laparoscopy: A survey of 100,000 cases. J Reprod Med 1977; 18:269-272.
11. Park SA, Giannattasio C, Tancer ML. Foreign body reaction to the intraperitoneal use of Avitene. Obstet Gynecol 1981; 58:664-666.
12. Peterson HB, Greenspan JR, Ory HW. Death following puncture of the aorta during laparoscopic sterilization. Obstet Gynecol 1982; 59:133-134.
13. Pring DW. Inferior epigastric haemorrhage: An avoidable complication of laparoscopic clip sterilization. Br J Obstet Gynaecol 1983; 90:480-482.
14. Shin CS. Vascular injury secondary to laparoscopy. NY State J Med 1982; 82:935-936.
15. White MK, Ory HW, Goldenberg LA. A case-control study of uterine perforations documented at laparoscopy. Am J Obstet Gynecol 1977; 129:623-625.

18 GASTROINTESTINAL INJURIES

Injury to the gastrointestinal tract is a serious complication of laparoscopy. Its incidence has been reported to range between 0.5 and 3.0 per 1,000 procedures. This is perhaps an underestimate of its true occurrence rate. Only large lesions or those complicated by disseminated peritonitis or manifestations of an acute surgical abdomen are usually reported. Smaller, self-limited minimal injuries quite often go undiagnosed.

Gastrointestinal injuries complicating laparoscopy can be classified either according to their causative factor (Verres needle, sharp trocar, electrical instrument) or by the type of injury sustained (lacerating or electrocoagulating). The latter categorization seems more appropriate for the clinician because it helps dictate the therapeutic management.

LACERATING INJURIES

Direct injury to the gastrointestinal tract is less common than is electrical injury. Thompson and Wheeless reported only 1 of 11 traumatic bowel injuries were the result of direct injury with the laparoscopic trocar.[9] Nevertheless, failure to recognize this type of lesion may allow it to progress to a serious, at times even life-threatening, complication.

Lacerating intestinal injuries can be produced at the time of insertion of the Verres needle, laparoscopic trocar, and auxiliary trocar. The last is rare because most accessory punctures are performed under laparoscopic guidance. Predisposing factors include previous abdominal surgery, peritonitis, bowel distention, and unsuspected intraperitoneal disease. Nevertheless, more than half the cases of reported bowel injury complicating laparoscopy are described in patients without any of these qualifications.

Gastrointestinal injury at the time of Verres needle insertion is not unusual. Anatomically, in the absence of ascites or accumulation of air (from a perforated viscus) the peritoneal cavity is a virtual space, not an actual one. The parietal and visceral layers of peritoneum are in close contact. Little or no space exists between the abdominopelvic organs as well. Consequently, any instrument entering a closed abdominal cavity comes into contact with an intraperitoneal structure.

The Verres needle comes equipped with an inner spring-loaded blunt stylet. This is designed to push away any freely mobile organ from its outer sharp sleeve. Unfortunately, the narrow diameter of the needle (1.7 to 2.2 mm) may allow it to act as a perforating instrument itself.

Injury to diverse portions of the gastrointestinal tract by the Verres needle have been reported.[1] They include stomach, jejunoileal segment, and sigmoid colon. As with all Verres needle injuries (see Chapters 15 and 17), early recognition and management are accompanied by uneventful recovery.

The sharp laparoscopic trocar can produce injuries similar to those created by the Verres needle. The seriousness of the laceration is in direct proportion to its extent, that is, depth and size. Tissue destruction may range from a pinpoint hole produced by the tip of the pyramidal or conical trocar to one that extends the full diameter of the instrument's stem. The therapeutic approaches will vary accordingly.

Gastric Perforation

The anatomic position of the stomach varies according to its content and the body's posture. While one should be able to disregard the variations due to the presence of solids and fluid (since elective surgical procedure should not be undertaken in a patient who does not have an empty stomach), one recognizes that there are times when emergency laparoscopy may have to be done in a patient who has eaten recently. The full stomach is at even greater risk of perforation than an empty one. In the erect female, the most caudal part of the greater gastric curvature is found below the interiliac line (thus below the level of the umbilicus) in 87 percent of radiographically studied cases.[4] In the horizontal position, the lower edge of the greater curvature of the stomach can be seen below the interiliac line in up to 25 percent of cases. The use of the Trendelenburg position further reduces the possibility that the stomach will be located just under the umbilicus.

Endler and Moghissi reported two cases of stomach perforation at the time of Verres needle insertion.[1] They suggested that gaseous distention of the stomach at the time of anesthetic induction was the most common predisposing cause. In both instances, the injury was recognized early, allowing removal and reinsertion of the Verres needle and thus completion of the laparoscopy.

Gastric perforation by the Verres needle at the time of insertion is suspected when gastric fluid can be recovered during the saline injection-aspiration test (Figure 18.1). Following insufflation of the distending gas, the appearance of eructation or stomach borborygmi is highly suggestive of intragastric placement of the Verres needle. Stethoscopic auscultation of intragastric air turbulence or production of eructation by pressing on the epigastric region further supports such a diagnosis.

When gastric perforation is suspected, passing a nasogastric tube decompresses the stomach at once. Displacement of the decompressed stomach may free it spontaneously from the perforating instrument. Removal and reinsertion of a new sterile Verres needle can then be accomplished.

In the course of a laparoscopy, it is essential to visualize the site of gastric perforation to assess the degree of damage and to determine if there is any bleeding. In the absence of active bleeding, the gastric musculature generally seals

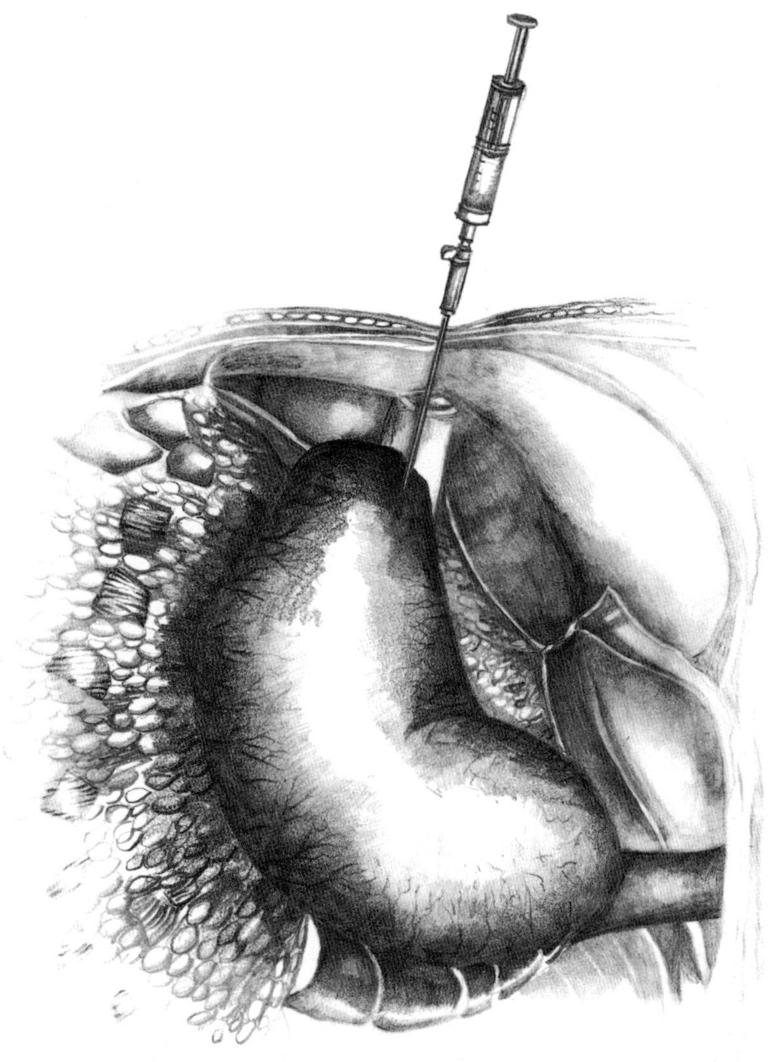

Figure 18.1 Gastric perforation, shown schematically in sagittal view. Distended stomach is located beneath the umbilicus. Insertion of the Verres needle in a routine manner enters the gastric cavity. Aspiration of gastric contents prior to carbon dioxide insufflation confirms the extraperitoneal location of the needle.

off the perforation spontaneously. The nasogastric tube is left in place to assist the healing process by continuous gastric decompression. This step avoids undesirable gastric distention and precludes leakage of gastric fluid into the peritoneal cavity.

Perforating injuries to the stomach can also be produced by the sharp laparoscopic trocar. In these circumstances, the traumatic opening in the gastric wall is of greater dimension and corresponds to the size of the laparoscope being used. An injury of 5 mm diameter or less is usually still amenable to conservative management since it is no larger than one produced by a gastrostomy tube. When the perforation through the stomach wall is larger, however, surgical closure is recommended.

Prevention and recognition of iatrogenic gastric distention is a responsibility shared by both the laparoscopist and the anesthesiologist. On some occasions gastric distention may precede the initiation of the laparoscopy altogether (as a result of aerophagia in a very anxious patient, for example). More often than not, inflation of the stomach occurs at the time of preoxygenation or during manual pulmonary insufflation between the induction of anesthesia and the endotracheal intubation. Failure to place an endotracheal tube for ventilation during laparoscopy (when done under inhalation anesthesia) is a predipossing factor for inadvertent inflation of the stomach.

Hirt and Morris reported another cause of altered anatomy that led to gastric puncture by the Verres needle.[5] They described adherence of the omentum to a ruptured right pyosalpinx. As a consequence, the stomach was brought downward to just beneath the umbilicus. Placing the patient in steep Trendelenburg did not displace the abdominal organs cephalad because the adhesions restricted their normal mobility. Whenever gastric distention is suspected prior to or during laparoscopy, insertion of a nasogastric tube is indicated. Difficulty in diagnosing this condition in the obese patient supports the recommendation for the use of a nasogastric tube in all these subjects as a preventive measure.

Small Bowel Perforation

Trauma to the small intestine complicating a laparoscopic procedure is one of the most serious accidents confronting the laparoscopist.[7] Injuries produced by the Verres needle usually go unrecognized. Nevertheless, it is most important to dwell on them at some length because of the life-threatening condition they may initiate.

Traumatic bowel injury at laparoscopy tends to occur more often under certain circumstances. These include the presence of dense intra-abdominal adhesions from prior surgery, disseminated carcinoma, and bowel distention. Nonetheless, absence of these predisposing factors does not ensure against this accident. For a more thorough description of these conditions and their potential impact on the procedure, see Chapter 6.

The small intestine extends from the pylorus of the stomach to the ileocecal valve. This measures approximately 22 ft (duodenum 2 ft, jejunum 8 ft, and ileum 12 ft). The duodenum is the most fixed part of the small intestine; it does not have a mesentery and is partially covered by peritoneum. The jejunoileum is mobile. It is attached to the posterior wall of the peritoneal cavity by its mesentery. The jejunoileum is covered by peritoneum (serosa) which is continuous with its mesenteric leaves. Two layers of muscle can be distinguished beneath the serosa: a thin longitudinal outer layer and a thicker circular inner muscle layer. Between these two muscle layers is located the myenteric nerve plexus of Auerbach. A connective tissue submucosa, a smooth muscle layer (muscularis mucosae), and the mucosa stratum complete the composition of the intestinal wall.

Perforation of the jejunoileum with the Verres needle can be promptly recognized when intestinal fluid is recovered during the syringe-aspiration test (Figure 18.2). This safety step ought to be performed routinely prior to the insufflation of distending gas. Intraluminal location of the insufflating needle is difficult to recognize during insufflation of gas. This is because the intraintestinal and intraperitoneal pressures are not significantly different from each other at the onset of insufflation. Several liters of gas are required to raise the insufflating pressure within the closed compartment of the intestinal lumen.

Perforation of the jejunoileum with the Verres needle is usually inconsequential. Intraperitoneal spillage of intestinal fluid is prevented by contraction of the bowel musculature that seals off such a small opening. Because the peritoneal cavity is a potential space prior to the insufflation of gas, it is believed that this type of piercing injury probably occurs more often than is currently known or reported. Lack of subsequent complications underscores the usually benign nature of this accident. Nevertheless, whenever an intestinal perforation is identified at the time it occurs, it is advisible to hospitalize the patient for a 24 to 48 hour observation period.

On occasion, injury to the bowel wall does not cause a complete perforation. Partial transfixation of the bowel with a Verres needle is usually inconsequential if the vascular supply has not been compromised. Failing to recognize the abnormal location of the needle and proceeding to insufflate with distending gas results in bullous distention of the intestinal wall (Figure 18.3). Early identification, to which one should be alerted by a rapid rise in insufflating pressure, is essential to prevent rupture of the bowel wall. Diagnosis of bullous distention does not require any therapy since the gas is promptly reabsorbed. Nevertheless, the patient should be admitted for observation because one cannot determine the degree of weakening of the bowel wall by direct visualization; thus, the potential for rupture is always present.

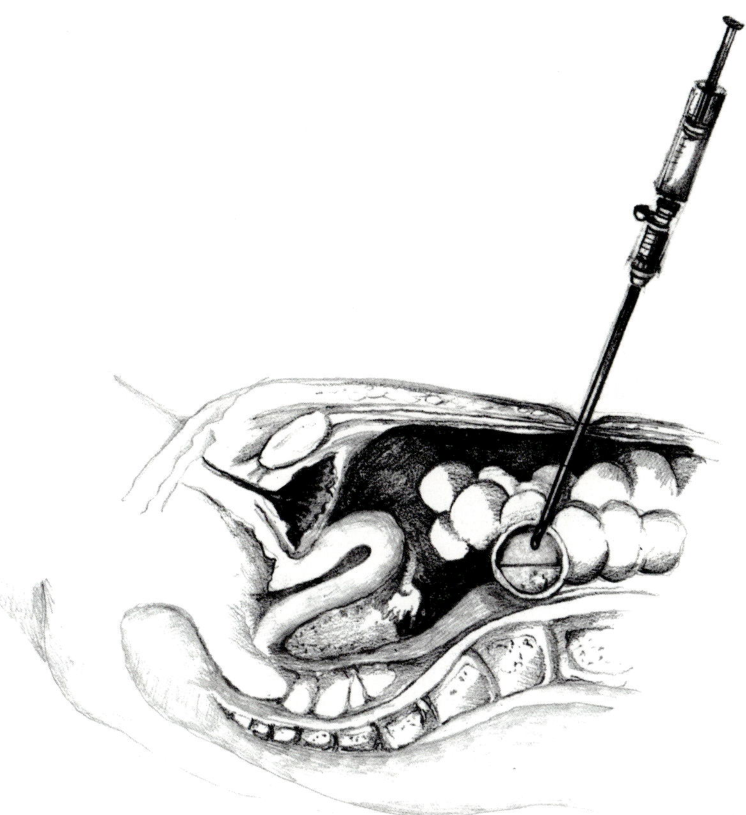

Figure 18.2 Bowel perforation. Aspiration of intestinal fluid confirms the abnormal location of the insufflating needle. Withdrawal and reinsertion (of a new sterile needle) is usually sufficient to correct this complication.

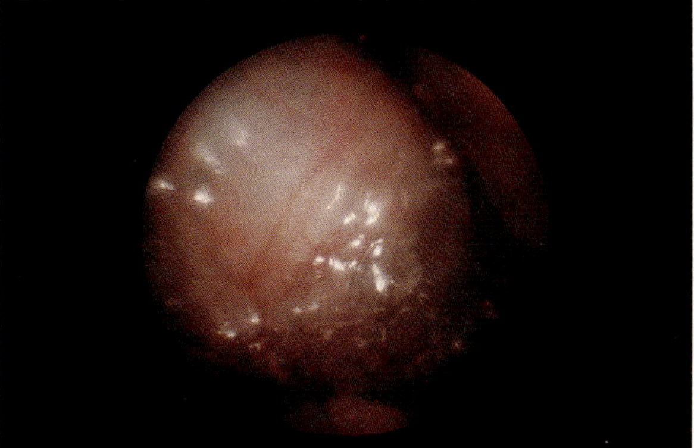

Figure 18.3 Bowel wall emphysema. Verres needle pierced the bowel serosa. Bullous distention of the intestinal wall resulted from carbon dioxide insufflation into the subserosa. Elevated insufflating pressure dictates discontinuing the insufflation. Spontaneous reabsorption of the gas within the bowel wall can be expected.

Perforation of the jejunoileum with the Verres needle does not make it necessary to stop the laparoscopy. Removal of the insufflating needle followed by reinsertion at a different angle usually suffices, permitting laparoscopy to be carried out in a routine fashion. Use of a new sterile Verres needle is recommended whenever feasible.

Whether to administer antibiotics or not during the observation period remains controversial. I feel their use is justified because most laparoscopies are performed in patients without prior preoperative bowel preparation. Coverage for enterobacteria and anaerobes must be included.

Patients undergoing second-look laparoscopy for cancer evaluation are at a higher risk of experiencing intestinal perforating injuries. The laparoscopist may consider the use of preoperative mechanical bowel cleansing in these cases. Prophylactic antibiotic administration may also prove advantageous.

Every effort should be made to identify the site of perforation. Whereas the risk of serious complications following a simple puncture of the small bowel is minimal, the potential for piercing a vessel in the bowel wall or its mesentery is always present. Laceration of a bowel vessel requires visual evaluation to ascertain the degree of bleeding or hematoma formation (Figure 18.4). If bleeding is not active and the hematoma is self limited, hospitalization for observation is required. Stable vital signs and lack of peritoneal signs for 48 hours following the initial injury are good prognostic factors.

To the contrary, evidence of active intraperitoneal bleeding or continuous enlargement of the hematoma requires a laparotomy for the purpose of providing hemostasis. Ligature of the injured vessel is, at times, all that is required. When a mesenteric vessel has been injured, resection of a segment of bowel and an end-to-end anastomosis may be indicated.

Injury to the intestine by the sharp laparoscopic trocar is more serious (Figure 18.5). Subsequent complications are related to the extent of damage (depth and size). The trauma may involve the small or large bowel.

Sharp trocar injuries to the bowel can be superficial (limited to serosa) or deep (entire wall thickness). Superficial lacerations that affect only the serosa need not be repaired. Observation must ensure adequate hemostasis of the surrounding tissues. Patients can be discharged on the day of surgery following the usual postoperative recovery. Notwithstanding the rapid healing of a serosal lesion, the strength of the bowel wall at the site of injury is weakened. Patients must be advised to report any untoward reaction occurring within the first 7 postoperative days.

Perforating injuries to the bowel wall must be evaluated individually on a case by case basis. Generally, small lacerations not greater than the Verres needle diameter can be managed conservatively. Continuous observation and antibiotic coverage is recommended. The patient should be kept without alimentation by mouth during the observation period. This reduces the amount of

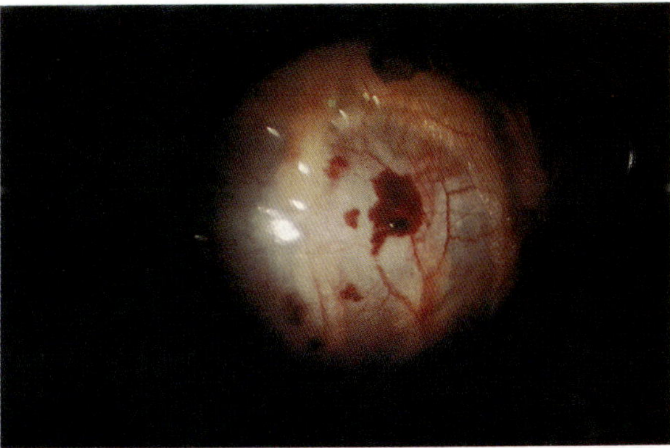

Figure 18.4 Subserosal bowel hematoma. An intestinal vessel was injured during insertion of the Verres needle. If the hemorrhagic diathesis remains subserosal, it is usually self limited. Prolonged observation (not less than 5 minutes) is indicated to ensure that there is no free bleeding into the peritoneal cavity. During this time, the operator must evaluate for continued expansion of the hematoma within the bowel wall.

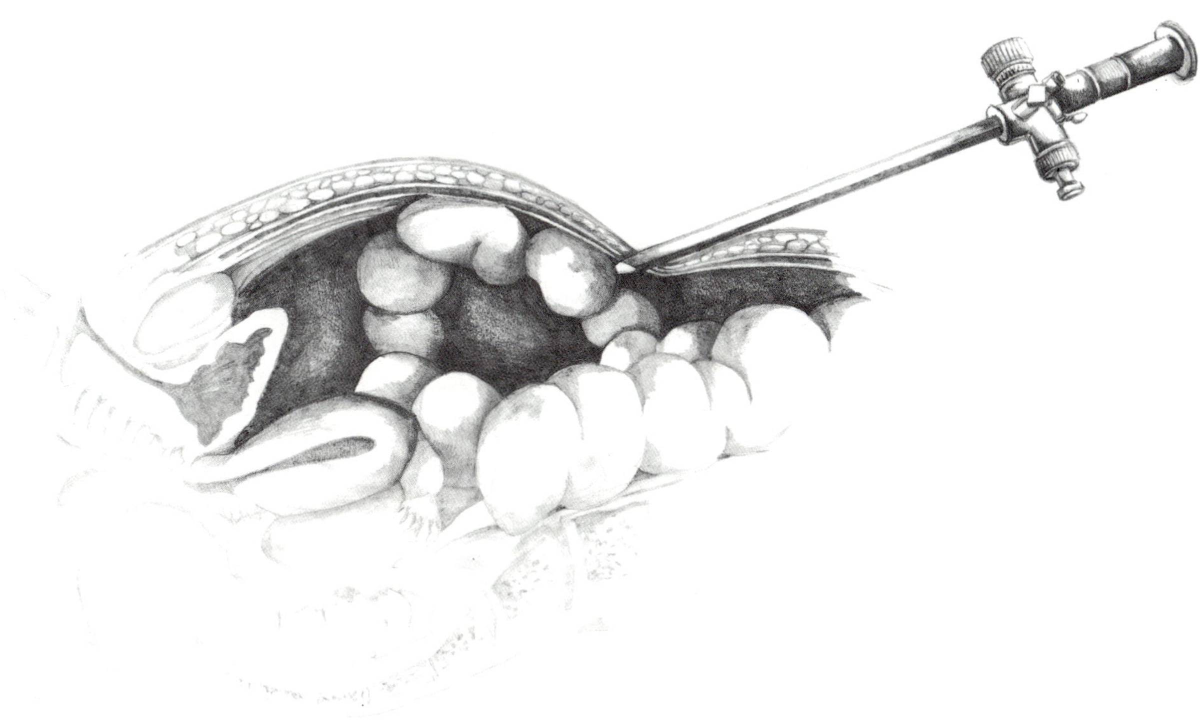

Figure 18.5 Bowel perforation with laparoscopic trocar. A loop of intestine is adherent to the posterior aspect of the anterior abdominal wall. The pneumoperitoneum has failed to displace the entire bowel from the subumbilical area. Visualization of intraluminal bowel content or a foul smell raises the suspicion of intestinal injury.

intestinal contents. In addition, the patient should be advised of the event and its complication so that she is prepared in the event of a major abdominal procedure being required under general anesthesia.

Irrespective of the size of the bowel perforation, any spilled intestinal contents into the peritoneal cavity identified at laparoscopy require reparative surgery. An initial row of absorbable interrupted sutures (3–0 chromic catgut) approximates the mucosa and muscularis layers. A reinforcing tier of nonabsorbable interrupted (3–0 silk) Lembert stitches brings the muscularis and serosal edges together. Longitudinal (axial) lacerations of the small intestine are repaired transversely. This prevents stenosis of its lumen.

Spilled intestinal fluid must be aspirated. Copious amounts of physiologic saline solution are used to lavage the peritoneal cavity. Antibiotic coverage for enteric aerobic and anaerobic bacteria is indicated.

Large lacerations of the intestinal wall require laparotomy for repair. Clean edged injuries can be handled in the same way as described for small penetrating lesions. Ragged lacerations require segmental bowel resection to restore intestinal continuity. A single layer (of through and through absorbable sutures), open intestinal anastomosis, (Gambee technique) was popularized by Wheeless for gynecologic surgery.[10] For a detailed description of bowel resection and reanastomosis techniques, the laparoscopist is referred to standard surgical treatises.

Large Bowel Perforation

Traumatic injury of the large bowel during laparoscopy is a rare event. It usually occurs in patients with some predisposing factor such as prior abdominal surgery. The high morbidity and mortality associated with penetrating colon injuries require prompt identification and management whenever this type of accident takes place.

The large bowel lies against the posterior abdominal wall. It extends from the end of the ileum to the anus. The ascending, transverse and descending portions of colon are positioned laterally and form a frame for the small intestine. Only its terminal portion (rectosigmoid) lies in the midline.

The cecum, ascending and descending portions of colon remain fixed to the posterior abdominal wall by short mesenteries. The transverse colon and sigmoid have longer mesenteries which give them more mobility. The rectum is entirely retroperitoneal in location. The muscular wall of the large intestine is composed by internal and external layers. The internal circular layer is found throughout the large bowel. The outer longitudinal layer covers the appendix entirely and then subdivides. It forms three narrow bands or tenia (mesocolica, omentalis, and libera). These bands coalesce at the rectosigmoid junction to cover the rectum with a full longitudinal muscular layer.

Perforation of the large bowel with the Verres needle can sometimes be promptly recognized by the saline aspiration test. Recovery of fecally stained fluid is pathognomonic. An additional characteristic is the fecal odor that can be detected following insertion of the insufflating needle. The needle should be promptly withdrawn.

Reinsertion must be done with another sterile Verres needle. Because the colon has the single most concentrated accumulation of bacteria, any instrument which has entered its lumen is highly contaminated. Utilization of a nonsterile insufflating needle may give rise to severe septic morbidity.

At the time of laparoscopy, one must attempt to identify the lacerated area. Because of the high bacterial concentration, minor leaks of fecal material into the peritoneal cavity can be the source of a large and hazardous inoculum. Aspiration of peritoneal fluid for bacterial culture and sensitivity studies is helpful.

Treatment of small colonic wounds associated with minimal contamination remains controversial. At present, laparotomy with primary suture closure is an accepted therapeutic modality. Copious lavage of the peritoneal cavity with physiologic saline solution is indicated prior to abdominal closure. Broad spectrum antibiotics against aerobic and anaerobic organisms must be administered.

Injuries to the large bowel created by the laparoscopic trocar require more extensive therapy. Trauma to the right colon is managed by resection of the lacerated segment of bowel. Primary anastomosis can be attempted under these circumstances since most injuries occur in stable patients. Diverting ileostomy is said to facilitate healing and thus reduce the morbidity and mortality associated with this type of lesion.

Injury of the descending colon, sigmoid, and rectum are not amenable to primary closure or resection with primary anastomosis. Diverting colostomy with resection of the injured portion is recommended. Primary closure with exteriorization of the colonic wound to prevent intra-abdominal leakage has also been suggested.[6] More experience is needed before this approach can be supported.

ELECTROCOAGULATING INJURY

The physiopathology of electrical injuries to the bowel will be described in detail in Chapter 23. What differentiates this type of injury from the lacerating ones is its subtle presentation. Patients usually remain asymptomatic for up to 72 hours postoperatively.[9] Signs and symptoms of disruption of bowel wall continuity may develop slowly. Vague complaints of abdominal discomfort initially are the norm rather than the exception.

Most intestinal burns complicating laparoscopic surgery follow an essentially uneventful procedure. This tends to delay the diagnosis. Occasionally, the operator identifies an area of blanching on the bowel serosa. This represents thermal trauma. If the lesion appears to be small (less than 5 mm) in diameter, expectant observation is acceptable. During the observation period which may extend 3 to 5 days, the laparoscopist should be alerted to the early manifestations of peritonitis. They include nausea, anorexia, vomiting, lower abdominal cramps, and low grade fever.

Some of the aforementioned symptoms may be present during the immediate postoperative period of an otherwise uncomplicated case. What enhances their significance is their interval appearance. Patients ordinarily should recover uneventfully for 1 to 2 days following the laparoscopy, and if complicated, they start experiencing the symptoms previously described. If appropriate therapy is not instituted, most of them go on to develop ileus and pelvic peritonitis. Most deaths attributed to complicating bowel burns after tubal sterilization describe a similar pattern.[8]

If the identified area thermally injured is larger than 5 mm, therapy must be instituted at once. Because one is unable to ascertain the true depth or lateral extension of such lesions, damage can be expected to exceed that seen. Therefore, these patients are at increased risk of bowel perforation. Repair can be accomplished by extirpation of the injured area followed by primary closure. Oversewing the area with adjacent healthy bowel muscularis and serosa has also been suggested. By utilizing either technique, the patient may be spared a bowel resection with or without a diverting procedure (ileostomy or colostomy).

Patients presenting with any of the aforementioned symptoms following their discharge from the surgical facility should be readmitted for observation. Failure to respond to conservative therapy (including intravenous antibiotics) for 24 hours warrants more aggressive intervention. Exploratory laparotomy is indicated for patients with persistent symptoms on the third or fourth postoperative day. Resection of the damaged portion of bowel and primary reanastomosis are the standard therapeutic approaches.

If peritonitis is already established, the surgical procedure may have to be modified accordingly. A diverting procedure may be required. In all instances, the peritoneal cavity should be cleansed with copious amounts of physiologic saline solution. The pelvis and abdomen should be liberally drained. Broad coverage antibiotic therapy is also indicated.

OTHER INJURIES

Traumatic injury to the bowel complicating a laparoscopy is not limited to lacerations produced by the Verres needle or the sharp trocar. Ancillary procedures performed under direct endoscopic observation can also result in undesirable intestinal wounds. Gentile and Siegler reported inadvertent biopsy of the small intestine during translaparoscopic salpingoneostomy.[3] The diagnosis was confirmed by histologic evaluation after 36 hours. Signs and symptoms of peritoneal inflammation were evident within 72 hours after surgery. At laparotomy, a small defect in the distal ileum was identified requiring an ileal resection with end-to-end anastomosis.

Esposito reported the incorporation of a knuckle of bowel within a silastic band applied to the fallopian tube.[2] The silastic ring was divided with translaparoscopic scissors and another band applied to the oviduct. The patient made an uneventful recovery.

Care should be exercised during translaparoscopic bowel manipulations. Displacement of small bowel from the pelvis by means of a metal probe is frequently performed to facilitate visualization of the pelvic organs. Such maneuvers should be carried out gently and always under vision. If bowel adhesions are present, it is recommended that additional auxiliary probes be inserted. Forceful displacement of adhered bowel may lead to blunt laceration of the intestinal wall.

References

1. Endler GC, Moghissi KS. Gastric perforation during pelvic laparoscopy. Obstet Gynecol 1976; 47(s):40s-42s.
2. Esposito JM. An unusual complication of tubal sterilization by silicone rubber banding under laparoscopic vision. Am J Obstet Gynecol 1976; 126:507-508.
3. Gentile GP, Siegler AM. Inadvertent intestinal biopsy during laparoscopy and hysteroscopy: A report of two cases. Fertil Steril 1981; 36:402-404.
4. Gray H. Anatomy of the Human Body. In: Goss CM (ed) 29th edition. Philadelphia, Lea & Febiger 1973:1225.
5. Hirt PS, Morris R. Gastric bleeding secondary to laparoscopy in a patient with salpingitis. Obstet Gynecol 1982; 59:655-657.
6. Kirkpatrick JR, Rajpal SG. The injured colon: Therapeutic considerations. Am J Surg 1975; 129:187-191.
7. Levinson CJ, Schwartz SF, Saltzstein EC. Complication of laparoscopic tubal cauterization: Small bowel perforation. Obstet Gynecol 1973; 41:253-256.
8. Peterson HB, DeStefano F, Rubin GL, Greenspan JR, Lee NC, Ory HW. Deaths attributable to tubal sterilization in the United States. Am J Obstet Gynecol 1981; 146:131-136.
9. Thompson BH, Wheeless CR. Gastrointestinal complications of laparoscopy sterilization. Obstet Gynecol 1973; 41:669-676.
10. Wheeless CR. The Gambee intestinal anastomosis in gynecologic surgery. Obstet Gynecol 1975; 46:448-452.

19 URINARY TRACT INJURIES

Close proximity between the urinary tract and the female genital organs makes the former susceptible to injury during a gynecologic surgical procedure. Knowledge about prevention, identification, and correction of such injuries is an integral part of the training of a gynecologist. Nevertheless, the incidence of injuries to the urinary tract has increased as new and more sophisticated operations are being performed.[9]

Trauma to the bladder and ureters has been described as a complication of laparoscopy and translaparoscopic surgery. The incidence of damage to the urinary tract during laparoscopy is low, generally totalling less than 0.5 percent. Nevertheless, failure to identify injury at the time of laparoscopy or in the immediate postoperative period may result in serious sequelae.

URINARY BLADDER INJURY

Traumatization of the urinary bladder is a rare complication in laparoscopy. It occurs primarily in patients in whom a congenital malformation and/or prior pelvic surgery has distorted the normal anatomic relationship of the organs in the area.[3] A similar predisposing condition can be created iatrogenically by failure to empty the bladder prior to the introduction of the laparoscopic instruments.

A brief description of the normal anatomy of the urinary bladder and its relation to the surrounding structures aids in the understanding and prevention of urinary tract injuries. The urinary bladder is a musculomembranous sac that acts solely as a reservoir for urine. In the adult, the bladder is located within the anterior half of the pelvis and lies between the symphysis anteriorly and the uterus posteriorly. Its multifaceted shape (tetrahedron) can, for didactic purposes, be divided into a posterior wall or base, a superior wall or dome, and an anterior wall. The bladder is an entirely extraperitoneal organ.

Functionally, the posterior bladder wall, including the vesical trigone, is relatively fixed when compared with the rest of the organ. The superior bladder surface is dome shaped, and is the only portion covered by peritoneum. The anterior wall extends from the urachal insertion at the top to the vesical neck inferiorly. The junction between the superior surface and anterior bladder wall (the area of urachal attachment) is called the vertex. Both the superior and the anterior bladder walls are freely mobile and vary in position and shape during the transition from the empty to the full state. The bladder is held in position by the pubovesical ligaments which attach the deep pelvic fascia to the pubic bone. These ligamentous attachments surround the posterior bladder wall (base), thereby supporting the entire organ. In the retropubic region, (space of Retzius), the bladder is attached to the pubis and the anterior abdominal wall by loose areolar tissue; this allows easy mobility, but little structural support.

In infants and small children, the bladder maintains an intra-abdominal position. The area covered by peritoneum is proportionally much larger than in the adult. This fact must be kept in mind when performing a laparoscopy in very young patients.

When empty, the bladder contains small amounts of urine (less than 30 cc). Its superior surface is concave in shape, and its peritoneal covering forms the anterior and inferior walls of the anterior cul-de-sac. The anterior wall of the bladder lies wholly behind the pubis.

Under normal conditions, the capacity of the bladder is 300 to 600 cc. Its inherent distensibility allows the bladder to accommodate up to 4 L of urine under abnormal conditions. The dynamic change in volume is accompanied by concomitant anatomic variations in position and interorgan relationships. As the organ gradually fills, the bladder vertex rises suprapubically. Under extreme filling conditions, it can even extend to the level of the umbilicus.

Conditions that predispose to injuring the bladder during laparoscopy are at times impossible to anticipate. Congenital malformation of the urinary tract (the urachal anomaly in particular) is an example of this type of hidden condition.[1] However, sometimes predisposing factors can be elicited preoperatively by obtaining a careful medical history. Antecedent abdomino-pelvic surgery (including cesarean section) may in some circumstances become a relative contraindication to laparoscopy. Preoperative failure to prepare the patient by neglecting to ensure that the bladder is empty also contributes to the risk of bladder injury during laparoscopy.

Congenital Anomalies of the Urinary Tract

Embryologically, the urachus or median umbilical ligament is the vestige of the obliterated allantois. Anatomically, the urachus is a midline structure extending from the umbilicus to the dome of the bladder. It is attached anteriorly to the transversalis fascia and posteriorly to the parietal peritoneum.

Urachal anomalies have four variants: (1) patent urachus with free communication between the bladder and the umbilicus; (2) urachal sinus with communication of the urachal lumen with the umbilicus; (3) urachal cyst in which proximal and distal urachal ends are obliterated, but in which there is a patent middle portion; and (4) vesicourachal diverticulum in which there is free communication of the lumen of the urachus with the urinary bladder.

Whereas laparoscopy is not specifically indicated for either of the first two conditions (patent urachus, urachal sinus), the last two are asymptomatic and may warrant laparoscopic evaluation. Nonetheless, these findings are usually incidental. Therefore, it is not difficult to envision the potential complication of perforating a urachal cyst or a vesicourachal diverticulum with the Verres needle or the primary or secondary trocar puncture during laparoscopy (Figure 19.1). Hematoma formation, leakage of urine, or the more dangerous intraperitoneal dissemination of the contents of an infected urachal cyst could ensue under such circumstances.

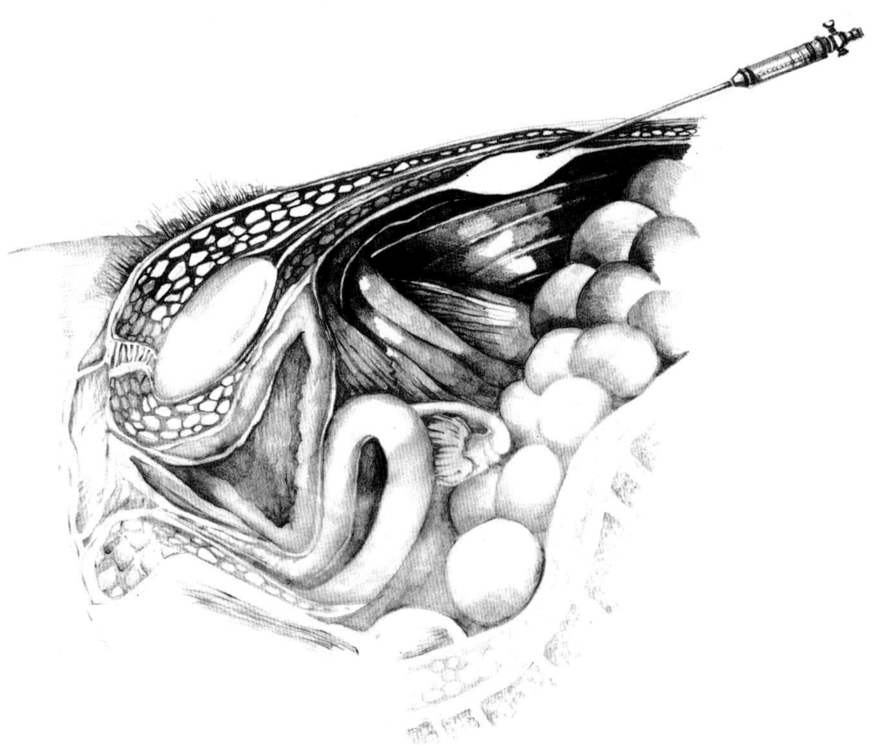

Figure 19.1 Urachal cyst perforation with Verres needle. Aspiration of urine through the Verres needle is possible. This is usually an incidental finding at the time of laparoscopy.

Previous Surgery

As described under anatomic considerations, the anterior and superior bladder walls are loosely attached to the surrounding structures. Easy mobility is important to the proper function of the organ. Structural changes arising as a consequence of surgery on or near the bladder can change its position. Commonly, following abdomino-pelvic surgery, the bladder is drawn upward by the healing process which may involve fibrosis of surrounding tissue (Figures 19.2 and 19.3). From the practical point of view, abnormal location of the urinary bladder should always be suspected in a patient who has had a previous infraumbilical laparotomy. This includes surgery for benign as well as malignant lesions.

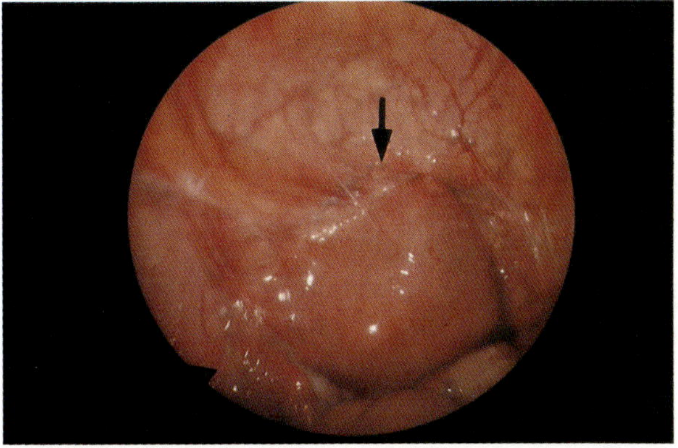

Figure 19.2 Cephalad displacement of urinary bladder. The bladder has become adherent to the anterior wall of the uterus after a cesarean section. Dark spots (arrow) indicate line of previously placed silk sutures.

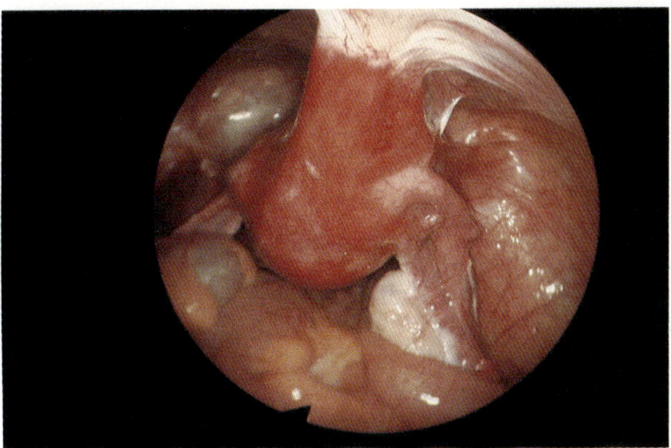

Figure 19.3 Obliteration of vesicouterine peritoneal fold. Patient had had a myomectomy several years prior to the laparoscopy (same case as Figure 4.2)

Failure to Empty the Bladder

By far the most common underlying condition predisposing the patient to bladder injury during laparoscopy is a distended bladder (Figure 19.4). A retained urinary volume as small as 100 cc can expose the bladder to an increased risk of trauma (Figure 19.5). Consequently, the most important precaution a laparoscopist can take to prevent trauma is to ensure that the urinary bladder is empty immediately prior to surgery. This is easily accomplished by straight catheterization of the urinary bladder just before vaginal examination of the patient and the placement of the uterine mobilizer. When additional surgery is contemplated, placement of a Foley catheter precludes the need for repeated catheterization. Knowledge of the intraluminal location of the Foley catheter balloon avoids confusion of it with an abnormal finding (Figure 19.6).

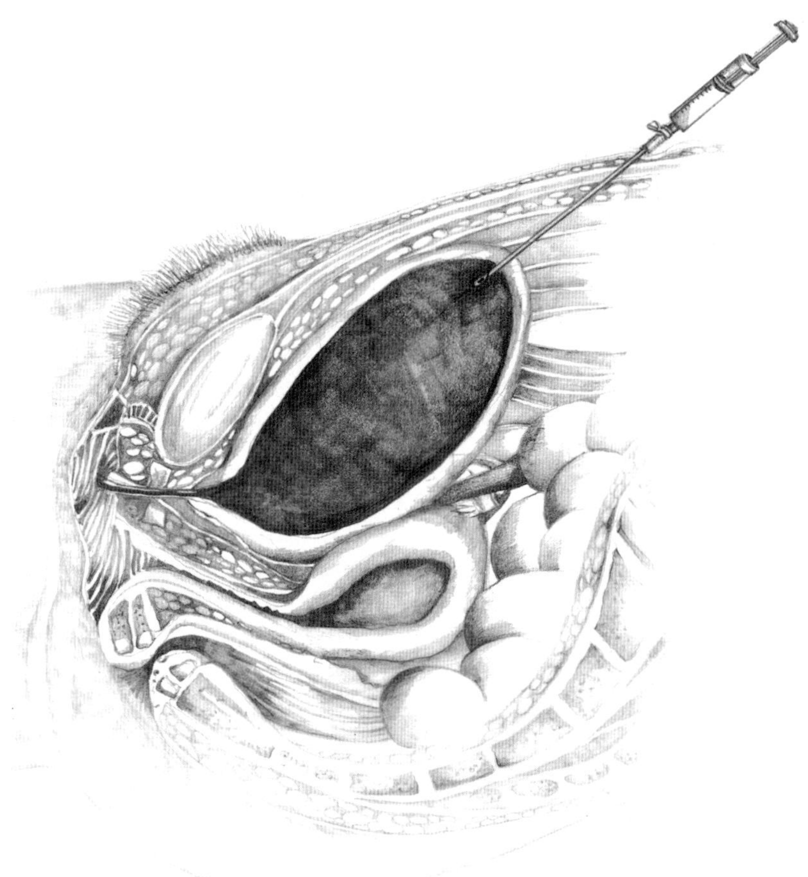

Figure 19.4 Bladder perforation with Verres needle. Urine can be retrieved by aspiration. Bladder catheterization before creating the pneumoperitoneum generally prevents this complication.

Some laparoscopists maintain that emptying the bladder by spontaneous voluntary voiding a few minutes prior to the procedure is a sufficient preventive measure. This has not proved to be effective in all cases. Anxiety may prevent a patient from voiding on demand while waiting for surgery. Additionally, the volume of residual urine which remains post voiding is variable among patients. Large volumes (100 to 200 cc) of urine can be found in women with incipient or established urinary stress incontinence and/or bladder dysfunction.

Injury to the urinary bladder may be produced by the Verres needle, the laparoscopic trocar, the laparoscope itself, the secondary puncture trocar, or by any auxiliary instrument used during laparoscopy.

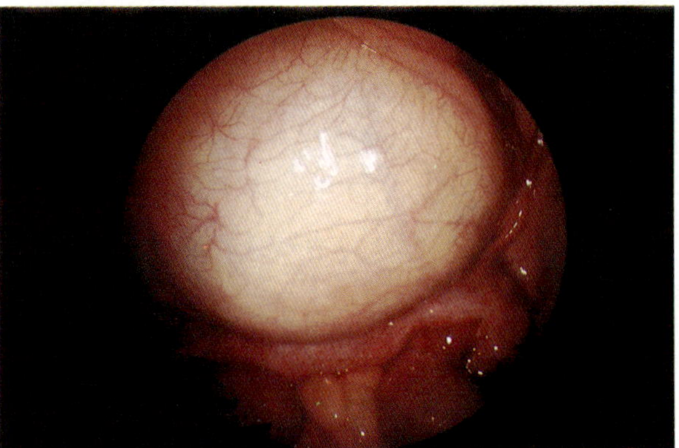

Figure 19.5 Urine filled bladder. As little as 100 cc of urine within the bladder predisposes the organ to injury. Obliteration of the vesicouterine fold precludes visualization of the anterior hemipelvis.

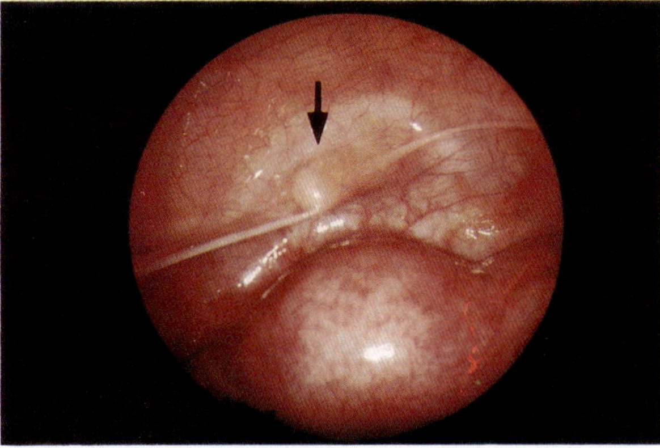

Figure 19.6 Catheter within urinary bladder. Being alert to the location of the catheter tip (arrow) avoids confusing it with an intrinsic pathologic condition.

Verres Needle

Damage to the bladder wall can take place at the time the Verres needle is inserted for creation of the pneumoperitoneum (see Figure 19.4). It usually occurs as a consequence of not emptying the bladder prior to the procedure and/or misdirection of the needle thrust at the time of insertion. Both of these situations are preventable by strict adherence to proper technique (see Chapter 2). Location of the urinary bladder varies according to the patient's stature and habitus.

The shorter the patient, the smaller the umbilico-pubic distance. Thus, in short patients, smaller amounts of urine are required to bring a distended bladder closer to the site at which the Verres needle enters. A similar condition exists in children and young adolescents.

When the bladder has been properly emptied, faulty angulation of the thrust for introducing the Verres needle is generally responsible for an injury. This results as a consequence of failing to direct the Verres needle towards the hollow of the sacrum. Advancing the Verres needle for the entire length of its shaft also predisposes to bladder injury. As discussed in Chapter 2, the thickness of the abdominal wall at the level of the umbilicus does not require the Verres needle to be introduced more than half way (approximately 3 to 4 cm). If the peritoneal cavity is not successfully entered by inserting the insufflating needle to only half its length, it should be withdrawn and properly reinserted.

Diagnosis of perforation of the bladder by the Verres needle is relatively simple. After the needle has been inserted into the abdomen, injection and reaspiration of normal saline yields urine or urine-like fluid if its tip is in the bladder cavity. Another indicator of mislocation is a rapid rise in pressure registered by the abdominal pressure manometer following the insufflation of small amounts of gas (1 L of carbon dioxide). This unexpected increment in pressure suggests the distention of a closed cavity instead of the large peritoneal sac.

When penetration of the urinary bladder with the Verres needle is suspected, withdrawal and reinsertion is indicated. The musculoelastic composition of the bladder wall seals off the site of entry of the small-bore Verres needle (1.7 to 2.2 mm), thereby making this type of injury inconsequential. Nevertheless, penetrating injuries to the bladder with the Verres needle should be avoided to ensure against rare, but serious consequences. For example, the presence of a urinary tract infection may lead to disseminated peritonitis. Hematoma formation in or around the bladder wall may prove difficult to manage.

Whenever gas (carbon dioxide or nitrous oxide) has been insufflated into the bladder lumen during laparoscopy, it should be allowed to escape through the same route by which it gained access, namely, the insufflating needle. If the needle has already been removed, straight transurethral catheterization immediately deflates the bladder. Catheterization can be avoided if the patient is sufficiently awake and can empty the bladder voluntarily.

Laparoscopic Trocar

Perforation of the bladder by the laparoscopic trocar is a rare event. It is usually the consequence of inappropriate selection of patients (for example, failure to eliminate those with a history of multiple abdomino-pelvic surgical procedures), misdirection of the entry route, and/or failure to empty the bladder prior to laparoscopy. Patients who have undergone repeated abdomino-pelvic surgery are likely to present anatomical distortions, such as fixed elevation of the bladder.

Bladder injury with the laparoscopic trocar usually occurs at the time of its insertion. If the bladder has been displaced by congenital abnormalities and/or prior surgery, the traumatic site can be located within the anterior abdominal wall. A similar type of injury can occur after the trocar has entered the peritoneal cavity. In this instance, excessive penetration of the sharp trocar may cause it to reach the posterior bladder wall, especially if the organ has not been completely emptied.

Georgy et al reported two cases of perforated urinary bladder complicating laparoscopy.[4] In one instance, no preoperative catheterization was performed. After uneventful creation of a pneumoperitoneum, the laparoscopic trocar was inserted and the interior of the bladder was visualized. In a second case, failure to enter the peritoneal cavity with the laparoscope was followed by anuria for 24 hours. Catheterization of the bladder produced only 50 cc of urine. Laceration of the bladder was diagnosed by means of cystography. Traumatic injury of the posterior wall of the bladder was confirmed at laparotomy.

Adherence to proper technique, as described in Chapter 2, should prevent this type of injury. With the exception of congenital abnormalities of the urachus, the bladder does not usually reach the periumbilical area in its empty state. Thus, entry of the laparoscopic trocar into the peritoneal cavity periumbilically, in a straight 60° angle pointed to the hollow of the sacrum, seldom, if ever, allows it to come into close proximity with the bladder edge.

Trauma to the bladder after the trocar has successfully traversed the abdominal wall is usually the consequence of the use of excessive force and uncontrolled thrust at the time of insertion. The limited thickness of the anterior abdominal wall at the level of the umbilicus requires the laparoscope trocar to be inserted no deeper than 2.5 to 3.5 cm. Only when the bladder is excessively overfilled can it advance sufficiently cephalad to come near the posterior aspect of the umbilicus (see Figure 19.4).

More often, poor control of the depth of trocar insertion brings this instrument very close to the superior bladder wall, even when the bladder is not distended. This situation can be avoided by limiting the extent of trocar penetration. This is accomplished by placing the extended index finger on the laparoscope trocar sleeve to the point of maximal insertion (usually 3.0 to 3.5 cm from its tip). It then acts as a backstop, preventing any deeper entry of the trocar.

Laparoscope

The laparoscope itself can perforate the thin bladder wall. Homburg and Segal reported such an occurrence during a laparoscopy for evaluation of pelvic pain.[5] Carbon dioxide was inadvertently insufflated into the prevesical space of Retzius. Insertion of the laparoscopic trocar was accompanied by the characteristic hiss of escaping gas. The initial view through the laparoscope was not clear. On searching for a clearer picture, the Foley catheter balloon was visualized, thus confirming the intravesical location of the laparoscope.

Fogging of the forward lens of the laparoscope is common upon entering the warm peritoneal cavity with an instrument that is at room temperature. Contact of the front lens with any organ at body temperature warms up the lens and clarifies the view (see Chapter 26). The possibility of bladder perforation demands that this maneuver be performed carefully and in a gentle manner. A more effective way of preventing the fogging is to immerse the laparoscope in warm saline before it is introduced into the peritoneal cavity.

Accessory Puncture Trocar

The accessory puncture trocar may also cause bladder injury because of its customary location of entry, which is in the midline suprapubically (Figure 19.7). This lower location makes the secondary trocar puncture theoretically more dangerous than that of the laparoscopic trocar for this type of trauma. Nevertheless, the literature contains no report of bladder injury produced by the auxiliary trocar. A possible explanation is that such a puncture is usually performed under direct laparoscopic visualization.

The ability to see the site of entry of the auxiliary trocar allows the instrument to be directed away from the bladder or other organs susceptible to damage (Figure 19.8). More important is the fact that visual exploration of the pelvis by way of the laparoscope eliminates the potential risk of inserting the trocar into a filled bladder. Whenever the bladder is suspected of containing more than 50 cc of urine, emptying by means of straight catheterization is indicated before the auxiliary trocar is inserted.

Notwithstanding its safety record, the suprapubic auxiliary trocar can be the source of damage in the presence of an undiagnosed congenital urachal anomaly. If such an abnormality is in direct continuity with the bladder lumen, the injury is manifested by signs and symptoms similar to those occurring after the bladder itself has been traumatized.

Superficial injuries to the bladder wall may go unnoticed owing to the small size of the auxiliary trocar used. When the bladder lumen has been entered by a sharp trocar, the injury must be evaluated. Usually a 5 mm trocar produces an opening not larger than the medium size Malecot or mushroom catheter used by urologists during suprapubic drainage. Nevertheless, continuous transurethral bladder drainage by means of a Foley catheter enhances the healing process and is thus recommended.

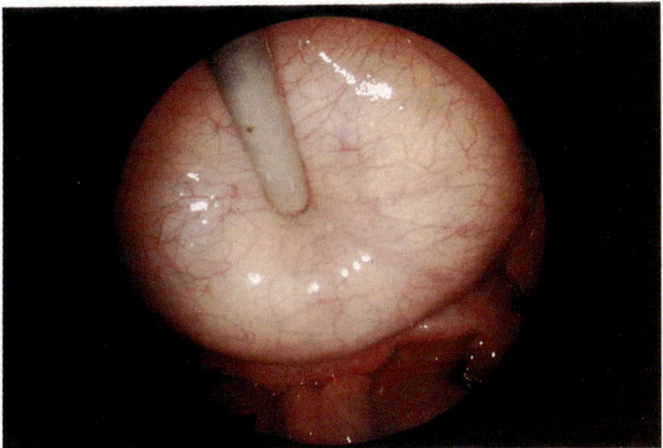

Figure 19.7 Bladder perforation by the auxiliary puncture trocar. Failure to empty the bladder predisposes it to injury. Whenever a distended bladder is identified, it must be evacuated by catheterization before introducing any additional instruments.

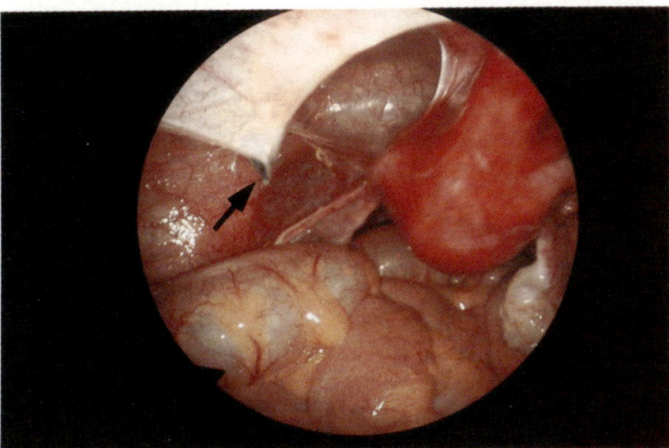

Figure 19.8 Lateral insertion of the auxiliary puncture. Midline obliteration by adhesions (same case as Figure 19.3) requires selection of a new site for the auxiliary trocar insertion. The sharp trocar (arrow) must be introduced under direct visualization.

Auxiliary Instrument

Trauma to the bladder wall may also result from the use of accessory instruments during laparoscopy. These injuries can be produced bluntly or as a complication of the use of electrical devices. Blunt trauma to the bladder may occur as a consequence of undue force employed when mobilizing the organ with a probe (Figure 19.9). This usually occurs when a moderately filled bladder obstructs the visual exploration of the anterior cul-de-sac. This type of complication is preventable. Straight catheterization, easily performed during laparoscopy deflates the organ, thus averting the need to mobilize it for better visualization. Excessive manipulation of a densely adherent fibrotic band may cause trauma to the bladder. Adhesions between the bladder and the anterior wall of the uterus should be electrocoagulated and sharply dissected.

Injuries to the bladder produced by electrocoagulating instruments are rare. Pakter and Budnick reported a case in which there was a 1 to 2 cm burn with a central area of perforation into the urinary bladder.[7] This was thought to have been produced by arcing of sparks within the abdomen from a unipolar coagulating device at the time of a tubal sterilization procedure. The patient was managed conservatively by continuous bladder drainage. Cystography performed 5 days later demonstrated no evidence of bladder perforation.

Deshmukh reported a similar complication.[3] The diagnosis of bladder perforation was not made until several hours following a laparoscopic tubal coagulation with a unipolar device. The patient complained of minimal abdominal discomfort postoperatively. An intravenous pyelogram revealed gross intraperitoneal spillage of contrast material. Cystoscopic evaluation confirmed a perforation of the bladder dome, and a laparotomy was required for excision and repair of the bladder wall.

Although most injuries caused by electrical coagulation occur as a result of inadvertent touching or grasping of an organ with the electrical instrument, arcing of sparks is a more likely cause (see Chapter 23). Diagnosis of such an injury is facilitated by visualization of a blanched area of the bladder at the time of laparoscopy. Conservative therapy by means of continuous bladder drainage is an alternative treatment in these cases in lieu of surgical repair.

More difficult is the evaluation of patients complaining of minimal abdominal discomfort several hours after a translaparoscopic electrocoagulative procedure in which no injury is suspected to have occurred. Similar to cases with electrical injuries of the bowel, several hours—and even days—may elapse between the procedure and the appearance of signs and symptoms of the visceral damage. This is due to the time required between the initial insult (burn), which devitalizes the affected tissue, and the actual disruption of integrity of the wall. The latter results from tissue necrosis.

Trauma to the urinary bladder complicating a laparoscopy ought to be suspected whenever the patient is unable to void spontaneously or urine is unobtainable by catheterization following surgery. During the immediate postoperative period, bladder injuries can be asymptomatic, depending on their location. If the disruption of the bladder wall is confined extraperitoneally, urine extravasates into a virtual space to form a mass (Figure 19.10). This lower abdominal fluid accumulation is usually painless at the outset. When it reaches large proportions or becomes secondarily infected, the patient complains of suprapubic pain. If the injury to the bladder communicates with the peritoneal cavity, vast amounts of urine can enter that space asymptomatically. Persistent oliguria/anuria is at times the only abnormality found.

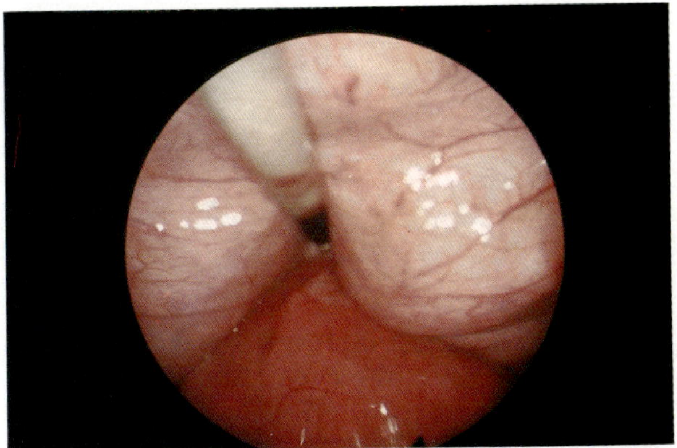

Figure 19.9 Displacement of a urine filled bladder by auxiliary probe. Risk of perforating the bladder is increased. Catheterization is indicated.

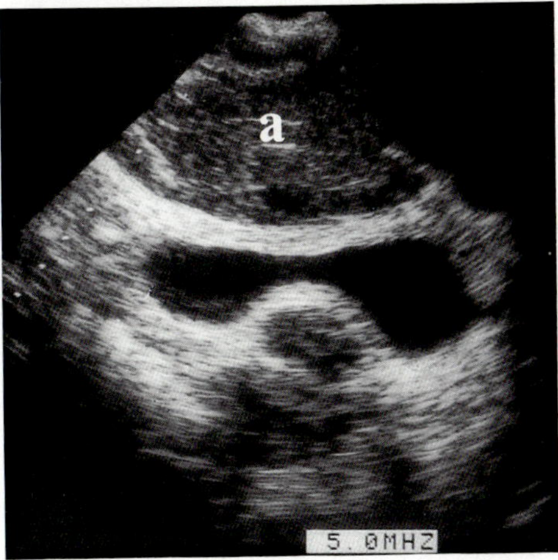

Figure 19.10 Prevesical mass on pelvic ultrasonogram. Hypoechoic area (a) anterior to the bladder represents urine or blood accumulated within the space of Retzius.

Diagnosis of an injury to the urinary bladder can be made during laparoscopy by visualization of the interior surface of the organ. If one is uncertain about the location of the laparoscope, passing a straight catheter into the bladder under translaparoscopic visualization helps confirm its intraluminal position. If damage to the bladder is suspected, but not overtly evident, filling the bladder transurethrally with a methylene blue solution will reveal intraperitoneal spillage. When there is doubt, such steps should always be taken since a small laceration identified at the time of laparoscopy responds to conservative treatment in the form of prolonged, continuous bladder drainage.

Postoperatively, diagnosis of a laceration of the urinary bladder wall requires a retrograde cystogram. Extravasation of contrast material confirms disruption of the bladder's integrity (Figures 19.11 and 19.12). Cystoscopy can be helpful in establishing a bladder perforation, but it is less accurate than a cystogram.

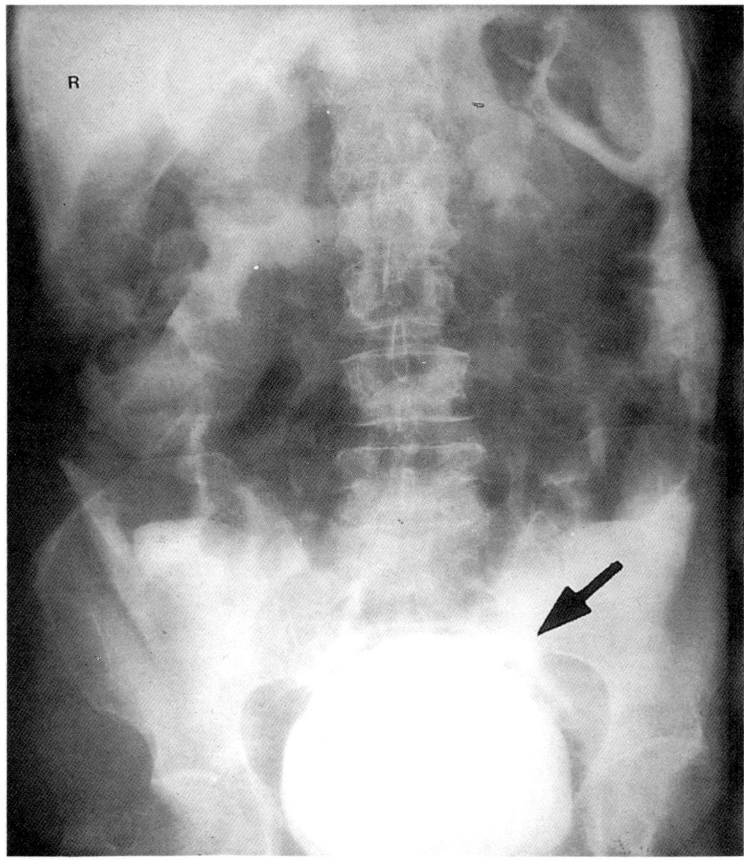

Figure 19.11 Postoperative retrograde cystogram showing spillage of contrast material outside the bladder (arrow). Disruption in bladder wall continuity is thus confirmed. Small perforations may only be identified by cystoscopic evaluation.

Treatment of a laceration of the urinary bladder wall complicating a laparoscopy varies according to the size of the lesion. Injuries produced by the Verres needle are usually of no consequence and require no special therapy. Small lacerations of the vesical wall (5 mm or less) produced by a small laparoscopic trocar or the auxiliary instrument trocar can be treated conservatively. Treatment consists of continuous bladder drainage for 4 to 5 days. Follow-up cystography is required before the indwelling catheter is removed.

Injuries to the bladder wall greater than 5 mm in diameter require transabdominal bladder repair. This can be accomplished by primary suture of the laceration site in layers or by cuneiform resection of the trauma site followed by similar repair.

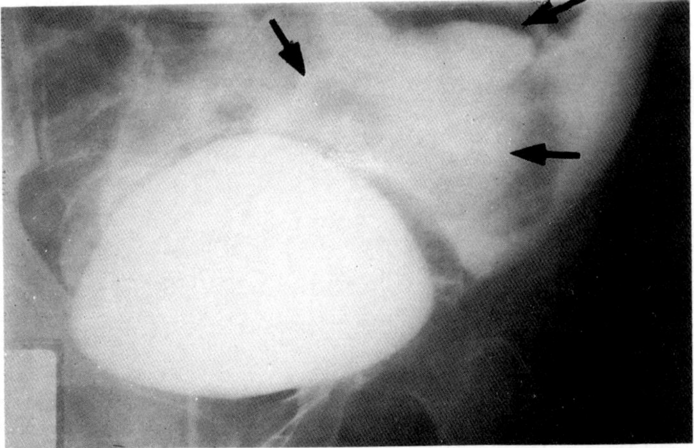

Figure 19.12 Intraperitoneal spillage of contrast solution on retrograde cystogram. The considerable amount of extravesical contrast material (arrows) suggests a large disruption of the bladder wall.

URETERAL INJURY

Injury to the ureter during gynecologic surgery has been reported to occur at a rate of 0.5 to 2.5 percent.[9] Because damage to the ureter can be asymptomatic, the larger figure probably reflects a more realistic rate of incidence. Injury to the ureter complicating laparoscopy is rather unusual. Nevertheless, it has been reported and carries the same serious implications as when it occurs during other surgical procedures.[2,6,8]

A short description of the anatomic configuration of the ureter and its relation to the surrounding organs serves to clarify the physiopathology of this type of insult. The ureter is a retroperitoneal structure which varies in length from 28 cm to 34 cm. It has an abdominal and a pelvic segment. The abdominal portion extends from the renal pelvis to the point where it enters the pelvic region and courses over the common iliac vessels. Injury to this portion of ureter arising as a complication of laparoscopy (albeit feasible) has not been described.

In its pelvic portion, the ureter continues retroperitoneally and is crossed by the ovarian vessels (in the infundibulopelvic ligament). The rectosigmoid also crosses it on the left. It continues caudad on the posterior leaf of the broad ligament, passing lateral to the uterosacral ligament, traversing the Mackenrodt ligament (lateral cervical ligament in the ureteral tunnel or canal), and running posterior to the uterine vessels before reaching the bladder.

The sites of ureteral injury at the time of laparoscopy include, from above to below, the pelvic brim, the peritoneal surface covering the lateral pelvic wall and broad ligament, and the uterosacral ligament. Injury to the ureter may be the result of direct trauma at the time of insertion of the Verres needle and the sharp laparoscopy or auxiliary trocar. More commonly reported are burn injuries produced by the use of electrocoagulating instruments for translaparoscopic surgery.[2]

Ureteral laceration produced by the Verres needle is a preventable complication. The appearance of this complication suggests that at the time of insertion the needle was directed toward the lateral pelvic wall rather than in the midline toward the hollow of the sacrum. Similarly, misdirection of the auxiliary trocar can cause injury to the ureter (Figures 19.13 and 19.14). The anatomic proximity of the ureter to the iliac vessels mandates that ureteral integrity should be explored whenever a retroperitoneal vessel is injured during laparoscopy (Figure 19.15). Likewise, the opposite holds true, that is, one should examine for vascular injury if the ureter is damaged.

Injury to the ureter at the time of diagnostic laparoscopy was reported by Shapira et al.[8] Three weeks after a laparoscopic investigation of secondary infertility, a woman was hospitalized with ascites. Laparotomy revealed a ure-

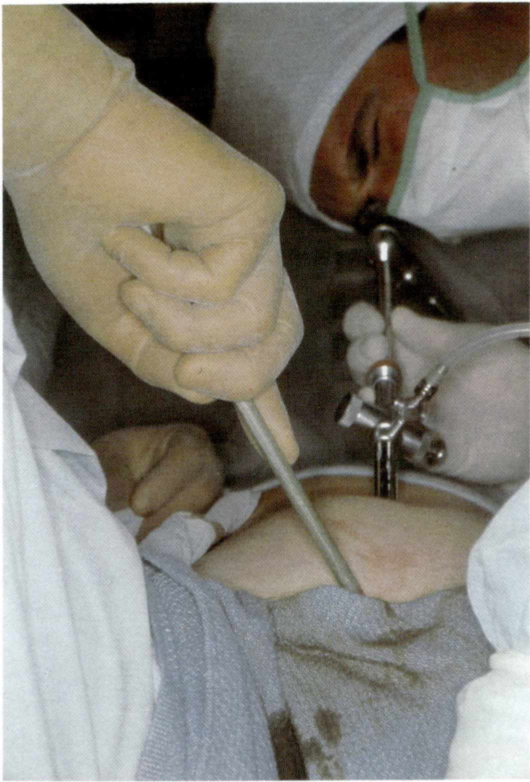

Figure 19.13 Misdirection of auxiliary puncture insertion. Deviation from the midline puts lateral pelvic organs and structures at risk of injury.

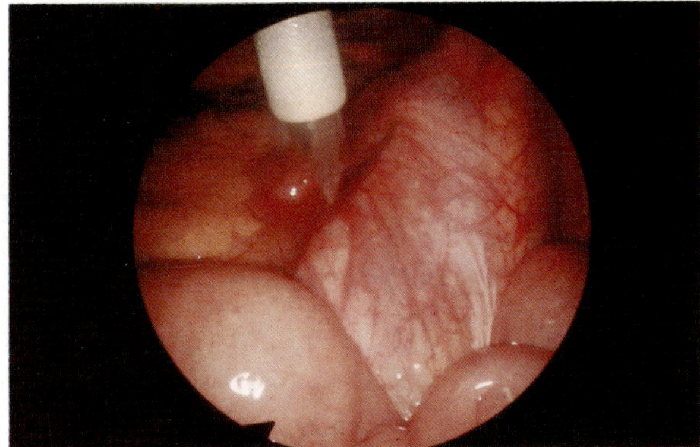

Figure 19.14 Misdirection of auxiliary puncture trocar. Sharp trocar in close proximity to right ureter. Controlled midline thrust during insertion reduces the risk of this type of injury.

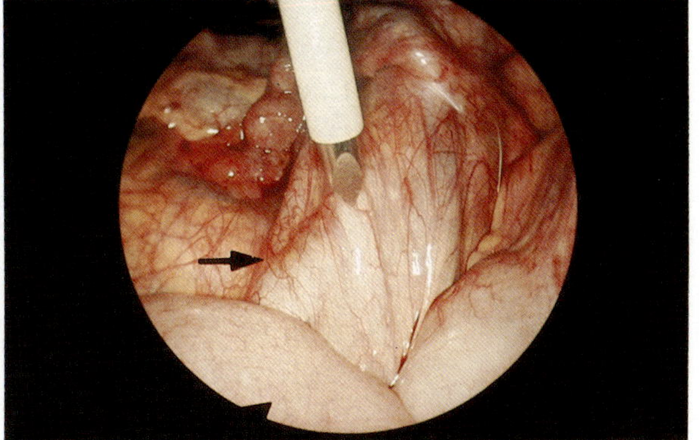

Figure 19.15 Ureteral injury by auxiliary puncture trocar. Close proximity of the ureter and the major retroperitoneal vessels requires surgical exploration of both when either has incurred an injury. Arrow indicates division of common iliac artery.

teroperitoneal fistula 5 cm above the ureterovesical junction with continuous extravasation of urine.

Irvin et al described ascites following a laparoscopic tubal electrocoagulation.[6] The ascitic fluid was actually urine emerging from a grossly dilated right ureter that had been transected at the time of sterilization. Accidental ureteral burn at the time of tubal fulguration is usually described as occurring at the level of the pelvic brim. It is believed to be the result of arcing of the electrical current while it is seeking the dispersive electrode (see Chapter 23). These lesions are usually not recognized at the time of laparoscopy. Postoperatively, diagnosis is based on the appearance of unilateral flank pain with or without oliguria and/or the formation of urinary ascites. Extravasation of radiopaque material as demonstrated by intravenous pyelography confirms the ureteral injury (Figure 19.16).

A factor contributing to this type of injury is believed to be the result of the technique of displacing the uterus in order to put the adnexa under tension. Stretching the infundibulopelvic ligament by this maneuver displaces the ureter medially bringing it closer to the primary site of fulguration. Ureteral adhesions may also transfer the ureter from its normal location (Figure 19.17).

Electrocoagulation of endometriotic lesions under laparoscopic control has been recommended as an acceptable method of managing patients with pelvic pain and infertility. Although technically simple, translaparoscopic fulguration of endometriotic nodules is potentially a hazardous procedure (Figures 19.18 and 19.19). Inability to control the depth and width of the cautery applied to a particular point places any adjacent structures at risk of accidental cauterization. This can occur by direct contact or by extension of the electrocoagulating current.

Cheng reported a ureteral injury resulting from the translaparoscopic fulguration of an endometriotic implant.[2] This consisted of the electrocoagulation of a single, small nodule of endometriosis on the uterosacral ligament about 1 inch from the uterus. Five days after the primary procedure, the patient developed lower quadrant abdominal and costovertebral angle pain, moderate fever, and hematuria. Intravenous pyelogram revealed delayed excretion of dye by an enlarged kidney and free extravasation of contrast material at the level of the pelvic brim where the ureter crosses the iliac vessels. The distance between the area originally treated and the ureteral lesion implicated electrical sparking as the cause of the ureteral damage.

In its downward path to reach the cardinal ligaments, the ureters travel in close proximity to the uterosacral ligaments for approximately 1.0 to 1.5 cm. The ureter can also sustain electrocoagulating injury because of its contiguity with endometriotic implants on the uterosacral ligaments, especially those located close to the uterus (Figure 19.19).

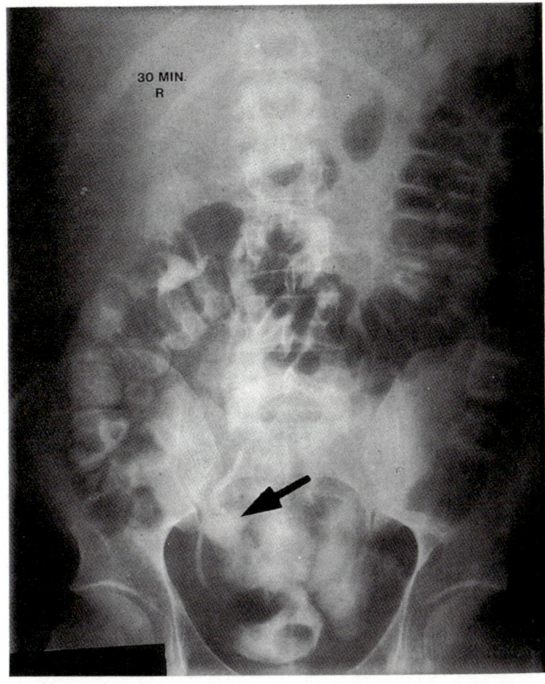

Figure 19.16 Ureteral injury seen on intravenous pyelogram. Extravasation of radiopaque material (arrow) confirms injury to ureteral wall.

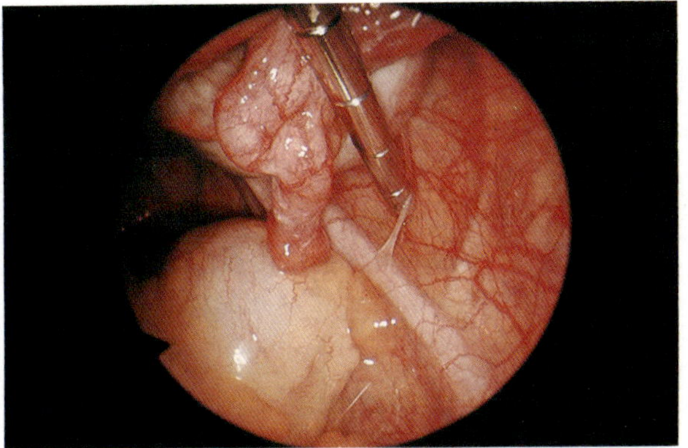

Figure 19.17 Uretero-ovarian adhesion. As a result of previous pelvic surgery, the ureter is drawn medially. Its proximity with the adnexal structures increased the risk of injury during translaparoscopic tubal or ovarian surgery (same case as Figure 3.39).

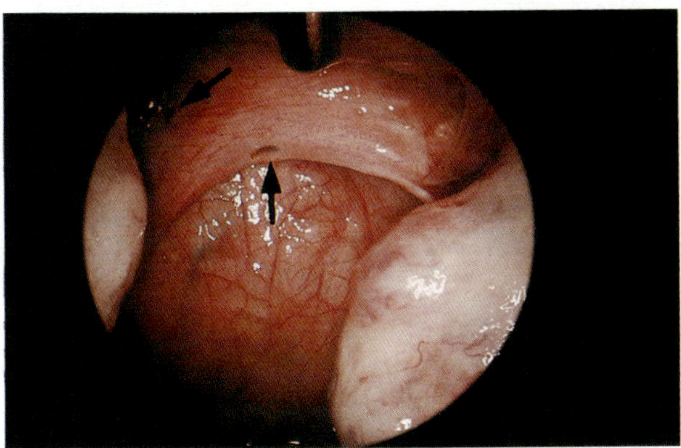

Figure 19.18 Endometriosis on the left uterosacral ligament. Electrocoagulation of this endometriotic spot risks electrical injury to the ureter passing nearby.

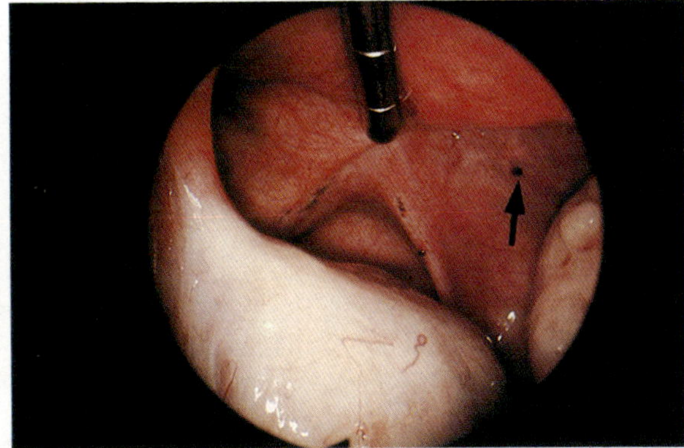

Figure 19.19 Endometriotic focus on the posterior leaf of the broad ligament. The ureter crosses in close proximity beneath the uterine vessels. Contact electrocoagulation could damage the ureter (same case as Figure 3.40B).

Unipolar cautery has been used in most instances in which there was a ureteral injury associated with fulguration of an endometriotic lesion. Use of bipolar forceps offers some protection in preventing the propagative cauterization to adjacent tissue. Nevertheless, one of the shortcomings of using bipolar forceps to treat these lesions is the fact that the foci seen through the laparoscope may not truly represent the entire extent of the disease. Thus, bipolar electrocoagulation may not destroy the entire endometriotic nodule, thereby leaving residual disease in deeper tissue planes. The recent introduction of translaparoscopic laser treatment of endometriosis may provide the control necessary to treat the disease adequately without excessive risk of injury to adjacent structures (see Chapter 4).

Repair of a ureteral injury sustained during laparoscopy must be undertaken as soon as it is identified. Nonelectrical injuries, such as lacerations resulting from trauma with the Verres needle or the sharp trocar, are amenable to primary closure, if small. Larger lesions may require resection and uretero-ureteral reanastomosis.

Electrical damage to the ureter is a more serious type of injury. Propagation of the electric current away from the area of maximal injury may result in additional devitalization of tissue not evident to the naked eye. Thus, the portion of ureter to be resected at the time of repair must extend beyond the injury actually visualized and identified until one reaches normal tissue. This may make uretero-ureteral reanastomosis impossible and necessitate a ureteroneocystostomy. The Boari flap technique has been successfully used when the injury is not too far away from the urinary bladder. Lesions of the extrapelvic ureter may be treated by uretero-ureterostomy or by replacing the damaged portion of ureter with an isoperistaltic segment of ileum.

References

1. Borten M, Friedman EA. Spontaneous prevesical (Retzius-space) abscess with extraperitoneal presacral dissemination. J Reprod Med 1984; 29:841-844.
2. Cheng YS. Ureteral injury resulting from laparoscopic fulguration of endometriotic implant. Am J Obstet Gynecol 1976; 126:1045-1046.
3. Deshmukh AS. Laparoscopic bladder injury. Urology 1982; 19:306-307.
4. Georgy RM, Fetterman HH, Chefetz MD. Complications of laparoscopy: Two cases of perforated urinary bladder. Am J Obstet Gynecol 1974; 120:1121-1122.
5. Homburg R, Segal T. Perforation of the urinary bladder by the laparoscope. Am J Obstet Gynecol 1978; 130:597.
6. Irvin TT, Goligher JC, Scott JS. Injury to the ureter during laparoscopic tubal sterilization. Arch Surg 1975; 110:1501-1503.
7. Pakter J, Budnick LD. Bladder perforation owing to a unipolar coagulating device. Am J Obstet Gynecol 1981; 141:227.
8. Schapira M, Dizersens H, Essinger A, et al. Urinary ascites after gynaecological laparoscopy. Lancet 1978; 1:871-872.
9. St. Martin EC, Trichel BE, Campbell JH, Locke CM. Ureteral injuries in gynecologic surgery. J Urol 1953; 70:51-57.

20 ABDOMINAL WALL COMPLICATIONS

Complications affecting the abdominal wall as a consequence of a laparoscopy are not common and rarely cause seriously adverse outcome. Nevertheless, every surgeon should know of their existence and should be familiar with measures needed to prevent them and to diagnose and manage them promptly.

Hemorrhage within the abdominal wall may, if unchecked, lead to the formation of a hematoma. Usually, this is not recognized at once. Anatomic variations specifically as related to vascular anatomy, and deviations from appropriate surgical technique are the usual contributory factors leading to this form of morbidity.

Infectious complications range from minor superficial wound infection to abscess formation and, exceptionally, serious necrotizing fasciitis (see Chapter 21). Failure to adhere strictly to sterile technique can be responsible for introduction of bacteria in an otherwise sterile field.

Wound dehiscence, with or without herniation of intra-abdominal structures, is rarely seen with laparoscopy. This is particularly so since small diameter laparoscopes and trocar sleeves have come into common use.

In the interest of completeness, congenital malformations in the surgical field will be described briefly. Some of these can cause unexpected morbidity. The presence of an umbilical hernia may favor undertaking an operation combining laparoscopy and herniorrhaphy. Transection of a urachal cyst by trocar puncture may lead to serious complications.

HEMORRHAGE

Hemorrhage with hematoma formation is most frequently produced in the course of laparoscopy by the laceration of the superficial epigastric vessel at the time the secondary trocar is inserted in the lower abdominal wall lateral to the midline (see Chapter 17). This type of complication is easily avoided by preliminary transillumination of the abdominal wall with the intraperitoneal laparoscopic light source. Identifying the large vessels in this way facilitates finding an avascular site for the secondary puncture.

Identification of the deep inferior epigastric vessels by transillumination is more difficult. The light refraction and transmission indices of both rectus abdominis muscle and adjacent vessels are similar. Clear delineation of the vessels is thus problematical. Laceration of a blood vessel in the abdominal wall can usually be prevented by strict adherence to the established technique for selecting an avascular area for trocar insertion. The linea alba is the safest site because it is not vascularized.

Diagnosis of a bleeding complication is not always obvious. One should be alerted if postoperative incisional or circumincisional pain is persistent and out of proportion to the magnitude and complexity of the laparoscopy incision. In retroperitoneal or preperitoneal hemorrhage, a substantial fall in hematocrit can occur without any clinical evidence of intraperitoneal bleeding. A rapid, but unexplained drop in hematocrit and/or unstable blood pressure and pulse should raise the suspicion of an intraparietal process. A suprafascial hemorrhage is usually self limited. It tends to stop spontaneously when the pressure from the extravasated compartmented blood exceeds the intravenous pressure within the injured vessel. With infrafascial hemorrhage, in contrast, there is no resistance to dissection by the peritoneal layer. This allows the extravasated blood to dissect laterally to reach the retroperitoneal space where it can accumulate silently in considerable amounts. Sonography and soft-tissue roentgenography of the anterior abdominal wall are helpful in diagnosing the presence of a parietal mass.

After bleeding has been correctly diagnosed, the therapy consists of exploration of the wound with ligature of the injured vessel and drainage of the accumulated blood. The practice of elevating the abdominal wall by means of periumbilical skin clips or clamps for inserting the Verres needle and laparoscopic trocar is mentioned only to be decried. From the technical point of view, the clips only lift the skin and superficial subcutaneous tissue. They do not reach the rectus fascial layer. Thus, they distort the normal anatomy and thereby increase the risk of subcutaneous-suprafascial emphysematous insufflation (see Chapter 15). As a consequence, one is not able to introduce the laparoscopic trocar into the peritoneal cavity.

In addition to these technical difficulties from use of skin clips for elevating the abdominal wall, there may be other complications. Periumbilical hematoma and postoperative periumbilical incisional pain that lasts for several days may result. The vessels forming the periumbilical venous network can be perforated or avulsed by these sharp instruments because of the exaggerated upward tenting of the abdominal wall.

WOUND DEHISCENCE

Umbilical hernia is a true congenital defect which occurs through a patent umbilical ring. Incarceration and strangulation of omentum or bowel are rare occurrences, but they do occur. Umbilical hernias are common in infancy, being diagnosed in 10 percent of caucasian infants and 40 to 60 percent of black infants. They close spontaneously in the majority of cases by the time the individual has reached adulthood. In women who develop diastasis of the rectus muscle in the course of pregnancy, an occult umbilical hernia may become evident.

In gynecologic laparoscopy, a subumbilical midline site of entry for the laparoscopic trocar is universally utilized. The avascularity of the linea alba makes this site safe because it avoids injuring nearby vessels. The same diminished vascularity, however, may have an adverse impact on spontaneous healing. Slower healing makes this incision site in the abdominal wall more susceptible to herniation.

Several secondary factors may inhibit the rate of wound healing and predispose to wound dehiscence. Diabetes, malnutrition, long-term use of steroid medication, alcoholism, cirrhosis, and chronic obstructive pulmonary disease are some of the problems most frequently encountered in patients undergoing laparoscopy. Separation of the wound edges immediately following the procedure increases the risk of later appearance of an incisional hernia.

HERNIATION

Herniation of intraperitoneal organs through a laparoscopic incision is a rare event complicating laparoscopy. Nevertheless, its appearance can be associated with severe morbidity. Wound dehiscence, infection, and utilization of large diameter instruments seem to be predisposing.

Wound infection (see Chapter 21) also exposes the patient to the risk of wound separation. Fisher and Turner found wound infection to be the cause of incisional hernia more often than inadequate closure of the incision.[4] Aggressive management of a wound infection is recommended (see Chapter 21) to reduce the hazard of wound dehiscence.

Patients presenting for laparoscopy with any of the aforementioned risks require special precautions to decrease the possibility of wound complications. Whenever possible, a small diameter laparoscope (5 mm) should be employed. Use of gas sterilized instruments is also recommended.

The presence of an umbilical hernia or history of its surgical repair should discourage the use of the umbilicus or periumbilical area as the site of entry for the laparoscopic trocar. Any of the accessory sites described in Chapter 2 becomes the area of choice for the insertion of laparoscopic instruments. The same applies when severe diastasis of the rectus muscles is encountered.

Bishop and Halpin reported a wound dehiscence following laparoscopic sterilization.[1] The laparoscope used had an outside diameter of 11 mm. They attributed the complication to an intractable episode of coughing for the initial 24 postoperative hours.

Omental protrusion through the laparoscopic trocar wound was reported to occur once in 172 puerperal laparoscopic sterilizations.[5] Exteriorization of a portion of omentum through the trocar site has been described;[3] it occurred following an episode of persistent coughing on the fourth postoperative day. In a large series of laparoscopies, Kleppinger reported omental protrusion through the laparoscopy puncture site in 0.07 percent of cases.[6]

Schiff and Naftolin described two patients who required bowel resection because of small bowel incarcerations following herniation through the fascial site of the laparoscopic puncture.[7] In one, the herniation communicated with a previously unrecognized congenital umbilical hernia. The presence of an umbilical hernia was considered a relative contraindication against the choice of the periumbilical area for insertion of the laparoscopic trocar. Corrective surgery was performed 14 to 21 days after the original laparoscopic procedure. Bourke recounted a case of small intestinal obstruction from a Richter's hernia at the insertion site.[2] The hernial defect was repaired 13 days later following reduction of the hernial sac contents.

Common to all of these cases were (a) the use of a large diameter laparoscope and trocar (11 mm and 12 mm), (b) the delayed appearance of gastrointestinal signs and symptoms (3 to 7 days), and (c) the long delay in undertaking laparotomy for bowel obstruction after the primary laparoscopy (13 to 21 days). Postponement of definitive surgery made it necessary to perform bowel resection because portions of intestine were no longer viable.

The principal measure for preventing this type of complication is use of small diameter laparoscope and trocar (5 to 8 mm) whenever possible. If a larger bore instrument is required, the fascia should be closed separately with interrupted sutures in the same fashion as a laparotomy incision. The trocar sleeve should always be removed with its lumen previously occluded by a solid instrument such as a probe or the laparoscope itself. If this precaution is ignored, the positive intra-abdominal pressure may cause a piece of omentum or a knuckle of intestine to protrude into the lumen of the trocar sleeve. As the sleeve is withdrawn, herniation of the entrapped tissue occurs (Figure 20.1). This does not necessarily produce major symptoms until several days later. If an umbilical hernia is known to preexist the procedure, an open laparoscopic procedure should be entertained. This can be followed by a hernia repair. An alternative site can be selected for trocar insertion instead.

Expectant management is usually inappropriate in cases with herniation of bowel or omentum. Spontaneous resolution seldom occurs. Evaluation and management here are the same as for bowel burns following a translaparoscopic electrosurgical procedure (see Chapter 23). Exploratory laparotomy should be performed promptly to limit the damage and shorten the duration of this morbid condition. Bowel resection may be required.

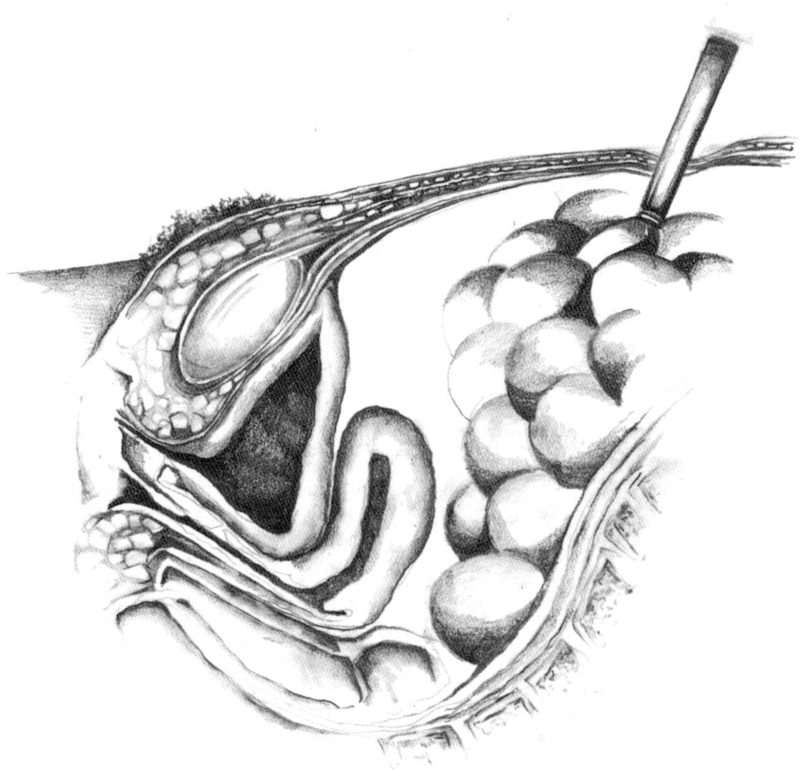

Figure 20.1 Knuckle of bowel within trocar sleeve. Positive intra-abdominal pressure may cause a piece of omentum or bowel to protrude into the trocar lumen. Withdrawal of the sleeve may herniate the aspirated tissue into or through the abdominal wall.

CONGENITAL MALFORMATIONS

The presence of congenital abnormalities of the anterior abdominal wall have to be considered when planning laparoscopy. One may have to modify the technique accordingly. The specific congenital defects that are most relevant here are umbilical hernias and urachal abnormalities. The latter include patent urachus, urachal cyst, and urachal fistula.

Umbilical Hernia

An umbilical hernia is a true congenital abnormality. It tends to close spontaneously in about 80 percent of cases during childhood. In the remaining cases, failure to heal normally, produces a permanent weakening of the umbilical ring. In most cases it is asymptomatic. Pregnancy can enlarge the fascial defect. Symptoms may appear subsequently for the first time.

It is common for the hernial sac to contain incarcerated omentum. On examination, this appears as a pea-size, irreducible, nontender lump.Under such circumstances, choosing a periumbilical site to enter the peritoneal cavity at laparoscopy risks perforating the omentum. More seriously, an omental vessel can be lacerated.

Patients with an umbilical hernia can benefit from a combined laparoscopy and hernia repair. The open laparoscopic technique permits the translaparoscopic pelvic procedure to be carried out as usual. At the conclusion of the laparoscopy, the original skin incision is extended to serve the needs of the herniorrhaphy. The umbilical skin must be completely dissected away from the hernia sac. A simple primary transverse closure is generally done and proves successful for repairing the defect in most cases.

Urachal Abnormalities

The urachus or median umbilical ligament is the embryological vestige of the obliterated allantois. Anatomically, it is a midline structure extending from the dome of the bladder to the umbilicus. It is attached anteriorly to the transversalis fascia and posteriorly to the parietal peritoneum. Fibrosis occurs after birth. It then becomes an integral component of the umbilicus.

Four types of abnormalities are encountered: (1) patent urachus with free communication between bladder and umbilicus; (2) urachal cyst, in which the proximal and distal ends are obliterated, but with a patent intervening portion; (3) urachal sinus, a communication between the urachal lumen and the umbilicus; and (4) vesico-urachal diverticulum, in which there is free communication of the urachal lumen with the urinary bladder.

Patent urachus and a urachal cyst are usually asymptomatic conditions found incidentally during surgery. With the advent of ultrasonography, they can sometimes be diagnosed prior to surgery. A urachal sinus should be evident upon close inspection of the umbilical fossa. With the exception of the vesico-urachal diverticulum, all other urachal anomalies should prompt a reconsideration of the indications for laparoscopy. Their presence constitutes a contraindication against blind perforation of the midline infraumbilical or suprapubic abdominal wall. An alternative site for the trocar puncture that can be used is one of the supraumbilical or infracostal quadrants.

Perforation of a patent urachus or a urachal cyst can result from the primary or secondary puncture. Hematoma formation, leakage of urine, or the more dangerous intraperitoneal dissemination of an infected urachal cyst could ensue under such circumstances. Immediate repair is recommended if this type of injury is diagnosed at laparoscopy.

References

1. Bishop HL, Halpin TF. Dehiscence following laparoscopy: Report of an unusual complication. Am J Obstet Gynecol 1973; 116:585-586.
2. Bourke JB. Small intestinal obstruction from a Richter's hernia at the site of insertion of a laparoscopy. Br Med J 1977; 2:1393-1394.
3. Cunanan RG, Courey NG, Lippes J. Complications of laparoscopic tubal sterilization. Obstet Gynecol 1980; 55:501-506.
4. Fischer JD, Turner FW. Abdominal incisional hernias: A ten-year review. Can J Surg 1974; 17:202-204.
5. Keith L, Webster A, Houser K, Procknicki L, Lash A, Barton J. Laparoscopy for puerperal sterilization. Obstet Gynecol 1972; 39:616-621.
6. Kleppinger RK. Laparoscopy at a community hospital: An analysis of 4,300 cases. J Reprod Med 1977; 19:353-363.
7. Schiff I, Naftolin F. Small bowel incarceration after uncomplicated laparoscopy. Obstet Gynecol 1974; 43:674-675

21 INFECTIOUS COMPLICATIONS

An infectious complication from a laparoscopic procedure is a rare occurrence. Phillips reported an incidence of 1.4 per 1,000 in over 100,000 surveyed laparoscopies.[19] Its rarity, however, is not an accurate indicator of its potential seriousness. Infectious morbidity can range from a mild superficial wound infection to a life-threatening disseminated peritonitis.

One must differentiate between infections complicating a diagnostic laparoscopy for pelvic pain or infertility and those following operative laparoscopy (such as tubal sterilization). Infectious morbidity associated with the former can be attributed to contamination of the instrument or deviation from acceptable technique. In the case of the latter, infection may have been present at a subclinical stage (in the form of salpingitis, for example) before the operation. The laparoscopic procedure may merely have facilitated dissemination of a preexisting process.

Laparoscopy is not inherently a completely sterile procedure. It belongs in the category of a clean-contaminated operation. Unavoidable breaks in aseptic technique occur universally. An example of the invariable contamination that occurs involves the contact between the operator's periorbital area with the laparoscopic eyepiece. Nevertheless, the laparoscopist must make every effort to minimize its impact on the patient.

Particular attention must be directed to avoiding contamination between the vulvovaginal and the abdominal fields. Introduction of organisms normally found in the vagina into the peritoneal cavity may produce serious morbidity. Strict adherence to proper technique (see Chapter 2) is essential.

INSTRUMENT PREPARATION

The most appropriate method for the aseptic preparation of the instruments required for laparoscopy remains controversial. The Centers for Disease Control states that sterilization is preferable to disinfection when preparing laparoscopic equipment for use.[4] In 1977, the Surgeon General's Office endorsed a recommendation issued by the United States Army for the sterilization of laparoscopic instruments.[21] The only acceptable methods were either a complete ethylene oxide cycle followed by an 8-hour aeration period or a 10-hour immersion in activated glutaraldehyde. A 10-minute to 20-minute soaking was to be considered a disinfecting process for emergency use only. It was further suggested that the surgeon ought to sign a release stating that he or she wished to operate under less than optimal conditions whenever the latter was used.

The aforementioned recommendations were issued without data to substantiate that disinfection of the instruments exposed the patient to a greater risk of infection than sterilization. Thus, the policy was based on theoretical hazards. Clinical experience has actually shown just the opposite.

Loffer reviewed over 10,000 laparoscopic procedures performed at a freestanding ambulatory surgicenter.[17] Sterilization was used for all the equipment except those items containing fiberoptics, rubber, plastic, or lenses (specifically, the laparoscope). The latter were immersed in 2 percent glutaraldehyde for 10 minutes. He found no cases in which an infectious complication could be attributed to the method used for the preparation of the laparoscopic equipment. He felt that surgical technique employed during laparoscopy is more important for preventing infectious morbidity than the instrument sterilization with its theoretical advantages over disinfection.

Attention to careful surgical technique cannot be emphasized enough. Because of the nature of the laparoscopic procedure (especially with the eyepiece in contact with the operator's periorbital region), contamination must always occur. The need to keep these breaks in aseptic method to a minimum by reducing deviations from proper technique is of utmost importance.

Corson et al bacteriologically evaluated the umbilical area, the pelvic serosal surfaces, and the laparoscope under ordinary conditions of clinical usage.[5] They first studied 100 cases in which the laparoscope was disinfected by immersion in activated 2 percent glutaraldehyde (Cidex). In 61 percent of cases, umbilical cultures yielded organisms after preparation with a 10 percent solution of povidone-iodine. All organisms cultured from the umbilical area were commonly found on normal skin (*Staphylococcus epidermidis, Bacillus corynebacterium*). Three types of fungi were also isolated (*Cryptococcus laurentii, Aspergillus and Penicillium*). Peritoneal cavity cultures were positive in 29 percent of patients. Cultures of the laparoscope following cold disinfection were positive in 22 percent of cases. The predominant organism cultured was *Staphylococcus epidermidis*. Cultures obtained from laparoscopes subjected to sterilization with ethylene oxide failed to grow any organisms. They were considered bacteriologically sterile.

Because the degree of contamination evidenced by colony counts fell within the range of the capability that the healthy peritoneum should be able to handle, Corson et al made the following recommendations: (a) To ensure deactivation of bacteria that have proliferated overnight, the laparoscope should be sterilized with ethylene oxide, autoclaved (seldom recommended), or immersed for 10 hours in activated 2 percent glutaraldehyde before its first use of the day. (b) A 15-minute immersion in activated 2 percent glutaraldehyde followed by rinsing with sterile water is sufficient for disinfection between cases. (c) If the equipment has been used in an overtly infected patient, it must undergo sterilization before it can be reused. (d) A sterilized instrument must be used in patients whose immune or bacterial defense mechanism is impaired.[6]

The aforementioned recommendations are practical and medically sound. Contrary to sterilization which destroys all living organisms, disinfection removes all common vegetative pathogens and viruses but does not affect bacterial spores. Activated 2 percent glutaraldehyde has some sporocidal activity, but it requires at least 3 hours to be effective.

The theoretical concern about transmission of hepatitis B viruses by disinfected laparoscopes has not been specifically studied. Experience with gastrointestinal endoscopy suggests that a 15- to 20-minute immersion in activated 2 percent glutaraldehyde is effective in preventing the transmission of the virus.[8]

More recently, the Centers for Disease Control analyzed data from a multicenter prospective study involving over 3,900 women undergoing laparoscopy.[16] The report compared the risk of wound and pelvic infection in women undergoing a tubal sterilization with disinfected (activated 2 percent glutaraldehyde) and sterilized (ethylene oxide) laparoscopes. No difference in relative risk of wound and/or pelvic infection was found between the two groups.

SYSTEMIC BACTEREMIA

Bacteremia associated with laparoscopy has not been reported. Zwelling et al studied 30 consecutive patients undergoing laparoscopy.[22] They obtained aerobic and anaerobic bacterial cultures before the operative procedure, within 2 minutes of the creation of the pneumoperitoneum, and at the conclusion of the operation before the instruments were removed. No positive cultures were obtained. They concluded that prophylactic antibiotics are not required prior to laparoscopy.

Bacteremia often accompanies surgery or instrumentation of the genitourinary tract. Because of the substantial morbidity and mortality associated with bacterial endocarditis, prophylactic antibiotics are usually used for patients at risk prior to undergoing operations that are likely to cause bacteremia. The American Heart Association classifies peritoneal endoscopy without biopsy as having a low risk of triggering transient bacteremia. They, too, do not recommend the use of prophylactic antibiotics unless the patient has a prosthetic heart valve or a surgically constructed systemic pulmonary shunt.

Several factors speak against the aforementioned recommendations. Transient bacteremia has been reported following nasotracheal intubation during general anesthesia.[2] Furthermore, mobilization of the small and large bowel (a common event during diagnostic laparoscopy) has been accompanied by bacteremia. This is confirmed by positive blood cultures obtained at the time of intestinal manipulation.

Aqueous penicillin G, 2 million U given intravenously or intramuscularly 30 to 60 minutes prior to the surgical procedure followed by 1 million U 6 hours later, is adequate prophylaxis. Patients allergic to penicillin can receive a single 1 g dose of Vancomycin intravenously. Because of the long half-life of this medication, no repeat dose is required.

WOUND INFECTION

Wound infections complicating a laparoscopic procedure are rare occurrences despite the obvious breaks in aseptic technique that often take place during laparoscopy. Brenner et al reported rates of wound infection following different techniques of laparoscopic sterilization in the range of 0.8 to 1.3 percent.[3] The few reported cases of infection at the laparoscopic entry site were due to *Staphylococcus aureus* and hemolytic streptococcus. Both of them are common skin pathogens.

Mild infections usually develop 48 to 72 hours after laparoscopy. Erythema around the primary or secondary puncture sites is a common early sign. During the initial stages of the infectious process, it is difficult to discriminate between normal postoperative incisional pain and pain due to the inflammatory reaction of local infection. Because laparoscopy is frequently performed as a same day outpatient procedure with early discharge, examination of the wound by the patient is recommended. Information to that effect must be included with the postoperative instructions (see Chapter 24). Evaluation by a nurse or physician is indicated at an early stage. It should not be delayed until the appearance of suppuration.

Once suppuration has taken place, one must remove the suture or sutures approximating the incisional wound edges. This helps to provide an external pathway for drainage. Secondary healing then occurs by formation of granulations from the depth of the wound. Systemic antibiotic therapy has little effect unless adequate drainage of the necrotic and purulent material is accomplished.

The opportunity to forestall wound infections begins in the preoperative period. The umbilical fossa is a common repository of contaminated material.

An important measure for preventing infection from this source is careful cleansing of the umbilical folds. This is done with several cotton tip applicators previously immersed in an antiseptic solution. Cleansing should always be carried out in a diligent manner in the process of preparing the abdomen as a sterile surgical field. The purpose of the surgical scrub is to remove dirt and bacteria at and around the incisional area. Equally important is the antibacterial residue left on the skin by these solutions. This residual layer acts as a barrier to bacterial growth. Its removal for cosmetic reasons immediately following the operation is counterproductive.

Shaving the incisional area is also controversial. Cruse and Foord reported that wound infection rates are highest when the skin is shaved 24 hours prior to surgery, lower when shaving is done immediately before the operation, and least when this step is omitted altogether.[7] The operator should not feel obligated to shave the peri-incisional region simply because it has been routinely done. Personal experience shows that skin shaving for laparoscopy is seldom required.

Because most operative wounds can be shown to contain some bacteria, the appearance of wound infection must relate to factors other than mere contamination of the operative field. Concomitant distant infectious process, virulence of the organisms involved (see the section on necrotizing fasciitis), and host resistance all seem to play important roles in the occurrence of wound infections.

Patients with established infections distant to the operative site, who undergo clean surgical procedures, are more likely to develop subsequent wound infection than noninfected subjects. Laparoscopy is no exception. Women in whom salpingitis or a tubo-ovarian abscess is found during diagnostic laparoscopy are at risk of developing wound infection at the site of trocar insertion. Because antibiotic therapy would necessarily be used in these patients to treat the established infection, no additional medications to prevent wound infection is required. A metal clip (or clips) to approximate the skin edges is preferred over absorbable suture material in these situations.

It is advisable to adhere closely to strict sterile technique during laparoscopy in subjects who are susceptible to infection. In diabetics and immune deficient patients, the use of gas sterilized instruments is recommended. In addition, antiseptic preparation of the skin surface should be done twice to ensure a sterile field. Similar precautions are appropriate for laparoscopy in malnourished, chronic alcoholic, and older patients in whom the host defense mechanisms might be impaired.

Inadequate levels of hemoglobin and organic iron can also diminish host resistance. The appearance of peri-incisional wound hematoma predisposes to subsequent wound infection. Careful hemostasis appears to be the best prophylaxis (see Chapter 20).

Any type of infection at the site of the incisional punctures should be followed closely. Aggressive management is in order to prevent development of the much more serious condition of necrotizing fasciitis.

NECROTIZING FASCIITIS

Necrotizing fasciitis, also known as Meleney's disease, gangrenous erysipelas, and necrotizing erysipelas, is characterized by extensive necrosis of the subcutaneous and fascial layers. Its nomenclature emphasizes its most constant feature, namely the fascial necrosis undermining the skin. It is typically accompanied by thrombosis of the microvasculature.

This condition may originate from a trivial injury in an operative wound. In gynecological surgery, the necrotizing cellulitis of the anterior abdominal wall is usually associated with laparotomy done for a septic intra-abdominal process. The clinical course of this disease has changed little since Meleney's original description.[18] However, the pathogenic organisms are no longer limited to beta-hemolytic streptococci or the synergistic combination of streptococci and staphylococci which were recovered from all of Meleney's patients.

Giuliano et al investigated the bacteriology of this disease utilizing Gram-stained smears and aerobic and anaerobic culture methods.[9] Bacteria cultured from cases of necrotizing fasciitis included streptococci (alpha- and beta-hemolytic, but not exclusively), staphylococci, enterobacteria (*Escherichia coli, Klebsiella*, and *Proteus enterobacter*) and *Pseudomonas aeruginosa*. Anaerobic Gram-positive bacteria included *Clostridium perfringens*, peptococci, and peptostreptococci, among others. Anaerobic gram-negative bacteria found were mostly of the *Bacteroides* family.

With the increased use of laparoscopy for diagnostic purposes in the presence of pelvic infections as well as in infection susceptible individuals, this condition should be considered in patients who develop a wound infection or unusual abdominal wall discomfort postoperatively. Sotrel et al reported such a case following an uneventful diagnostic laparoscopy in an elderly diabetic patient.[20] They suggested that the indication for laparoscopy should be carefully considered and prophylactic antibiotics given in these patients.

No therapeutic modality can ever replace good preventive measures. Once this complication arises, it can spread in a fulminating fashion in less than 24 hours. Management must be aggressive. Evaluation should include blood, urine, and wound cultures. In addition, smears are obtained, promptly stained, and examined microscopically. After the patient is stabilized, extensive operative debridement is done in the operating room with excision of all necrotic tissue. It is essential that no affected tissue be left behind. Because of the extensive microvascular thrombosis, it is important to continue to evaluate the viability of the remaining tissues during the immediate postoperative period. The wound should be generously irrigated with normal saline and with a solution of neomycin and bacitracin. Penicillin is still the most effective antibiotic agent for systemic use, but the presence of synergistic aerobic and anaerobic bacteria mandates broad spectrum coverage for both Gram-negative and anaerobic organisms.

Mortality from this condition remains high. It is strongly influenced by delay in diagnosis. Movereover, death may reflect the presence of associated diseases and complications.

PERITONITIS

The incidence of peritonitis complicating a laparoscopic procedure is difficult to establish. The main hindrance to determining its true incidence is the fact that often laparoscopy is not the only procedure performed. Maneuvers carried out as part of the endoscopy operation (bimanual examination, insertion of the uterine manipulator) or additional surgical procedures (dilation and uterine curettage, partial salpingectomy) are themselves known to cause peritonitis when carried out alone.

Infectious morbidity associated with the manipulation of the uterus to facilitate visualization of the pelvic viscera can be serious. Goodnough et al reported a case of severe gonococcal peritonitis arising 24 hours after an uneventful diagnostic laparoscopy.[12] At laparotomy, no evidence of bowel perforation was seen and *Neisseria gonorrhoeae* was cultured from the peritoneal cavity.

Care should also be exercised when manipulating a uterus containing an intrauterine device (IUD). Goldacre et al reported an increase in anaerobes in the vaginal microbial flora in young women wearing an IUD.[11] Dissemination of a localized uterine or tubal infectious process can occur as a result of transcervical instillation of a dye solution. This is similar to pelvic peritonitis developing after hydrotubation with radiopaque solutions during hysterosalpingography. It is thus recommended that no solution be injected transcervically if pelvic inflammation is present or suspected.

Infectious morbidity associated with diagnostic laparoscopy is usually a complication of another surgical procedure carried out concurrently. The recommendation to perform a dilation of the cervix and curettage of the uterine cavity (D&C) with all laparoscopies (except when a desired pregnancy is suspected) is unsubstantiated. Infectious complications associated with a diagnostic D&C range from 3 to 5 per 1,000 procedures. Grimes and Peterson suggested that adding a D&C to laparoscopy may increase the morbidity of the operation twofold.[13] They concluded that routine performance of a D&C at the time of laparoscopy is an unwarranted practice.

Disseminated peritonitis may result from inadvertent injury of the gastrointestinal tract. These traumatic lacerations can be produced at the time of insertion of the Verres needle, laparoscopic trocar, and auxiliary instruments (see Chapter 18).

House reported a case of abdominal actinomycosis following a diagnostic laparoscopy for pelvic pain.[15] The patient presented 3 months later with abdominal pain. A 6 cm diameter mass was diagnosed by sonogram. At laparotomy, the large inflammatory mass was densely adherent to the anterior abdominal wall at the site of insertion of the Verres needle used during the previous laparoscopy. Histologic examination showed several small abscesses containing actinomyces.

INFECTION FOLLOWING LAPAROSCOPIC STERILIZATION

Pelvic infections complicating laparoscopic sterilizations are rare events. Huezo et al reported pelvic infection following laparoscopic tubal occlusion in 0.3 to 0.4 percent of cases.[16] Nevertheless, the potential life-threatening character of such complications deserves attention.

The low incidence of salpingitis and pelvic infection following laparoscopic sterilization is to be expected. It has long been suspected that upper genital tract infections have an ascending origin. Organisms gain access to the tubes and peritoneal cavity by surface spread during or immediately after menses. The presence of blood and retrograde flow of the menstruum facilitates the passage of bacteria into the upper genital tract. Tubal obliteration thus interrupts the upward dissemination of the infectious process.

Hajj reported no hospitalization for acute pelvic inflammatory disease in any of over 3,500 patients who have undergone laparoscopic sterilization at his institution.[14] He suggested that a search for another cause must be entertained when a previously sterilized woman presents with symptoms of acute pelvic inflammation. This is not entirely accurate.

Badra et al reported three cases of suppurative salpingitis following tubal electrocauterization.[1] In two instances, the infectious process had progressed to form pelvic abscesses. These required extirpative surgery for therapy. In all cases, they noted a delay of at least 4 days between the laparoscopic procedure and the onset of symptoms.

In all of the aformentioned cases, tubal cauterization was preceded by removal of an IUD and a uterine curettage. The histologic evaluation of the endometrial curettings yielded chronic endometritis. They speculated that the endometrial inflammatory response seen with IUDs, uterine curettage, and tubal electrical injury combined to cause suppurative salpingitis.

Glew and Pokoly described the appearance of unilateral tubo-ovarian abscess in 2 women who had undergone tubal occlusion with silicone bands.[10] Both patients required treatment by surgical drainage. In both instances the sterilization procedures were performed in close temporal relation to a pregnancy interruption, the relevancy of which was questioned by the authors. Bacterial cultures obtained at the time of surgical treatment grew *Corynebacterium vaginale* and *Bacteroides* species; both organisms are found in normal vaginal and cervical flora. This observation suggested that the abscesses developed by way of an ascending infection rather than as a consequence of intraoperative wound infection.

Serious infection following laparoscopic sterilization can occur shortly after the procedure is performed or appear weeks thereafter. Early infectious complications seem to be associated with electrocoagulation. Delayed abscess formation is more commonly reported with silastic band procedures.

The reason for the temporal variation in appearance of the infectious complication is unknown. Both techniques produce necrosis of a portion of fallopian tube which could predispose the area to bacterial colonization. Further studies are required to elucidate the pathophysiology of this entity.

Whether or not pelvic infection occurs more frequently when the sterilization procedure is performed immediately after the removal of an IUD remains controversial. Nevertheless, some facts are undisputed. Women using an IUD for contraception have a high incidence of chronic endometritis. Endosalpingeal inflammation is also frequently present. Given the elective nature of a sterilization procedure, it makes sense to avoid operating on inflamed or infected tissue whenever possible. Thus, a 6-week interval between removal of the IUD and the tubal occlusive operation is recommended.

The appearance of a unilateral tubo-ovarian abscess as a complication of laparoscopic sterilization performed concurrently with pregnancy termination raises questions about the soundness of this combined procedure. Glew and Pokoly suggested that pregnancy may impair the local defense mechanisms predisposing to this complication.[10] The recommendation to allow an interval of not less than 6 weeks between procedures is also applicable to this situation.

References

1. Badra PL, Young JR, Laros RK, Peterson EP. Suppurative salpingitis after laparoscopic tubal cauterization. Obstet Gynecol 1973; 42:511-514.
2. Berry FA, Blankenbaker WL, Ball CG. A comparison of bacteremia occurring with nasotracheal and orotracheal intubation. Anesth Analg 1973; 52:873-877.
3. Brenner WE, Edelman DA, Black JK. Laparoscopic sterilization with electrocautery, spring-loaded clips and silastic bands: Technical problems and early complications. Fertil Steril 1976; 27:256-266.
4. Centers for Disease Control. Guidelines for hospital environmental control: Cleaning, disinfection, and sterilization of hospital equipment. Infect Control 1981; 2:131-134.
5. Corson SL, Block S, Mintz C, et al. Sterilization of laparoscopes: Is soaking sufficient? J Reprod Med 1979; 23:49-56.
6. Corson SL, Dole M, Kraus R, et al. Studies in sterilization of the laparoscope: II. J Reprod Med 1979; 23:57-59.
7. Cruse PJE, Foord D. A five-year prospective study of 23,649 surgical wounds. Arch Surg 1973; 107:206-210.
8. Gerding DN, Peterson LR, Vennes JA. Cleaning and disinfection of fiberoptic endoscopies: Evaluation of glutaraldehyde exposure time and forced-air drying. Gastroenterology 1982; 83:613-618.

9. Giuliano A, Lewis F, Hadley K, Blaisdell FW. Bacteriology of necrotizing fasciitis Am J Surg 1977; 134:52-57.
10. Glew RH, Pokoly TB. Tubo-ovarian abscess following laparoscopic sterilization with silicone rubber bands. Obstet Gynecol 1980; 55:760-762.
11. Goldacre MJ, Watt B, Loudon N, et al. ''Normal'' vaginal microbial flora in normal young women. Br Med J 1979; 1:1450-1453.
12. Goodnough JE, O'Shaughnessy R, Shoff D. Gonococcal peritonitis following uterine manipulation at laparoscopy. Am J Obstet Gynecol 1981; 139:218-219.
13. Grimes DA, Peterson HB. Should dilatation and curettage be performed routinely at the time of laparoscopy? J Reprod Med 1982; 27:213-216.
14. Hajj SN. Does sterilization prevent pelvic infection? J Reprod Med 1978; 20:289-290.
15. House MJ. Abdominal actinomycosis complication of laparoscopy. Br J Obstet Gynaecol 1981; 88:459-460.
16. Huezo CM, DeStefano F, Rubin GL, Ory HW. Risk of wound and pelvic infection after laparoscopic tubal sterilization: Instrument disinfection versus sterilization. Obstet Gynecol 1983; 61:598-602.
17. Loffer FD. Disinfection vs sterilization of gynecologic laparoscopy equipment: The experience of the Phoenix Surgicenter. J Reprod Med 1980; 25:263-266.
18. Meleney FL. Hemolytic streptococcus gangrene. Arch Surg 1924; 9:317-320.
19. Phillips JM. Complications in laparoscopy. Int J Gynaecol Obstet 1977; 15:157-162.
20. Sotrel G, Hirsch E, Edelin KC. Necrotizing fasciitis following diagnostic laparoscopy. Obstet Gynecol 1983; 62:67s-69s.
21. Sterilization Policy for Laparoscope. Washington, DC. Surgeon General's Office, February 25, 1977.
22. Zwelling LA, Mandell GL, Young RC. Peritoneoscopy: An invasive procedure without bacteremia. Ann Int Med 1977; 87:454.

22 COMPLICATIONS OF STERILIZATION

Laparoscopic tubal occlusion has to a large extent become the most frequently utilized method of female sterilization. Its increased use has been accompanied by its own special group of complications. After 20 years of widespread use, it is becoming clear that many complications can be avoided by strict adherence to the basic technical principles as detailed in Chapter 2.

Phillips et al, reporting the results of a survey of the American Association of Gynecologic Laparoscopists (AAGL), demonstrated that the rate of complications is inversely proportional to the experience of the operator.[20] Most laparoscopic mishaps occur during the early stages of learning by the laparoscopist. This is to be expected and parallels that associated with mastery of any other surgical procedure.

While laparoscopic sterilization appears to be a safe procedure overall, serious morbidity and mortality related to this procedure still occur. No accurate estimate of the rate of minor complications associated with the procedure can be obtained. Problems solved without sequelae usually go unreported. In this chapter, only those complications encountered with the common laparoscopic sterilization methods will be described.

Complications associated with laparoscopic sterilization can be classified according to their temporal occurrence. Those occurring intraoperatively or in the immediate postoperative period show a more direct cause and effect relationship than those appearing months or years later. Some of the reported complications are common to all methods for laparoscopic tubal occlusion, such as mesosalpingeal bleeding, pain, and poststerilization pregnancy. Others are peculiar to particular techniques. The latter encompass those in which technical difficulties are especially seen or in which the amount of tissue damage can be expected to be considerable. Because the gynecologist must be familiar with most, if not all, translaparoscopic sterilization techniques, a description of the most frequent complications common to all and those idiosyncratic for certain techniques are included in this chapter.

MESOSALPINGEAL BLEEDING

Tubal or mesosalpingeal hemorrhage is a feared complication of laparoscopic sterilization. It is the result of uncontrolled injury to vessels of the region. Hemostasis can at times be achieved only by identification and ligation of the lacerated vessel at laparotomy. Knowledge of the regional anatomy is essential. A review of the normal vascular supply, its origin and anastomosis is beneficial not only to help prevent hemorrhagic diathesis but also to aid in achieving hemostasis successfully.

Vascularization of the fallopian tube can be quite variable; nevertheless, the distribution of vessels is often fairly standard (Figure 22.1). The arterial supply to the oviduct derives from two sources. Its intramural and isthmic portions are supplied by the ascending uterine artery. The ampulla, infundibulum and fimbria are nourished by branches of the ovarian artery.

The ascending uterine artery supplies a branch to the cornu and interstitial portion of the tube before entering the mesosalpinx. A short distance beyond, it dichotomizes into its final branches, the tubal and utero-ovarian arteries. The former feeds the medial portion of the tube; the latter goes on to anastomose with the ovarian artery.

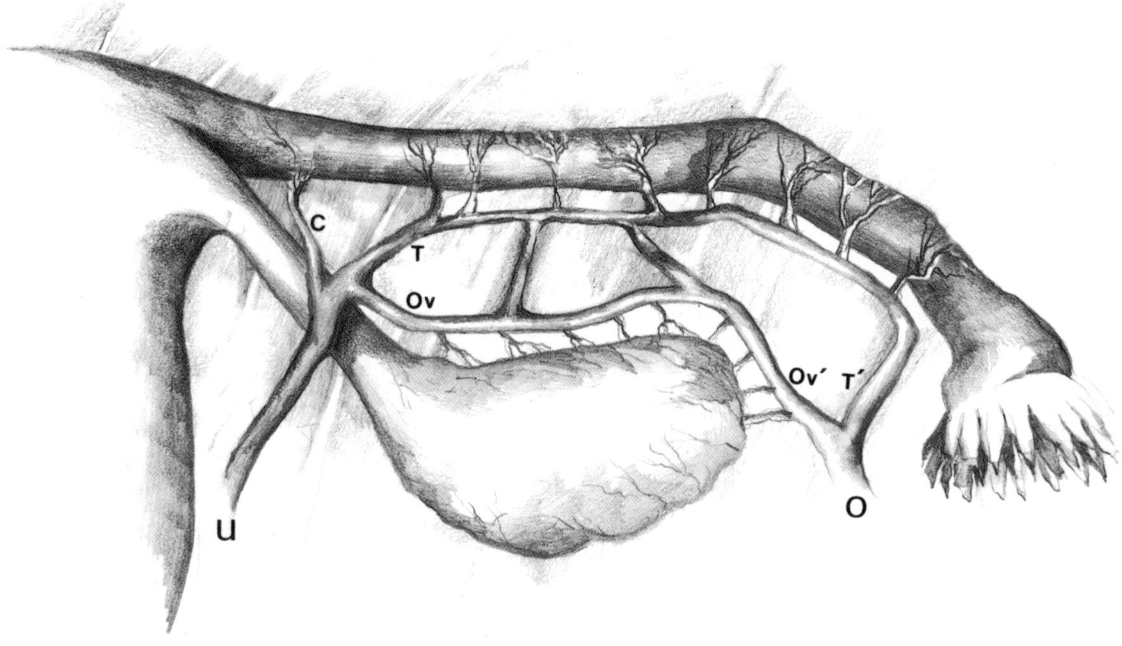

Figure 22.1 Vasculature of the fallopian tube. Uterine and ovarian vessels are depicted. *Key*: *u* = uterine artery with its *c* = cornual, *t* = tubal, and *ov* = ovarian branches, *o* = ovarian artery with its *t′*, tubal and *ov′* = ovarian branches. t and t′ join to form the tubal artery; ov and ov′ supply the ovary.

The ovarian artery enters the abdominal cavity within the infundibulopelvic ligament. Before it furnishes any blood supply to the ovary, it gives off its tubal subsidiary. The tubal branch supplies the fimbria, infundibulum, and ampulla before it anastomoses with its tubal counterpart originating from the ascending uterine artery.

The tubal artery traverses the mesosalpinx on the inferior border of the oviduct. It provides multiple small arteries to each section of the tube. These branches intercommunicate with each other after reaching the serosa and muscularis layers. The tubal artery also gives off intermediate size branches that cross the mesosalpinx to join the ovarian artery which nourishes the ovary. The venous drainage follows the arterial supply in close proximity.

Injury to the oviductal vasculature is not limited to a particular modality of laparoscopic sterilization. Mesosalpingeal hemorrhage has been reported to complicate unipolar and bipolar electrocoagulation as well as silastic band procedures (Figure 22.2).

Unipolar Electrocoagulation

Mesosalpingeal hemorrhage complicates unipolar electrocoagulation of the tubes only when accompanied by division or resection of a portion of the oviduct.

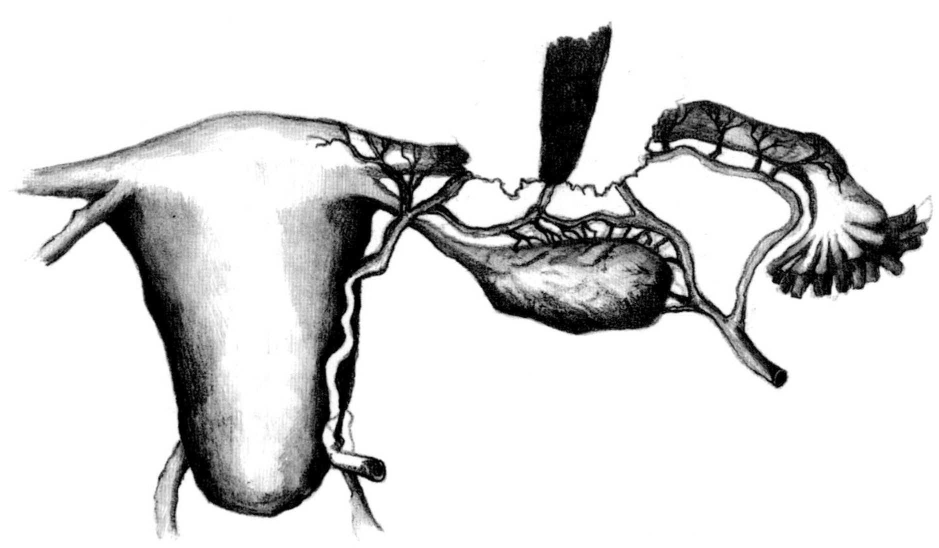

Figure 22.2 Mesosalpingeal hemorrhage. Laceration of the tubal artery is the most common source of bleeding. Smaller vessels which cross the mesosalpinx (tubo-ovarian anastomosis) can also be the source of a serious hemorrhagic diathesis, as shown.

Inadequate high frequency coagulation of the oviductal vasculature prior to incision of the tube is the most likely underlying cause.

Usually, unipolar electrocoagulation is carried out with a single application of the forceps. The current will spread radially away from the instrument searching for the dispersive electrode (return plate). The operator is unable to estimate the exact extent of tissue destruction by visual inspection.

A measure of adequate unipolar electrocoagulation of tube and mesosalpinx is gained with experience. Rotating the tube grasped within the forceps while twisting down the cutting sleeve of the Palmer forceps indicate insufficient tissue desiccation. Additional cauterization is indicated.

If removal of a portion of oviduct is attempted following tubal electrocoagulation, resection should be limited to the fallopian tube itself. Division of the dessicated mesosalpinx is not required. Reabsorption of the injured portion of mesosalpinx occurs postoperatively. This results in spatial separation of the remaining uninjured tubal stumps.

If adequate electrocoagulation of the tube and the underlying mesosalpinx has been achieved, resection of a segment of oviduct is fairly simple. This is accomplished by positioning the unipolar forceps perpendicularly to the mesosalpingeal plane before the cutting power is applied. This prevents inadvertent incision into the mesosalpinx (Figure 22.3).

Incomplete electrocauterization can also occur when the electrical generator is set at high levels. Blanching of the serosa and portions of the muscularis layer give the operator a false impression of sufficient tissue dessication when in fact the vasculature remains unaffected (that is, still patent). Complete tissue dessication within and surrounding the unipolar forceps is indispensable. Use of low settings on the electrogenerator is recommended.

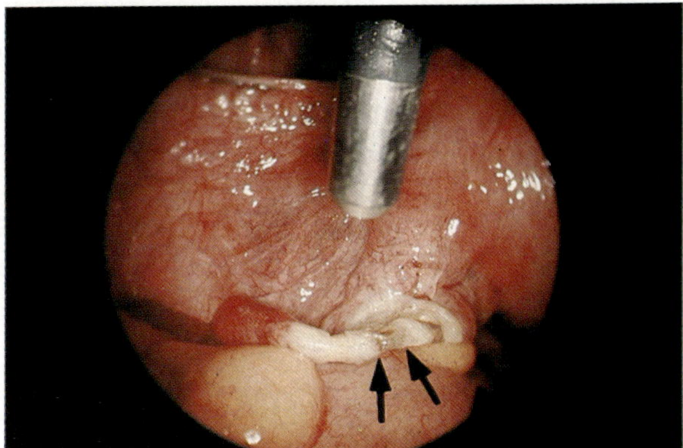

Figure 22.3 Tubal resection following electrocauterization. The amount of tissue dessication must extend beyond the resection margin. Cutting must be limited to the fallopian tube itself. Division of the mesosalpinx is unnecessary.

Bipolar Electrocoagulation

Sterilization by bipolar electrocoagulation does not usually include division or resection of the fallopian tube. Nevertheless, mesosalpingeal hemorrhage can occur when this instrument is used. This can be seen when the forceps remains attached to the burned tissue, making its separation difficult (Figure 22.4). This difficulty results as a consequence of the accumulation of carbonized debris on the inner surface of the forceps tongs.

The operator must avoid using excessive traction or jerky movements to dislodge the adherent tissue. The instrument and cauterized portion of tube and mesosalpinx should be allowed to cool. This facilitates their separation and spontaneous detachment usually occurs. If the tissue remains affixed to the forceps tongs, disengagement is accomplished by gently pushing the adherent tissue off the forceps with the front end of the laparoscope. This maneuver ought to be carried out under direct visualization. Sometimes, contact of the front laparoscopic lens with the warmed cauterized tissue helps sharpen the view by defogging the viewing lens (see Chapter 26).

Management of mesosalpingeal hemorrhage during unipolar or bipolar electrocoagulation consists of additional cauterization of the contiguous portions of tube. Further desiccation of the vessels both proximal and distal to the injured area is usually sufficient. A small proportion of patients will require laparotomy for hemostasis.

The operator should not hesitate to insert an additional auxiliary puncture if needed. This could be used to place a hollow cannula for the purpose of aspirating the extravasated blood. The area to which further coagulation is to be applied should be kept dry to enhance the hemostatic capability of additional electrocoagulation.

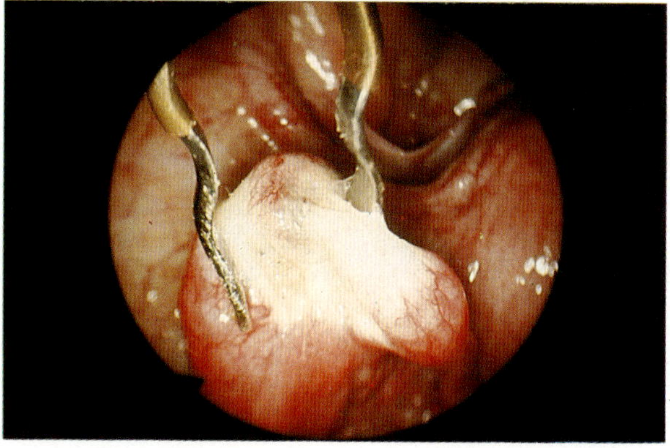

Figure 22.4 Adherence of bipolar forceps to cauterized tube. Excessive carbonized debris on the forceps tongs is the underlying cause. Excessive traction or jerky motions must be avoided to prevent laceration of the affixed tissue.

Spring loaded clips and silastic bands have also proven useful in controlling mesosalpingeal hemorrhage. They are applied to the proximal and distal segment of the tube near the bleeding site to interrupt circulation to the injured area. The use of such clips or bands requires the insertion of a 7 mm sleeve to accommodate the passage of their applicators.

Silastic Bands

Mesosalpingeal hemorrhage is the most common complication associated with the use of silastic bands (Falope ring) for tubal occlusion. Laceration of the fallopian tube and underlying mesosalpinx occurs at the time of application of the ring over the loop of tube. Transection of the tube can be partial or complete.

Partial transection usually occurs at the time the distended Falope ring is fired over the tubal knuckle. Notwithstanding the lack of knuckle formation, the band may still obliterate the blood supply to the lacerated tube (Figure 22.5). Observation for adequate hemostasis is all that is generally required.

Formation of a blood clot over the transected portion of oviduct may be misleading. Irrigation of the injured section with physiologic saline solution elucidates any point of persistent hemorrhage (Figure 26.6).

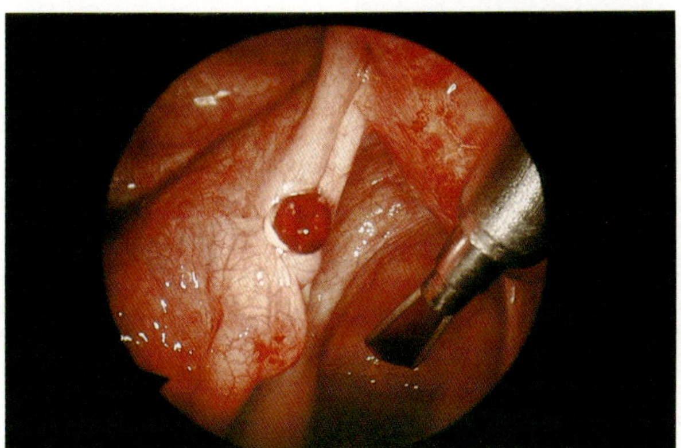

Figure 22.5 Transection of fallopian tube. Division of the tube occurred when the Falope ring was fired over the tubal knuckle.

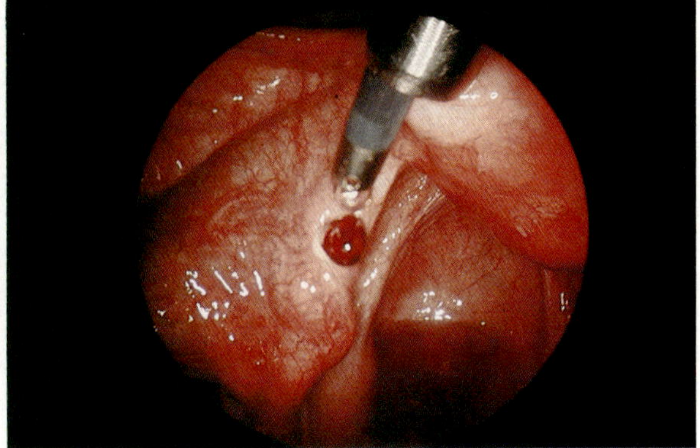

Figure 22.6 Evaluation of lacerated fallopian tube. Formation of a blood clot may mislead one to believe adequate hemostasis has been accomplished. Profuse irrigation with physiologic saline solution demonstrates a source of persistent bleeding, if present.

If the transection occurs on the first tube to be operated on, application of the silastic band on the contralateral side should proceed as usual. This allows some time to transpire prior to the conclusion of the operation and removal of all instruments. If by then no evidence of continuous bleeding from the injured area is seen, hemostasis can be considered adequate (Figure 22.7). If the transection arises during application of the band to the second oviduct, the operator must observe the area for no less than 5 minutes after hemostasis has been achieved to ensure that bleeding has been controlled.

Persistence of the tubal loop following Falope ring application is not essential. Ansari et al, in an attempt to reduce the failure rate of this technique, intentionally severed the tubal knuckle following adequate placement of the silastic rings.[1] No bleeding complications were reported in their series.

Complete transection of the oviduct tends to happen during the formation of the tubal knuckle. Withdrawal of the forceps tongs before adequate encasement of the tubal loop is accomplished within the applicator's inner cylinder usually severs the tube. The lacerated ends of the tube retract away from the forceps tongs and bleed freely.

Conditions that predispose to tubal transection include: grasping the tube close to its cornual implantation; thick or swollen tubes; peritubal adhesions, and technical considerations related to individual dexterity.

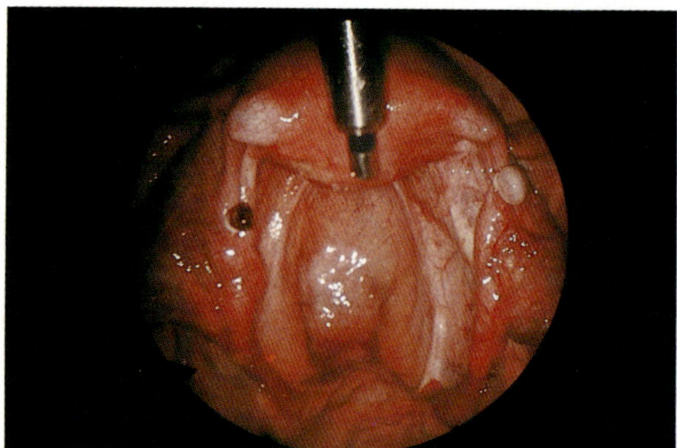

Figure 22.7 Panoramic view at the conclusion of silastic band application. Evidence of adequate hemostasis is confirmed by continued observation for several minutes. Clearing the posterior cul-de-sac of blood and saline by aspiration permits one to confirm the absence of any active bleeding.

Grasping the Tube Close to its Cornual Implantation. Application of the forceps tongs less than 2 cm from the interstitial portion of the tube increases the risk of tubal transection. Such proximity to the uterus prevents the formation of an adequate tubal loop. The proximal portion of the tube is unduly stretched. Full retraction of the forceps tongs lacerates the tube and the underlying mesosalpinx. Division of the tube at this site is particularly prone to result in hemorrhage. It occurs because of the rich vascularity of the cornual region cularity of the cornual region (see Figure 22.2).

This particular cause of tubal transection is avoidable. Forceps tongs should not be applied to the tube closer than 3 cm from its uterine origin. The tubal loop is thus formed free of tension. Avoid firing the silastic band over a tubal loop that appears to overstretch the adjacent portions of oviduct.

Large Diameter of the Fallopian Tubes. Abnormally distended oviducts are prone to be transected at the time of band application. Severing the tube results because one is mechanically unable to fit the enlarged tubal loop into the applicator's central cylinder. The narrow forceps tongs cut through the grasped tissue when the instrument is retracted into their close position.

This complication is also a preventable one. Evaluation of tubal thickness must be carried out before any attempts are made to apply a Falope ring. Distance between the forceps tongs in their open position (completely extruded) must be greater than the diameter of the oviduct (Figure 22.8). When large diameter tubes are unexpectedly encountered at the time of laparoscopy, it is advisable to switch to an alternative method of sterilization such as bipolar electrocoagulation (Figure 22.9).

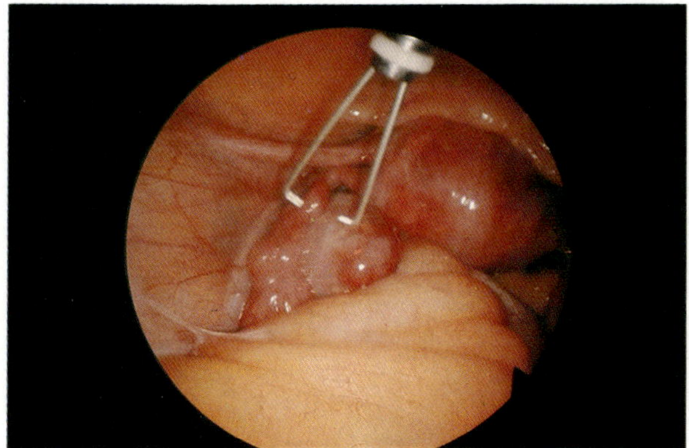

Figure 22.8 Assessing for tubal thickness. With the Falope ring loaded on the outer cylinder, the inner forceps tongs are extended into their open position under direct vision. The distance between the forceps tong tips must be greater than the diameter of the oviduct.

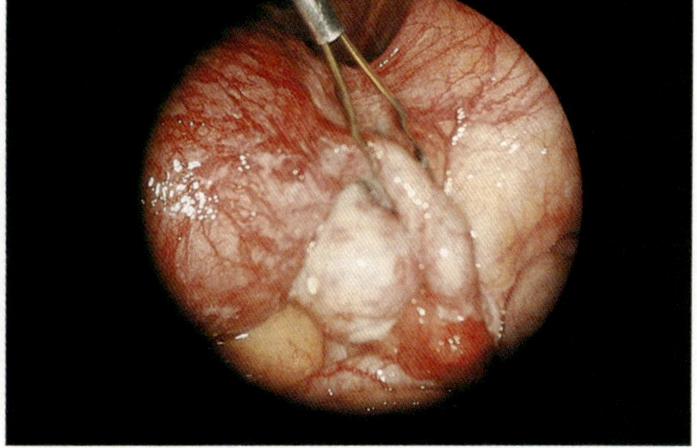

Figure 22.9 Bipolar electrocoagulation of a thick oviduct. Unexpected finding of a wide tube in a case for which silastic band sterilization was planned. The fallopian tube also appears to be foreshortened. This would preclude the formation of an adequate tubal knuckle. Use of bipolar electrocautery averted the risk of tubal transection from use of the silastic bands.

Peritubal Adhesions. The presence of peritubal adhesions increases the likelihood of transecting the tube during silastic band application. This appears to be due to the relative immobility of the oviduct which prevents elevation of the tube into the applicator's inner cylinder to form a knuckle (Figure 22.10). Excessive stretching of the fixed tube and its mesosalpinx also predisposes to laceration by the pointed forceps tongs. Occasionally, mobilization of the uterus (by manual or instrumental means) in a cephalad and lateral direction may facilitate formation of a loop without undue tension. Placement of a silastic ring, even in the presence of tubal adhesions, then becomes possible.

Technical Considerations. Transection of the fallopian tube during application of a silastic band can occur even in the presence of normal oviducts with no apparent predisposing factor. The cause is usually a departure from the standard technique (see Chapter 5). Withdrawing the tubal knuckle too rapidly into the applicator's central cylinder may damage it. This swift motion does not allow the tube time to accommodate to the lumen of the applicator, resulting in transection of the tube.

A similar situation may result from an inadequately cleaned applicator forceps. This yields a series of jerky, unsteady movements at the time the stretched silastic band is slid over the tubal loop. Levinson et al described a characteristic "click" sign when the tube is transected.[12] It is explained by the sudden loss of elastic resistance by the tube.

Beck and Gal reported an unusual complication.[4] During a procedure, while the tube is being held within the forceps, misfiring of the silicone band locked the tongs. This event prevented release of the tissue within the forceps prongs.

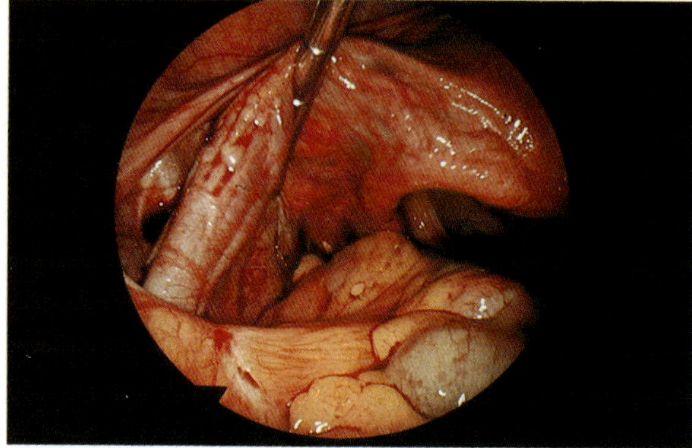

Figure 22.10 Peritubal adhesion. Left fallopian tube is dipping down into the posterior cul-de-sac and is adherent to the posterior leaf of the ipsilateral broad ligament. Displacement of the left infundibulopelvic ligament reveals fixation of the oviduct with stretching of the mesosalpinx. Anastomotic vessels between the tubal and ovarian arteries can be seen.

It is possible for this problem to be further aggravated by mesosalpingeal hemorrhage occurring because of tubal transection.

They recommended that firing the instrument in the usual manner may advance the band over the tip of the forceps. If unsuccessful, sharp division of the silastic band is required. This is accomplished by the introduction of sharp scissors through a tertiary puncture.

PAIN ASSOCIATED WITH STERILIZATION

Evaluation of pain during or following a sterilization procedure is difficult. The subjective nature of the complaint makes it subject to a variety of underlying factors not readily measurable objectively. Preoperative counseling, patient selection, and the physician's experience must be taken into account.

Pain associated with a sterilization procedure can occur intraoperatively (in the case of surgery under local anesthesia), during the immediate postoperative period, or months to years after the original surgery. This temporal classification is important. The appearance of intraoperative pain may affect the overall safety of the procedure. Inadvertent reactive movements by the patient may lead to serious complications (such as bowel injury and mesosalpingeal bleeding). Short-term or long-term postoperative discomfort may in turn require hospitalization and/or increased analgesia.

Intraoperative Pain

The extent of pain experienced at the time of sterilization varies among patients and by techniques. Pelland evaluated 150 patients undergoing sterilization by tubal fulguration and Falope ring banding under local anesthesia.[19] The type of tubal occlusion performed was unknown to the patients at the time of postoperative evaluation. Use of silastic bands was associated with more pain during application and for the subsequent 24 hours than with electrocoagulation.

The application of 4 percent lidocaine to the oviducts at the time of fulguration greatly diminished the discomfort reported by patients. Such topical anesthesia is also helpful for reducing (but not eliminating) the pain experienced during banding sterilization. The major differences in effect of local anesthesia between fulguration and band sterilization may reflect its mode of administration.

For electrocoagulative tubal surgery, the anesthetic solution can be injected directly into the tubal wall at the site of forceps application. This is feasible, but inappropriate, during silastic ring tubal occlusion. Injection of anesthetic solution into the tube results in swelling of the oviduct and thus prevent the formation of the tubal knuckle. For the application of silastic bands, the preferred method is to drip the anesthetic solution over each tube and mesosalpinx.

Postoperative Pain

Pain is often reported by patients following a sterilization procedure. The extent and duration varies with the technique employed. One must be careful to distinguish the pain associated with a laparoscopic procedure from the pain related to surgery of the oviduct.

Chi and Cole determined the incidence of pain among women undergoing laparoscopic sterilization by electrocoagulation, the spring loaded clip, and the silastic band.[5] Their data was a compilation of five comparative studies conducted at three separate medical centers. Each individual study compared two techniques randomly assigned to 300 patients.

Silastic bands were associated with the highest rate of abdominal and/or pelvic pain during the procedure and the immediate postoperative period. Intraoperative pain was reported during electrocoagulation of the tubes, but no discomfort was experienced postoperatively in this group. On the contrary, spring loaded clips were least likely to produce pain at the time of their application, but they were the source of postoperative pain comparable to that experienced postoperatively by the silastic band group.

Several theories have been advanced that attempt to explain this difference in postoperative discomfort with each technique. Destruction of the tubal sensory receptors during electrocoagulation would account for the absence of postoperative pain in this subset of patients. Tubal ischemia and edema of the tubal knuckle devascularized by the silastic band is thought to be the reason for the increased pain associated with this method. There is no clear explanation for the enhanced postoperative pain reported by women sterilized with spring loaded clips.

The appearance of postoperative pain following silastic band or spring loaded clip application cannot be prevented or predicted. Proper counseling and preoperative preparation facilitates a patient's acceptance of these side effects. Treatment is symptomatic. Pain relief medication and reassurance that the pain is self limited (24 to 36 hours) is usually sufficient.

Because laparoscopic sterilization is mainly an outpatient procedure, same day discharge is customary. Patients must be advised to communicate to the physician any lack of improvement or persistence of postoperative discomfort beyond 36 hours. To prevent overlooking a more serious complication, reevaluation of patients with persistent symptoms is indicated.

Whether or not prolonged persistence or de novo appearance of pelvic pain can be anticipated following laparoscopic sterilization remains controversial. Baggish et al reported that 45 percent of their patients either developed dysmenorrhea or experienced more severe pain following the procedure.[3] Contrariwise, Edgerton found no significant difference in the incidence of pelvic pain or dysmenorrhea in patients followed for up to 7 years after electrocoagulative tubal occlusion.[8] Additional prospective studies are needed to resolve this controversy.

POSTSTERILIZATION PREGNANCY

Unplanned pregnancy following laparoscopic sterilization is a serious complication of this technique. Its occurrence has social, medical, and legal implications, all of equal importance.

Social Implications

Frequently, the socioeconomic considerations surrounding sterilization are not part of the process of counseling patients. It is safe to assume, however, that they play a very important role in the decision-making process in each case. It is thus not difficult to understand the social implications of a failed sterilization.

Proper counseling of a patient requesting a sterilization includes a thorough explanation of the nature and consequences of the procedure. Notwithstanding the recent advances in microsurgical tubal reanastomosis following elective tubal occlusion, certain conditions must be met before sterilization is undertaken. One prerequisite is for the patient to have a clear understanding of the irreversibility of the procedure. This implies that she must have made the decision not to bear any more children before she can consent to being sterilized.

An in-depth evaluation of the socioeconomic ramifications of an unwanted (that is, unplanned) gestation is beyond the scope of this book. Nevertheless, one must be aware of their existence and include them as part of the discussion that precedes the operation.

Medical Implications

The exact incidence of failed laparoscopic sterilization is difficult to assess. Reported rates vary from as low as 2 per 1,000 to as high as 22 per 1,000 procedures.[14] This wide range is due in part to the nonuniform method of reporting this complication.

Some studies have a short follow-up period (1 year or less) from the time the operation was performed. Others do not include patients lost to follow-up, assuming on dubious grounds that the procedure must have been successful. Further complicating matters is the lack of differentiation between technical and true method failures. The former include luteal phase pregnancy and misidentification of pelvic structures.

Luteal Phase Pregnancy. Luteal phase pregnancy is not sterilization failure. Fertilization and tubal transport have already taken place by the time the oviducts are occluded. It results from inappropriate timing of the surgical procedure. Loffer and Pent reported a range of 2.2 to 3.0 per 1,000 incidence among laparoscopic sterilizations.[14]

Attempts to prevent this problem include the routine performance of a concomitant uterine curettage and preoperative measurement of serum human chorionic gonadotropin (hCG). Neither has proved to be universally successful.

Partial disruption of the endometrial lining during curettage does not prevent implantation of the conceptus. Evaluation of the extent of uterine scraping following sharp curettage reveals that less than 40 percent of the endometrium is removed in more than half the cases. Implantation may thus occur in any portion of undisturbed endometrial lining.

Preoperative measurement of serum hCG may also be inadequate. Tubal transport of the fertilized egg takes place within the 72 hours after fertilization. The conceptus then remains free within the uterine cavity for up to 96 hours before it implants. Production of hCG by the trophoblast follows implantation. Thus, surgical occlusion of the oviducts may be done following the passage of the fertilized egg into the uterine cavity, but before implantation has taken place. Under these circumstances, no detectable amount of hCG is present at the time of sterilization. This would explain the appearance of a luteal phase pregnancy even though there was a negative serum pregnancy test at the time of tubal occlusion.

An effective way to prevent a luteal phase pregnancy is to limit all sterilization procedures exclusively to the proliferative phase of the menstrual cycle. While this may present a logistic and programmatic problem, every attempt should be made to time the procedure accordingly. In addition, the patient should be counseled to continue the contraceptive method she has been using, without interruption, until the procedure has been carried out. Alternatively, the woman may choose to abstain from sexual intercourse from the time of her last normal menstrual period until the operation is performed.

Misidentification of Pelvic Structures. Misidentification of any pelvic structure for the fallopian tubes is clearly an operative error. Its incidence ranges between 0.6 and 2.4 per 1,000 laparoscopic sterilizations.[14] Analogous to luteal phase pregnancies, the resulting gestation should not be attributed to the method but should instead be classified as an operator error.

The structures most often mistaken for the tube are the round and the infundibulopelvic ligaments. In the absence of anatomical distortion due to pelvic adhesions, deficient visualization (due to suboptimal illumination or fogging of the laparoscopic lens) is the usual cause.

A complicating factor, which also predisposes to this type of operator error, is failure to mobilize the uterus adequately. Lateral displacement of the uterine fundus places the adnexal structures on stretch. This facilitates proper differentiation of round and infundibulopelvic ligaments from the fallopian tube.

The complication should be entirely preventable. Before proceeding to obliterate the tube, one must carefully identify the fimbriated end. Do not hesitate to utilize additional accessory punctures to aid in visualizing all relevant anatomical structures.

Furthermore, one cannot consider the operation to be satisfactorily completed before verifying that the fallopian tubes have been occluded. Misapplication of a silastic band or electrocautery to the round or the infundibulopelvic ligaments does not preclude repeating the procedure on the tubes to accomplish the technique correctly. If in doubt, transcervical instillation of a dye solution (such as methylene blue) must be carried out to test tubal patency.

Method Failure

When luteal phase pregnancies and misidentification of pelvic structures are excluded, the true failure rate for laparoscopic sterilizations ranges between 0.9 and 6.0 per 1,000.[14] This rate is similar to that of nonlaparoscopic sterilization methods. Incidence varies with the technique used for tubal occlusion. The lowest rate is found with electrocauterization (unipolar and bipolar) and the highest with the spring loaded clip; silastic band sterilizations have an intermediate rate of failure.

Several explanations have been advanced to explain a sterilization method failure. They include inadequate technique, recanalization, and fistula formation.

Inadequate technique can be associated with both electrical and mechanical methods. Pregnancies following insufficient electrocauterization were reported by Thompson and Wheeless in up to 8 per 1,000 cases when unipolar electrocautery was used.[22] The most common finding seen at repeat laparoscopy was a superficial unilateral defect along the top of the tube (antimesosalpingeal border) with an intact lumen (Figure 22.11). Patency is confirmed by hysterosalpingography and/or transcervical injection of indigo carmine (Figure 22.12).

Incomplete cauterization of the oviduct has also been reported with bipolar tubal cautery.[2] The risk of inadequate electrocoagulation with a bipolar forceps is reduced when a bipolar generator with an electron flowmeter is used (see Chapter 5). When electrons no longer pass between the forceps tongs, it indicates maximal resistance secondary to complete tissue cauterization.

Ayers et al reported that 90 percent of pregnancies after bipolar electrocoagulation occurred within the first 3 months following the operation.[2] They suggested that bipolar electrocoagulation occludes the fallopian tubes by delayed fibrosis and not by immediate destruction of tubal tissue. Maximal fibrosis does not occur until 8 to 12 weeks postoperatively.

Imperfect tubal occlusion has been advanced as the most likely cause of failed sterilization with spring loaded clips.[11] Application of these clips to large oviducts may not completely encompass the tubal wall within the arms of the clip (Figures 22.13 and 22.14). Earlier failures were attributed to decreased tension of the occlusive spring that left the lumen sufficiently patent to allow sperm to traverse it.[13–15]

Recanalization of the tubal lumen has also been offered to explain tubal patency following a sterilization procedure. This appears to be related more to inadequate cauterization, as reported by Thompson and Wheeless,[22] than to actual recanalization of fibrotic tissue. The degree of tissue destruction observed in segments of tube removed following electrocauterization makes it highly improbable that a lumen can reform.

A more likely explanation for the tubal patency observed following a sterilization procedure is the formation of a tuboperitoneal fistula. McCausland evaluated the histology of different portions of the oviducts to determine how they respond to electrocoagulation injury.[17] He found that cauterization of the midisthmic portion of tube yields fibrosis. When the proximal portion of the isthmus is similarly injured, however, the endosalpinx becomes activated (in the process of endosalpingiosis). The risk of fistula formation here is greatly increased.

Rock et al demonstrated endometriosis and tuboperitoneal fistulas in patients who had had a sterilization procedure.[21] Such fistulas were encountered more often after laparoscopic cauterization than after other sterilization methods. Destruction of the oviduct within 4 cm of its uterine implantation was felt to predispose to the development of endometriosis and fistulization of the proximal tubal stump.

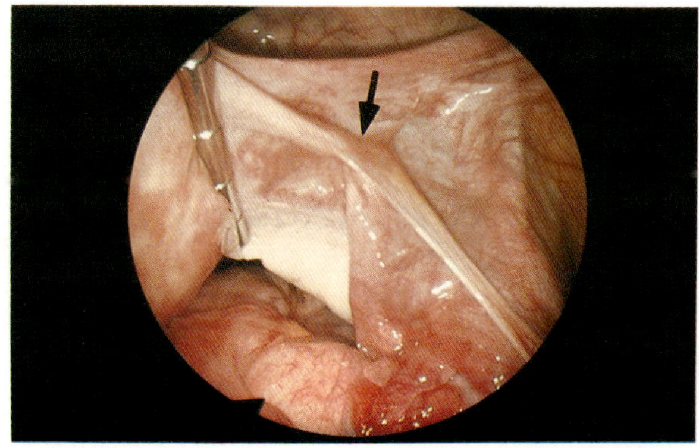

Figure 22.11 Failed sterilization. Site of previous electrocoagulation is marked by a newly formed peritoneal fold (arrow). Fibrotic distortion of tubal contour can be seen beneath the adhesion.

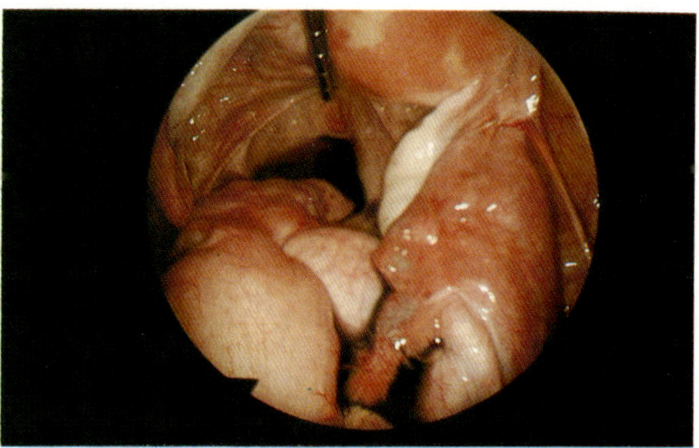

Figure 22.12 Patent tube post sterilization (same case as Figure 22.11). Transcervical instillation of methylene blue reveals free flow at the fimbrial end on the right. Repeat electrocauterization of the right fallopian tube was carried out concurrently with evacuation of an intrauterine gestation.

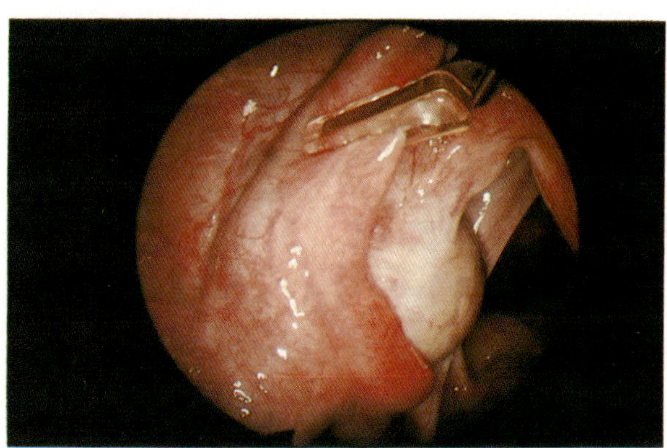

Figure 22.13 Misapplication of spring loaded clip. The clip fails to encompass the entire tubal circumference. The tube is too broad to ensure that the small clip will obliterate the tubal lumen completely.

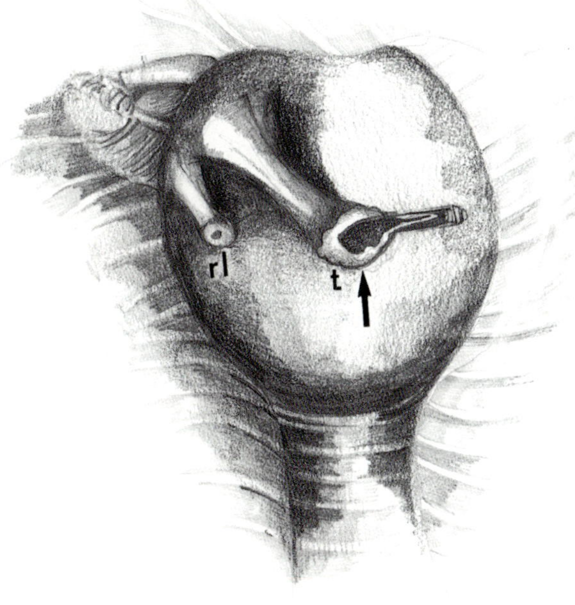

Figure 22.14 Schematic representation of incomplete tubal occlusion with spring-loaded clip. *Key: t* = tube, *rl* = round ligament. Longitudinal section at the level of clip application reveals unoccluded tubal lumen (arrow).

Type of Pregnancy

Failed sterilization resulting from a luteal phase pregnancy or misidentification of pelvic structures is generally intrauterine in location. This is not the case for gestations associated with a true method failure. Ectopic pregnancy is not unusual after an otherwise successful sterilization.

The incidence of ectopic gestation in failed sterilizations appears to be higher after laparoscopic operations than after nonlaparoscopic procedures.[6] McCausland, in a literature review, reported a 12.3 percent rate of ectopic pregnancies following nonlaparoscopic tubal ligation.[16] A comparable review of failed sterilizations subsequent to laparoscopic sterilization revealed 51 percent ectopic gestations. Because many sterilization failures resulting in intrauterine gestations may not be fully reported in the literature, this ectopic-to-intrauterine pregnancy ratio may not be accurate.

Cunanan et al reported a failure rate of 2.2 per 1,000 laparoscopic sterilizations performed over an 8.5 year period.[6] All the failures followed laparoscopic cauterization and resection of a segment of tube. Of the 11 pregnancies in this series, 7 were ectopic in location. All of them were found in the distal portion of the tube. Based on this experience, it was suggested that cauterization should not be accompanied by division or resection of the coagulated oviduct.

McCausland attributed the high incidence of ectopic gestation to the formation of uteroperitoneal fistulas.[17] Sperm thus gain access to the peritoneal cavity where fertilization occurs. The zygote is then picked up by the fimbria of the distal tubal remnant but is unable to enter the uterine cavity because the proximal end of this tubal segment is occluded. Ectopic implantation thus results (Figure 22.15).

Implantation in the distal remnant of the fallopian tube has special clinical significance. The large ampullary lumen and increased distensibility enables the gestation to develop to a more advanced stage (often up to 10 to 12 weeks from last menstrual period) before tubal rupture ensues (Figures 22.16 and 22.17). The pronounced delay may be diagnostically misleading at times.

Because of the relative high incidence of ectopic gestation among pregnancies following a laparoscopic sterilization, certain precautions are recommended. A missed menstrual period ought to be evaluated for pregnancy always, using the more sensitive serum beta-subunit hCG. Demonstration of hCG in serum should be assumed to reflect an ectopic gestation until proven otherwise. The identification of an intrauterine gestation by means of a pelvic ultrasonogram is a useful finding that helps to rule out tubal pregnancy. When in doubt, a laparoscopy is indicated to exclude the diagnosis definitely.

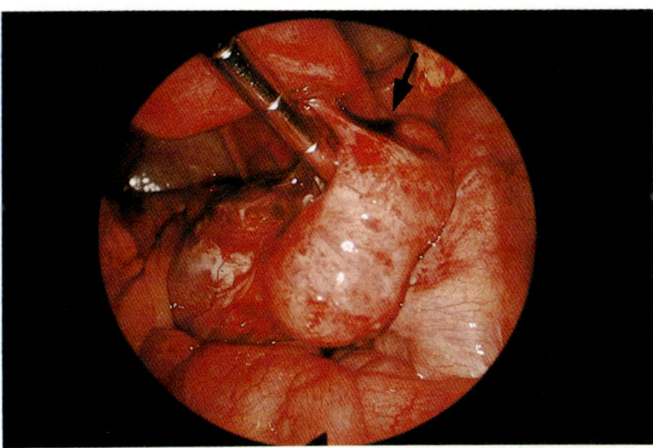

Figure 22.15 Poststerilization ectopic pregnancy (unruptured). Eccyesis is located in the ampulla of the distal remnant of the fallopian tube. The site of prior electrocauterization is marked by the arrow.

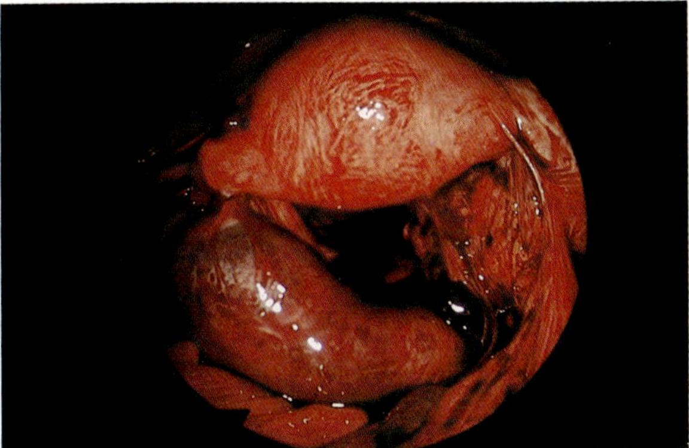

Figure 22.16 Poststerilization ectopic gestation (unruptured). Ampullary implantation enables the pregnancy to grow rather large before it disrupts the tube. Late appearance of clinical manifestations may be a misleading diagnostic factor in these cases.

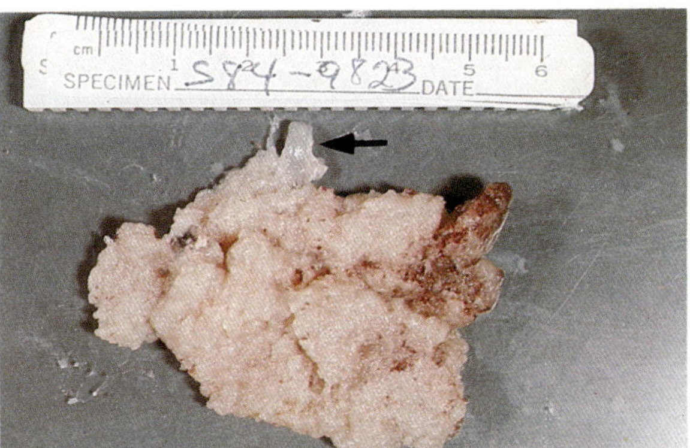

Figure 22.17 Placenta from ectopic gestation (same case as Figure 22.16). Ampullary location of the eccyesis allowed growth to continue beyond the usual time for symptoms to develop. The placenta weighed 28 g; the umbilical cord can be seen (arrow).

Legal Implications

Pregnancy following laparoscopic sterilization has legal implications that can affect the physician performing the operation and the hospital at which it was done. Contradictory decisions by courts in different states are further complicated by indiscriminate use of confusing terminology. Terms such as wrongful conception, wrongful life, and wrongful birth have been differently defined and dissimilarly applied in a number of cases. These are defined in Chapter 25 and their implications discussed. Conflicting court decisions prevail thus far.

As courts continue to accept or reject actions for wrongful birth following unsuccessful sterilization procedures, physicians cannot and should not rely on past decisions. Patients must be informed prior to undergoing a tubal ligation about its failure rate. Futhermore, information concerning the type of gestation that may ensue and the alternative treatment available for it must also be shared with the patient.

A truly informed consent must include documentation so that the prospective candidate for a tubal ligation understands that the procedure is not infallible. Reassurance about the nature of the operation and its risks must not be permitted to constitute a warranty or to be construed as such by the patient.

POSTSTERILIZATION MENSTRUAL ABNORMALITIES

Whether tubal sterilization increases the risk of subsequent menstrual disturbances has been controversial for many years. Popularization of laparoscopic tubal cauterization in the 1970s brought with it a renewed interest in the evaluation of possible late complications related to the procedure. Some even suggested the existence of a post-tubal ligation syndrome characterized by dysmenorrhea and irregularity in length and severity of menstrual bleeding.

Neil et al compared a group of women sterilized by laparoscopic cauterization with a control group whose husbands had a vasectomy.[18] They found increased menstrual blood loss and dysmenorrhea in the former. They postulated that destruction of the mesosalpinx during electrocauterization disrupts the utero-ovarian blood supply. These findings, coupled with the increased rate of later hysterectomy in these patients, led them to recommend the use of less destructive means for tubal occlusion.

Donnez et al evaluated the luteal function in women following laparoscopic sterilization and compared them with a control group of similar age.[7] The sterilized women were further subdivided by sterilization method (electrocoagulation versus spring loaded clips). Progesterone levels were below 10 ng per milliliter in 54 percent of those sterilized by electrocoagulation, in 20 percent with spring loaded clips, and in only 12 percent among controls. These data suggested that the utero-ovarian artery blood flow to the ovary was altered and thereby adversely affected the function of the corpus luteum.

In a similar study, Hargrove and Abraham evaluated 29 women who developed dysmenorrhea, increased menstrual bleeding and premenstrual tension following Pomeroy sterilization.[10] The midluteal phase endocrine profile revealed higher serum estradiol and lower serum progesterone levels than normal controls. The abnormal luteal function was felt to be responsible for the clinical manifestations. In addition, luteal dysfunction observed in these women may have served to explain the poor conception rates after successful tubal reanastomosis.

El-Minawi et al studied pelvic vein anatomy following different types of tubal sterilization procedures by means of transuterine pelvic phlebography.[9] Contrast material studies were performed preoperatively and subsequently after the first and sixth postoperative menstrual periods. In one group of patients, a Pomeroy tubal occlusion was performed unilaterally; the contralateral oviduct was suture ligated, preserving its blood supply intact. Uterine congestion, uterovaginal and ovarian varicosities, and generalized pelvic venous stasis was found to be common in patients whose sterilization procedure interfered with the mesosalpingeal vasculature. Those patients undergoing only suture ligation of the tube had no venographic abnormalities on that side, although they did show uterovaginal and ovarian varicosities on the contralateral side where the Pomeroy tubal occlusion had been done.

I have personally seen and recorded many instances of poststerilization pelvic congestion that had not previously been present (Figure 22.18 and 22.19). Until controlled, prospective studies are carried out, pelvic congestion and its attendant menstrual disorders and recurrent pelvic pain pattern must be considered a potential after effect of sterilization. It is, therefore, advisable to share the information concerning this possible risk with prospective candidates for laparoscopic sterilization.

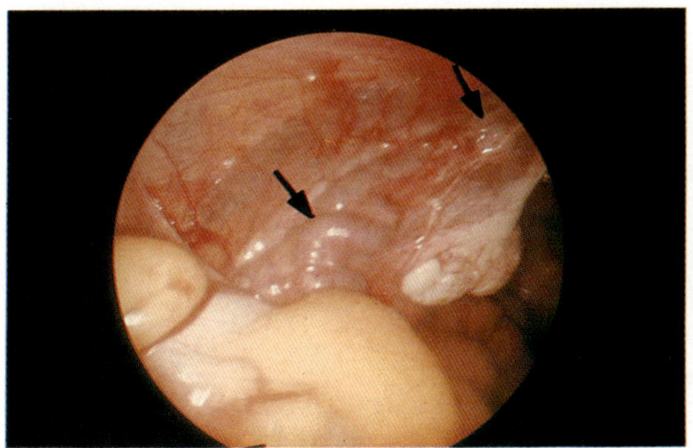

Figure 22.18 Poststerilization pelvic varicosities. Unipolar electrocoagulation was performed several years prior to this laparoscopy. Proximal tubal stump (right arrow) can be distinguished from dilated mesosalpingeal vessels (left arrow).

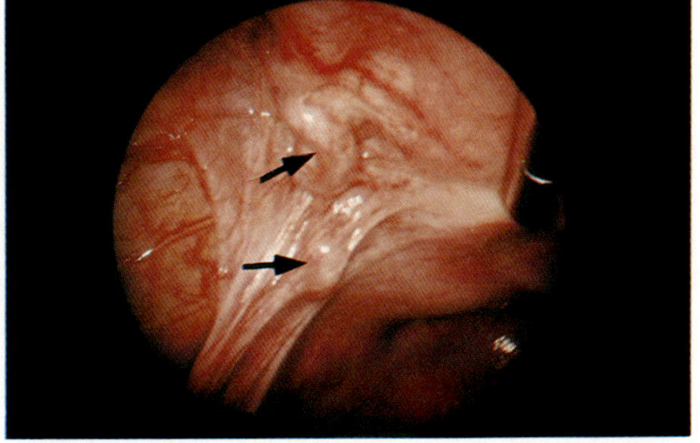

Figure 22.19 Poststerilization uterine varicosities. Metal probe displaces the uterus forward. Dilated and tortuous uterine vessels are seen (arrows) at follow-up laparoscopy several years after sterilization.

References

1. Ansari AH, Sealey RM, Gay JW, Kang I. Silicone rubber band for laparoscopic tubal sterilization. Fertil Steril 1977; 28:1306-1309.
2. Ayers JWT, Johnson RS, Ansbacher R, et al. Sterilization failures with bipolar tubal cautery. Fertil Steril 1984; 42:526-530.
3. Baggish MS, Lee WK, Miro SJ, et al. Complications of laparoscopic sterilization: Comparison of two methods. Obstet Gynecol 1979; 54:54-59.
4. Beck P, Gal D. Silicone band technique for laparoscopic tubal sterilization in the gravid and nongravid patient. Obstet Gynecol 1979; 53:653-656.
5. Chi EC, Cole LP. Incidence of pain among women undergoing laparoscopic sterilization by electrocoagulation, the spring-loaded clip, and the tubal ring. Am J Obstet Gynecol 1979; 135:397-401.
6. Cunanan RG, Courey NG, Lippes J. Complications of laparoscopic tubal sterilization. Obstet Gynecol 1980; 55:501-506.
7. Donnez J, Wauters M, Thomas K. Luteal function after tubal sterilization. Obstet Gynecol 1981; 57:65-68.
8. Edgerton WD. Late complications of laparoscopic sterilization, II. J Reprod Med 1978; 21:41-44.
9. El-Minawi MF, Mashhor N, Reda MS. Pelvic venous changes after tubal sterilization. J Reprod Med 1983; 28:641-648.
10. Hargrove JT, Abraham GE. Endocrine profile of patients with post-tubal-ligation syndrome. J Reprod Med 1981; 26:359-362.
11. Hulka JF, Mercer JP, Fishburns JI, et al. Spring clip sterilization: One-year follow-up of 1,079 cases. Am J Obstet Gynecol 1976; 125:1039-1043.
12. Levinson CJ, Daily HI, Marko MW, Richardson DC. Nonelectric laparoscopic sterilization: Experience with a silastic band. Obstet Gynecol 1976; 48:494-496.
13. Lieberman BA, Gordon AG, Bostock JF, et al. Laparoscopic sterilization with spring-loaded clips: Double-puncture technique. J Reprod Med 1977; 18:241-245.
14. Loffer FD, Pent D. Pregnancy after laparoscopic sterilization. Obstet Gynecol 1980; 55:643-648.
15. Madrigal V, Edelman DA, Henriquez E, Goldsmith A. A comparative study of spring-loaded clips and electrocoagulation for female sterilization. J Reprod Med 1977; 18:41-45.
16. McCausland A. High rate of ectopic pregnancy following laparoscopic tubal coagulation. Am J Obstet Gynecol 1980; 136:97-101.
17. McCausland A. Endosalpingiosis (''endosalpingoblastosis'') following laparoscopic tubal coagulation as an etiologic factor of ectopic pregnancy. Am J Obstet Gynecol 1982; 143:12-24.
18. Neil JR, Noble AD, Hammond GT, Rushton L, Letchworth AT. Late complications of sterilisation by laparoscopy and tubal ligation. Lancet 1975; 2:699-700.
19. Pelland PC. Patient acceptance of laparoscopic tubal fulguration versus falope-ring banding. Obstet Gynecol 1977; 50:106-108.
20. Phillips JM. Complication in laparoscopy. Int J Gynaecol Obstet 1977; 15:151-162.
21. Rock JA, Parmley TH, King TM, Laufe LE, Su BC. Endometriosis and the development of tuboperitoneal fistulas after tubal ligation. Fertil Steril 1981; 35:16-20.
22. Thompson BH, Wheeless RR. Failures of laparoscopic sterilization. Obstet Gynecol 1975; 45:659-664.

23 ELECTRICAL COMPLICATIONS

Complications related to the use of electrosurgical instruments in a laparoscopic procedure are not as uncommon as previously thought.[9] Although only major morbidity—such as skin burns, electrical burns to intra-abdominal structures (usually bowel), and burns sustained by the operator—is reported in the literature, minor complications occur more often during translaparoscopic electrosurgery. This is because the effect of electrical current on the human body is not necessarily benign, and local, occult extension of tissue coagulation can cause distant minor skin or muscle burn.

To understand fully the pathophysiology of an electrically induced tissue burn, the reader should refer to Chapter 1 on electroinstrumentation and Chapter 12 on failure of electrical instruments. Just as a physician must have pharmacologic knowledge about a medication he or she will use, so the surgeon must be familiar with the origin of the energy, the mechanism by which the energy is produced, the pathways of its dissipation, and the potential damage it may produce.

Without appropriate understanding of the transmission and dispersion properties of electrical current, one is not able to appreciate the necessity for there to be direct contact between the electrode tip and adjacent tissue for an intestinal or bladder burn to occur. Neither cutting nor coagulating current requires such contact to produce free jumping of the electric spark to nearby structures.

The most commonly occurring electrical complications will be described here. Their prevention and management will also be dealt with in detail. This material should prove useful to the physician performing translaparoscopic electrosurgical operations.

ELECTRICAL CIRCUIT

A discussion of the complications of translaparoscopic electrosurgery would not be feasible without prior understanding of the electrical circuitry. It is necessary to know the operational aspects and potential hazards before one can expect to be successful in preventing a complication or in recognizing a complication that has occurred. The two most common circuits in use today are incorporated into electrical instruments of the unipolar and the bipolar types. It is important to differentiate them.

Unipolar Circuit

The electrical current of a unipolar or monopolar circuit proceeds from one of the forceps elements (i.e., the active electrode), to a dispersive electrode or plate attached to the patient's skin.[4] The latter is usually placed in the vicinity of the operative field. The high frequency current concentrates on the small active electrode and destroys the tissue at the point of contact. It is here that the main difference between the two types of circuits exists. In the unipolar system, the current passes through the tissue and seeks a path of least resistance to reach the return electrode. It thus completes the electrical circuit. Deficiencies in the design of the return electrode, and the use of high voltage spark-gap generators explain most of the electrical burn accidents that have occurred during laparoscopy in the past.[5]

Return Electrode. The heat and coagulation created by the high current density at the tip of the active electrode diminishes as the resistance of the burned tissue increases. The current density falls quickly as the current is dissipated through the body in search of the dispersive electrode by way of which it returns to the generative instrument. The current seeks out an area of surface contact at which low power density exists. This site serves as the dispersive electrode. The ability to contain and to control this return pathway of electrons provides the safety needed to prevent unexpected burns.

The dispersive electrode or return plate should be of sufficient size to provide a large area of contact with the patient's skin.[8] It is not the size of the return plate, but rather the extent and quality of the contact between the patient's skin and the dispersive electrode that attracts the returning current to the electrode for completion of the electrical circuit. Bony prominences or irregular skin surface contact can build up sufficient heat at the contact point to produce a local skin burn (to be discussed).

Tissue in contact with the dispersive electrode should be well perfused. This is essential because water and salt ions are necessary in order for tissues to be able to conduct electricity efficiently. The use of conductive gels remains controversial. Nonetheless, they are recommended for the following reasons: (a)

They fill the void between the return plate and any irregular areas of the skin that are not in complete contact. (b) They reduce the possibility that the disinfectant solution used to prepare the surgical field will enter the area of the dispersive plate by capillary action. (c) They reduce the accumulation of perspiration pooling on and around the return plate. Caution should be exercised to avoid substituting a nonconductive substance such as petroleum jelly for a more appropriate dispersive gel specifically designed to improve electrical conductivity.

Bipolar Circuit. In the bipolar circuit, the return or dispersive electrode is incorporated into the forceps. This isolates the electrical current pathway between the forceps blades. The electrons are impelled from the generator to the active electrode jaw, thereby passing through the grasped tissue and returning to the originating instrument by the return electrode or the opposite jaw of the forceps. The objective of the bipolar circuit is to limit the area of damage to the tissue held between both forceps jaws. To limit the flow of electricity in this manner, the current generator must be isolated from the ground.

If the tissue adjacent to the forceps blade is being fulgurated, it means that the generator is not well isolated so that in reality it is operating in part as a monopolar circuit.[7] Although the practice is not specifically required in a truly bipolar circuit, one is well advised to use a dispersive return plate in all cases in which electrosurgery is being used. This measure also provides the operator with the capacity to utilize some monopolar instruments to perform procedures not otherwise feasible with available bipolar instruments.

SKIN BURNS

The use of electrocautery during a laparoscopic procedure can cause unexpected and distant skin burns. This complication is usually associated with an abnormal return pathway for the electrosurgical current because of inadequate contact between the patient and the dispersive plates. The extreme heat created at the tip of the electrode by the high current density is dissipated through the body. The dispersive electrode acts as a site of low current and power density. The design and location of the return electrode helps dissipate the current while minimizing tissue heat at the point of contact.

Design of the Return Electrode

The size of the return electrode is not as important as the size of the contact area between the patient's skin and the dispersive return electrode. A bony prominence or a wrinkled irregular skin surface results in concentrated heat build-up in the smaller contact areas. This provides the opportunity for localized burns to occur. A flexible return plate electrode allows maximal contact between patient and plate. Inherent characteristics of high-frequency electrical current attracts flow to the edges and corners of the dispersive plate. This creates unequal current densities that could have the same adverse effect by allowing accumulation of extreme heat over small areas of the return electrode with burns resulting at those points of contact. The use of plates without corners and the addition of a conductive gel or paste to maximize the area of dispersive contact should prevent this complication from occurring.

When utilizing a conductive gel or paste, one should pay attention to the duration of the procedure. During extensive laparoscopies, the initial coupling between the patient and the return electrode may be good, but with time the coupling will be disrupted as the interposing material dries.

Location of the Return Plate

Studying the location of electrosurgical burns, Becker et al found the most common sites to be those areas to which the electrocardiographic leads were attached.[1] The importance of the relative distances between the active electrode, the dispersive plate, and the electrocardiographic leads was shown. There was a seven-fold decrease in radiofrequency current flow through the electrocardiographic electrodes when they were positioned distally to the dispersive plate, that is, further away in relation to the active electrode.

The tissue in contact with the dispersive electrode should be well perfused. Blood facilitates electrical conductivity and provides an additional pathway for heat dissipation. Second only to the vessels themselves, the muscles offer the best peripherally perfused tissue over which a dispersive elecrode can be attached.

If a skin burn occurs, a local antibiotic unguent is applied and the lesion is merely observed. The original size of the white skin burn does not convey the full extent of the underlying lesion. As will be described in greater detail later in this chapter, electrical current is best conducted along blood vessels. Thrombosis of the subcutaneous microvasculature produces additional necrosis. Sloughing of the dead tissue reaches its maximum within 48 to 72 hours after the injury. Only then should debridement and excision of the devitalized tissue be undertaken. Secondary healing by granulation can then be allowed to take place. At times, the size of the defect may require the use of skin grafts to promote complete recovery.

BOWEL BURNS

Electrical injuries to the intestine resulting from the translaparoscopic use of electrocautery is perhaps the most serious complication of laparoscopy.[10] Whereas some bowel burns may be attributed to the operator's inexperience or to faulty equipment, most reported cases occurred in experienced hands during an essentially uneventful laparoscopic operation. This type of complication was once thought to be related only to the use of unipolar electrocautery. However, it has been reported to occur with bipolar instruments although much less frequently. Despite the recognized hazard, monopolar coagulation is still a common method used worldwide for laparoscopic sterilization. The attention given to the complication of bowel burn is well deserved. Although rare in occurrence, it is responsible for most of the fatalities associated with laparoscopic procedures.[11]

The generally accepted incidence of unexpected burns to bowel during translaparoscopic electrosurgery is 1 to 2 percent, but this is probably underestimated. Thompson and Wheeless noted that some bowel burns identified at the time of surgery, if managed conservatively by observation did not require any additional surgical therapy.[15] Some bowel burns are not necessarily recognized or even suspected at the time of the original procedure, and not all become evident postoperatively. Thus, the true incidence of thermal injury to the intestine is greater than usually reported.

The fact that this type of injury is not always diagnosed at the time it occurs can make it difficult to pinpoint the cause. The possible mechanisms advanced to explain this phenomenon include: (a) inadvertent direct contact of the bowel by the active electrode; (b) intraperitoneal arc of the sparks from the active electrode across to the nearby bowel wall; and (c) transformation of a nonconductive instrument into an active electrode as a result of its capacitance property.

Direct Contact

Inadvertent touching of the bowel with the active electrode occurs if an inexperienced operator fails to coordinate foot-switch activation with placement of the operating forceps. It is inappropriate to allow electrical current to continue flowing after the tissue being operated on has been released by the forceps. This error is also seen in procedures where a single puncture operative laparoscope is used. As described previously, there is an unavoidable blind spot encompassing approximately 60° of the circumferential field behind the forceps. Because the field of vision is incomplete, bowel may unexpectedly come in contact with the charged instrument without the operator being aware of it.

Spark Arc

Arcing of sparks may occur within the peritoneal cavity as the electrons seek the return or dispersive electrode. In the monopolar electrocautery technique, the fallopian tube is usually grasped in a single preselected location and current is applied until the extent of the desired tubal cauterization is achieved. The current searching for the dispersive electrode spreads radially away from the area being held by the forceps. As coagulation occurs, the resistance to conduction rises in the tissue that is already burned. Such an increase in resistance can interrupt the electrical circuit between the active electrode and the return plate that is in contact with the patient's skin. As a consequence, arcing of sparks may occur.

In the multiple burn technique performed by means of unipolar cautery, another pathway has been described by which sparks can jump from the forceps or the burned tube across to the adjacent bowel.[7] Initially, cauterizing the tube close to the uterus isolates the salpinx electrically so that current cannot flow toward the myometrium in search of the return electrode. Instead, the current is conducted toward the fimbrial end of the tube. This creates a significant voltage difference between the salpinx and the bowel, thereby facilitating the appearance of sparks between them. To prevent this situation from developing in the course of the unipolar multiple burn technique, the distal portion of the tube should be cauterized first; this can be followed by cauterization of the tissue nearer the uterine cornu.

Capacitance

A nonconductive, hollow metal tube, within which an active electrode is transferring current, can act as a capacitor to store electrical energy.[2] By this capacitance mechanism the tube transforms itself into an active electrode. Thus, any unexpected contact of the laparoscope with the intestine may cause a burn. This injury may not be visible to the operator. The use of nonconductive trocar sheaths further isolates the nonconductive laparoscope, thus enhancing the opportunity for capacitance to take place. Metal trocar sheaths were reintroduced after this phenomenon was recognized. Conductive sheaths allow the stored current to be dissipated over a large area of surface contact. If a thermal burn does occur, it only affects the tissue of the abdominal wall surrounding the sheath.

After cauterization, there is a possibility that the fallopian tube will remain extremely hot for a brief period. Direct contact between the hot tissue and the bowel serosa may cause unwanted thermal injury. This hypothetical risk was put into perspective by Stewart et al who showed that the cauterized tube cooled rather rapidly.[14] Thus, only trivial injuries are sustained even if the burned tissue makes contact with peritoneal tissue immediately after cauterization.

If an electrical injury to bowel is discovered during surgery, the degree and extent of the burn dictates the therapeutic approach. A small, superficial serosal burn can be observed expectantly. One must keep in mind that what is seen may not actually represent the full extent of the lesion (see below). If the injury is of sufficient gravity (involving a burn of the muscularis layer, for example) as to require an exploratory laparotomy, bowel resection is the procedure of choice. It should encompass and extend 3 cm into healthy tissue on each side. The reason for such wide resection is the possible subserosal extension of the injury by way of the vasculature of the intestine. Subserosal extension occurs in a manner similar to that for electrical skin burns.

The bowel injury is usually unrecognized at the time of surgery. Signs of peritonitis from spillage of intestinal contents are often the first indication of a serious problem. These generally appear from 3 to 6 days after the procedure. Abdominal pain, nausea, vomiting, and fever occur. Physical signs of an acute surgical abdomen or abdominal distention secondary to paralytic ileus are found. Most laparoscopic sterilizations are currently being performed in an ambulatory surgical setting and even if done in a hospital unit the patient is usually released shortly after the procedure is concluded. Under these circumstances, patients should be instructed to report any untoward manifestations that develop 24 hours or more postoperatively. Within the first day, patients may experience a variety of unrelated symptoms. Because most bowel burns follow an uneventful laparoscopic procedure, there is a tendency to delay making the diagnosis. This further complicates an already dangerous situation. If bowel injury is suspected following an electrosurgical laparoscopic procedure, exploratory laparotomy with bowel resection, if indicated, is the most appropriate course of action.

Nowhere better than in this specific type of complication does the value of preventive measures outweigh therapy. Whereas the use of a bipolar electrode does not eliminate the danger of bowel burn, it can markedly reduce it. Thus, its use is highly recommended. When obliged to use unipolar cautery, one must control the current flow at all times. Cauterization has to be carried out under direct vision with the tissue to be coagulated and the adjacent bowel in full view. These precautions reduce the incidence of electrical injury to the intestinal tract.

OCCULT ELECTROSURGICAL DAMAGE

As previously mentioned, electrical conductivity is dependent upon the presence of water and salt ions. Therefore, it is easy to appreciate that any patent blood vessel is a good conductor of electrical current. This explains why it is necessary to wait several days after a minimal skin burn is diagnosed to evaluate its full extent. Only at that time will the microvasculature damaged by the occult extension of the electrical current manifest further skin necrosis.

A similar example of occult electrosurgical damage is demonstrated by microscopic evaluation of the endosalpinx of a fallopian tube which has recently been electrocauterized. Damage to the tubal lumen, extending well beyond that seen translaparoscopically or on direct observation with the naked eye can be seen on the serosal surface. Even under ideal electrosurgical conditions, the high water content of the epithelium and the endosalpingeal mucus secretions are believed to be responsible for facilitating electrical conductivity which can cause imperceptible additional damage.

When using unipolar electrocautery for tubal sterilization, one must exercise caution with respect to the type of instrument used for uterine manipulation. Freilich suggested that the use of a metal instrument to manipulate the uterine position may stimulate electrons to jump to the close conductive object rather than to travel the longer course to the dispersive grounding plate.[6] In the occasional patient in whom a metal curet or sound is left in the uterus, this may cause burns of the buttocks, vulva, vagina, cervix, and endometrium.

Whereas the skin is a better conductor of electrical current than is the underlying subcutaneous fatty tissue, muscle is better. For example, a hypervascularized postabortal uterus can sustain an extensive degree of damage from this source. Contrary to previous recommendations for the use of nonconductive trocar sheaths, recently a Food and Drug Administration advisory panel recommended that conductive metal trocar sheaths be used for unipolar translaparoscopic electrosurgery. The aim is to avoid capacitance of the laparoscope. If this were to occur, it would become the cause of unwanted burns. A metal trocar sleeve acts as another pathway for the dispersion of accumulated electrical energy that can substitute a minor form of tissue damage in the trocar channel of the abdominal wall for the potentially more devastating and unexpected intraperitoneal burn. Nevertheless, such abdominal wall burns have to be considered a form of occult electrosurgical damage. Laparoscopists should be aware of their existence.

BURNS TO THE OPERATOR

The surgeon or ancillary operating room personnel may also incur electrical burns. These usually occur as a result of the transmission of high-frequency current through a conductive instrument. The mechanism is direct contact with either the active electrode or an instrument which is acting as a capacitor. These injuries occur exclusively with unipolar electrosurgical instruments.

Direct contact with the active electrode takes place if the operator activates the current flow before it is required for tissue cauterization. Accidentally stepping on the foot-switch transmits electrical current to any instrument connected to the generator. If the instrument is in contact with the surgeon or assistant, he or she will be burned. In order to prevent this accident, there should be audible signals to indicate electrode activation. One must ensure that the generator is not turned on until it is actually needed.

In the past, the use of noninsulated laparoscopes caused operator burns. Such burns can occur as a result of direct contact of the electrocauterizing instrument with the laparoscope itself. The metal casing of the laparoscope acts as a conductive and dispersive electrode and can thus burn any tissue it contacts, including eyelids, cornea and hands. The surgeon's rubber gloves form an insulating protection. However, any break in the gloves enhances the possibility of burning his or her hands.

The laparoscope can also act as a capacitor, charged by the process of capacitance. Thus any tissue coming into contact with the laparoscope at any level receives the discharge of accumulated energy. This condition is believed to be the source of burns to bowel as well as to the surgeon. The problem arises especially during single puncture operative laparoscopy. It is further aggravated by the use of an insulated, nonconductive laparoscopic trocar sheath. The reintroduction of the metal trocar sheath takes advantage of its conductive ability to disperse the current produced by capacitance over the tissue of the anterior abdominal wall. It thus produces minimal heat dissipated over a greater contact surface. These types of accidents can be substantially reduced in frequency or completely eliminated by use of insulated laparoscopes, conductive metal trocar sheaths, isolated electrosurgical units, and bipolar type instruments.

EXPLOSIONS AND FIRES

Discontinuation of flammable anesthetics has considerably reduced the hazard of fires and explosions in the operating room. Nevertheless, the use of electrical current in the surgical field means that the risk is not completely eliminated. Currently, fires and explosions generally involve fuel materials, such as alcohol-based antiseptic solutions and aerosol sprays containing highly flammable propellants which may remain suspended in the air for long periods of time.

It has long been known that intraoperative explosions may occur in cases in which diathermy is used for bowel surgery. Intestinal gas contains high concentrations of hydrogen and methane gases. If these gases are mixed with oxygen, a highly volatile gas mixture is generated. Hydrogen is present in intestinal gas in proportions up to 47 percent by volume, methane in up to 26 percent by volume. These concentrations are probably within the range of flammability.[12] An evaluation of intraoperative intestinal methane and hydrogen concentrations in patients who had not had preoperative bowel preparation showed 42 percent had explosive concentrations of one or both. Inadvertent puncture of the bowel, although usually uncomplicated if managed expectantly, may cause methane and hydrogen to diffuse into the abdominal cavity. The use of electrosurgical instruments under these conditions can result in fires and explosions in the operating room.

Drummond and Scott determined that the use of nitrous oxide is not a significant hazard during laparoscopy unless the wall of the intestine is punctured.[3] They evaluated the intraperitoneal gas content in a small number of patients and found it to be too low to create a dangerous situation. Steptoe reported that the incidence of known bowel puncture produced by the insufflating needle is approximately 2 percent.[13] He suggested that this figure may even be higher because punctures are not always identified at the time of surgery.

Nitrous oxide has been recommended for creating the pneumoperitoneum in order to prevent cardiac arrhythmias and reduce the discomfort experienced by patients undergoing laparoscopy under local anesthesia. However, it must be remembered that nitrous oxide can sustain combustion and it can yield highly explosive mixtures when mixed with the intestinal gases. Therefore, it would seem advisable not to use this gas to distend the peritoneal cavity in cases where any form of electrocautery is used. The risk, no matter how small, can be a serious one. In view of the ready availability of carbon dioxide to achieve a suitable pneumoperitoneum, it would be imprudent to subject any patient to such risks. With controlled ventilation, the side effects of carbon dioxide insufflation are easily handled. Furthermore, even under local anesthesia, it is preferable to deal with the consequences of an increase in $PaCO_2$ and mild patient discomfort than to have to contend with the damage to internal organs caused by an intra-abdominal explosion.

References

1. Becker CM, Malhotra IV, Hedley-White J. The distribution of radio-frequency current and burns. Anesthesiology 1973; 38:106-122.
2. Di Novo JA. Radio frequency leakage current from unipolar laparoscopic electrocoagulators. J Reprod Med 1983; 28:565-575.
3. Drummond GB, Scott DB. Laparoscopy explosion hazards with nitrous oxide. Br J Med 1976; 1:586.
4. Engel T, Harris FW. The electrical dynamics of laparoscopic sterilization. J Reprod Med 1975; 15:33-42.
5. Esposito JM. The laparoscopist and electrosurgery. Am J Obstet Gynecol 1976; 126:633-637.
6. Freilich TH. Possibility of burns during laparoscopic tubal sterilization. Am J Obstet Gynecol 1977; 129:708-709.
7. Harris FW. Electrosurgery in laparoscopy. J Reprod Med 1978; 21:48:52.
8. Hays CV. Making laparoscopy electrically safer: An engineer's approach. J Reprod Med 1979; 23:91-93.
9. Hulka JF. Relative risks and benefits of electric and nonelectric sterilization techniques. J Reprod Med 1978; 21:111-114.
10. Neufeld GR. Principles and hazards of electrosurgery including laparoscopy. Surg Gynecol Obstet 1978; 147:705-710.

11. Peterson HB, Ory HW, Greenspan JR, Tyler CW. Deaths associated with laparoscopic sterilization by unipolar electrocoagulating devices, 1978 and 1979. Am J Obstet Gynecol 1981; 139:141-143.
12. Reagans H, Shinya H, Wolff W. The explosive potential of colonic gas during colonoscopic electrosurgical polypectomy. Surg Gynecol Obstet 1974; 138:554-556.
13. Steptoe P. Laparoscopy explosion hazards with nitrous oxide. Br J Med 1976; 1:833.
14. Stewart KS, Pearson JF, Docker MF, Harvey LP, Rushton DI. A possible hazard of laparoscopic sterilization. Am J Obstet Gynecol 1973; 115:1154-1157.
15. Thompson BH, Wheeless CR. Gastrointestinal complications of laparoscopy sterilization. Obstet Gynecol 1973; 41:669-676.

24 POSTOPERATIVE COMPLICATIONS

For the last decade, the tendency has been to perform most laparoscopies on an outpatient basis. This means that the patient is not admitted the evening before the operation. More important is the fact that early discharge, within 3 to 6 hours following surgery, is expected.

What can be expected during the short postoperative period during which the patient remains within the surgical facility has been described previously (see Chapter 11). Similarly, discharge instructions were also detailed. In this chapter, a variety of postoperative complaints associated with laparoscopy, usually developing at some time after the patient is discharged, are discussed. Some of these complications are not specific to the laparoscopic procedure itself. Nevertheless, because they result from the spectrum of ancillary maneuvers required to perform the procedure, familiarity by the operator is advantageous.

POSTOPERATIVE PAIN

Following laparoscopy, a certain amount of discomfort should be expected by patients. Common complaints include incisional pain, diffuse abdominal malaise, and referred shoulder pain. Patients receiving general anesthesia may, in addition, experience sore throat and generalized muscle pain.

Incisional Pain

Incisional pain following laparoscopy is common. Peri-incisional aches may persist for 2 to 3 days. The degree of discomfort is in direct proportion to the size of the incision.

Uncomplicated incisional discomfort responds quite well to mild analgesic medication. Lack of progressive abatement of circumincisional soreness may signal localized bleeding with hematoma formation (see Chapters 11 and 17). Patients must be advised to contact their physician if incisional pain lingers for more than 48 to 72 hours. Prompt evaluation is indicated.

Diffuse Abdominal Pain

Some diffuse abdominal sensitivity can be expected following most laparoscopies. This applies to diagnostic as well as operative endoscopic procedures. It is usually the result of irritation from the peritoneal stretching of the pneumoperitoneum. In patients in whom carbon dioxide is used as a distending gas, additional discomfort is often experienced. Carbonic acid produced from the combined carbon dioxide and peritoneal fluid ($CO_2 + H_2O \rightleftarrows H_2CO_3$) is thought to be the offending agent. Less tenderness is reported when nitrous oxide is used.

Abdominal pain following an uncomplicated laparoscopy usually subsides in a progressive fashion over 24 to 48 hours after the procedure. Mild analgesic medication usually suffices to relieve this discomfort. Patients should be advised and reassured about the benign and self-limited nature of this side effect of laparoscopy. Persistence or reappearance of abdominal soreness requires prompt reevaluation.

Shoulder Pain

Referred shoulder pain is a characteristic manifestation of the presence of free gas within the peritoneal cavity. It is believed to reflect irritation of the peritoneum underlying the diaphragm (see Chapter 11). Control of this pain following an uncomplicated laparoscopy rarely requires more than mild analgesics.

If shoulder pain lasts beyond 48 hours following surgery or recurs thereafter, it requires a more thorough work-up. The patient should be admitted to the hospital for observation.

Sore Throat

When general anesthesia is administered for laparoscopy, tracheal intubation is the norm. Postoperatively, therefore, it is not uncommon for the patient to have a sore throat. Use of special endotracheal tubes with variable cuff designs, in conjunction with lubricants, may reduce the frequency and severity of this complaint.

Capan et al reported sore throat symptoms in patients receiving intravenous succinylcholine who were not endotracheally intubated.[2] These women did have a nasopharyngeal airway, however. The peak incidence (68 percent) occurred 24 to 30 hours following surgery. The late appearance of sore throat means it may not be reported before the patient is discharged from the surgical facility. Discharge instructions to the patient should forewarn her of the probability of a sore throat and of the self-limited nature of this process. Symptomatic treatment is beneficial.

Generalized Muscle Pain

Postoperative muscle pain is another common complaint of patients who have had laparoscopy under general anesthesia. It can last from 12 to 48 hours. It is more marked in patients who engage in early ambulation.

This form of pain is believed to be a side effect of succinylcholine administered for neuromuscular block. The pathophysiology of this untoward effect is not fully understood. Although postoperative muscle pain cannot be directly correlated with the degree and duration of muscular fasciculations observed during anesthesia, it is believed to represent a continuation of uncoordinated muscle contractions. While fasciculations can be suppressed by the administration of a competitive agent such as d-tubocurarine, the postoperative muscle pain cannot be completely eliminated.

Patients must be made aware of the frequent appearance of postoperative muscle pain. Concurrently, they can be reassured about its benign nature and self-limited duration.

NAUSEA AND VOMITING

Nausea and vomiting are the most common complications following general anesthesia. Their appearance following laparoscopy may be enhanced by the diaphragmatic irritation produced by the pneumoperitoneum. In the majority of patients, complete improvement with disappearance of symptoms is evident within 4 to 6 hours following surgery.

A small number of patients will experience persistent nausea and intermittent emesis following laparoscopy. Antinauseant and antiemetic medication may be beneficial. Intravenous fluid administration may have to be administered in some cases to prevent or correct dehydration. Discharging such patients should be delayed until recovery is complete.

NEUROLOGIC COMPLICATIONS

The incidence of neurologic complications associated with laparoscopy is remarkably low. Nevertheless, they cannot be ignored. Central nervous system impairment generally only follows a severe hypoxic episode from a major cardiorespiratory event. Contrariwise, peripheral nerve damage can sometimes appear following an essentially uneventful procedure.

Inappropriate positioning of the patient on the operating table may cause pressure injury on the peripheral nerves. The type of nerve fibers affected determines the symptoms that develop. These range from sensory limitations to complete motor paresis.

Shoulder-Hand Syndrome

Shoulder pain following laparoscopy is a common complaint. As described earlier in this chapter and in Chapter 11, it is benign and self limited in nature. It frequently abates in a progressive fashion within the first 12 to 24 hours. Persistence for over a day or reappearance following improvement deserves a more thorough evaluation.

Low et al reported the occurrence of shoulder-hand syndrome in a woman following an uneventful laparoscopic sterilization.[4] This condition is characterized by painful restriction of shoulder movements with radiation down the arm. Swelling, temperature variations in the arm, and increased perspiration of the arm and hand may also accompany the pain.

The exact physiopathology of this syndrome is unknown. Pain which leads to immobility with impairment of venous return and sympathetic innervation is thought to help trigger it. Treatment is symptomatic. Analgesics, physiotherapy, and diathermy have proved helpful. Although this syndrome is extremely rare, patients should be advised to report a persistence of shoulder pain of over 24 hours to their physician.

Brachial Palsy

Paresis of the upper brachial plexus has also been observed in patients who have been placed in steep Trendelenburg position for prolonged periods of time. Use of a shoulder brace to prevent the patient slipping cephalad on the operating table increases the risk. Appropriate padding helps prevent pressure paresis. Limitation of the head down tilt and minimization of the duration of the procedure are also helpful in avoiding this difficulty.

Discontinuing the use of shoulder braces substantially decreases the frequency of positional brachial plexus injuries. To reduce the risk during laparoscopy further, the patient's arms should be adducted laterally against her trunk. If anesthetic needs (for obtaining blood pressure or maintaining intravenous lines) require one arm to be extended, hyperextension must be avoided.

When obese patients or those of short stature are placed in the lithotomy position, the space allowed the operator is limited. This is further aggravated by the Trendelenburg position. Both operator and assistant must refrain from leaning on the patient's extended arm.

Whenever space is limited, the laparoscopist may inadvertently lean on the patient's chest (Figure 24.1) and his or her back may rest on the extended arm. This is easily avoided by the operator switching from one side of the operating table to the other (Figure 24.2). The change is not necessary if the surgeon is ambidextrous and can operate equally well from either side of the patient.

Sciatic Nerve Injury

Laparoscopy requires the patient to be placed in the lithotomy or semilithotomy position. For that purpose, special stirrups have been designed (see Chapter 2). Their use carries the potential risk of sciatic and/or peroneal nerve damage.

Loffer et al first reported a sciatic nerve injury in a patient undergoing laparoscopy.[3] The operation was performed under general anesthesia. Free hanging stirrups were used to place the patient, who was of normal height and weight, in the lithotomy position. She complained of weakness and numbness in her left leg upon awakening from anesthesia. The patient's symptoms were attributed to stretching of the left sciatic nerve.

Batres and Barclay described unilateral sciatic nerve injury in two patients who were operated on in the semilithotomy position.[1] One had been in stirrups for only 35 minutes and the other for 85 minutes. They also attributed the nerve damage to overstretching of the sciatic nerve.

The sciatic nerve arises from the fourth and fifth lumbar roots and the first, second, and third sacral roots. At the level of the thigh, the nerve trunk divides into the common peroneal and tibial nerves. The peroneal branch (lateral popliteal) is more susceptible to damage than the tibial division (medial popliteal). The peroneal nerve innervates the extensor muscles of the ankle and the abductor muscles of the foot. Its injury gives rise to foot drop and inversion. The tibial nerve innervates the calf muscles.

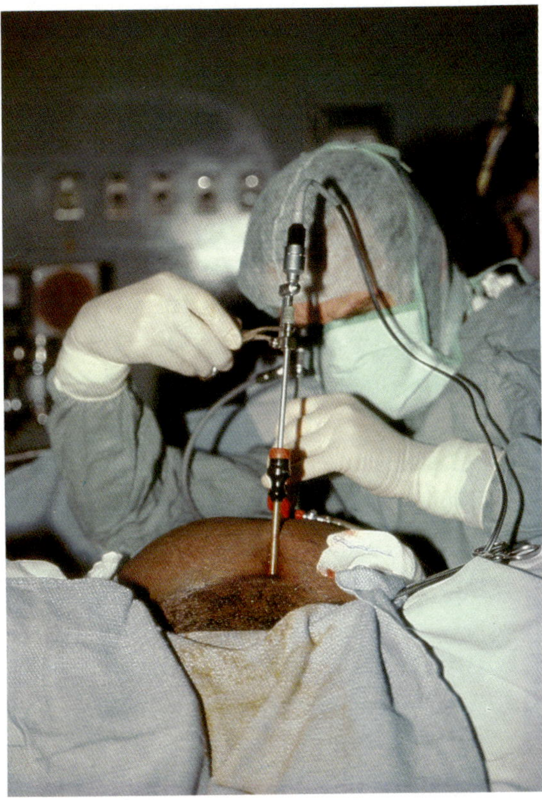

Figure 24.1 Inappropriate position of the operator. The surgeon's right arm rests on patient's chest. Decreased thoracic compliance and increased intraabdominal pressure may result.

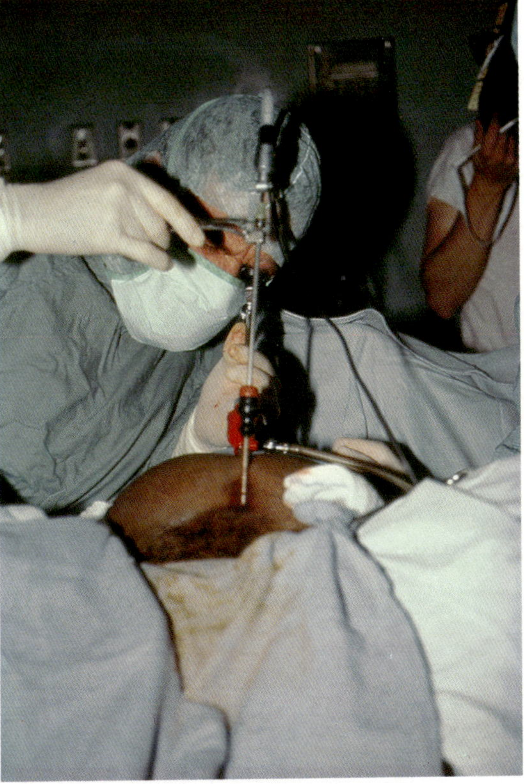

Figure 24.2 Correct position of operator. Changing one's position to the opposite side of the patient avoids inadvertently leaning on the patient's chest or the surgical field.

Stretching of the sciatic nerve occurs as a result of extension of the leg with a flexed hip. Additional tension is placed on the nerve by external rotation of the thigh with the hip and knee flexed. Hyperflexion of the hip joint aggravates this condition.

Tall patients with long extremities are particularly prone to external rotation of the hip joint and thigh. This is accentuated when free hanging stirrups are used. A similar problem can be iatrogenically created by an assistant or nurse resting an arm on the inner aspect of the patient's thigh. Another cause of peripheral nerve injury is direct pressure anywhere along its course. The short operative duration among most cases in which sciatic nerve injury has been reported makes it unlikely that this factor plays a predominant role.

Motor and sensory sciatic nerve deficits are usually evident immediately following recovery from anesthesia or shortly thereafter. The full extent of the neural impairment may not become manifest until 3 to 4 weeks after surgery. It is not until then that complete degeneration of the distal portion of the injured nerve has taken place.

The stretching type of peripheral nerve injury does not preclude regeneration. Sciatic nerve damage sustained during laparoscopy is usually self limited. Spontaneous resolution over time (3 to 9 months) can be expected. Analgesics and physiotherapy to prevent muscle atrophy are helpful and necessary. One should obtain neurologic and orthopedic consultations to optimize care.

As with other avoidable complications, prevention is critical. Suggested guidelines include the following:

- Use knee supporting stirrups for the semilithotomy position.
- Complete the positioning of the patient after the induction of anesthesia.
- Raise both legs simultaneously to place them in stirrups.
- Flex the knees prior to flexing the hip joints.
- Allow only limited external hip rotation.
- Ensure that assistants refrain from leaning on the inner aspect of the thigh, thereby causing excessive external hip rotation.
- Verify that the entire vertebral spine is resting on the operating room table to avoid accentuating the natural lordotic curvature.
- At the conclusion of the procedure, lower both legs at the same time and carefully extend the hip and knee joints.

Obese patients present an additional challenge. Acute flexion of the thigh at the groin can lead to compression and traumatic injury of the obturator nerve. Weakness and paralysis of the adductor muscles of the thigh may result.

VENOUS THROMBOSIS

Thromboembolic accidents are rarely associated with laparoscopy. This may be due to the short duration of the procedure and the fact that it is done most often in a young and healthy population of women. As the popularity and applicability of laparoscopy spreads, older and more compromised patients are being subjected to this operation. As a result, more thromboembolic complications can be expected.

Deep vein thrombosis is a prime precursor of embolic phenomena. Three major factors that contribute to the formation of venous thrombosis are (a) alteration in blood coagulation factors, (b) damage to the vessel wall, and (c) venous stasis. The latter is of particular significance for the gynecologist.

Venous stasis in the lower extremities has long been recognized as a complication of the lithotomy position. Elevation of the legs increases the venous drainage by gravity at first. As the operation proceeds, however, the legs being supported in hanging stirrups tend to accumulate blood. During laparoscopy, creation of the pneumoperitoneum increases the intra-abdominal pressure. This in turn compresses the pelvic veins and slows the venous return.

Immobilization of the patient also predisposes to venous stagnation. It is always desirable for the patient not to move during the surgical procedure; however, the contrary applies postoperatively. Early ambulation should be encouraged. Activity should also be recommended preoperatively as well. Whenever possible, the patient should be up and about until shortly before the laparoscopy is to be undertaken.

Prolonged or intense pressure may injure the walls of vessels. The hanging stirrups were developed to minimize this type of lesion during protracted gynecologic operations. As described in Chapter 2, knee support stirrups help to avoid the problem by positioning the patient more favorably for laparoscopy. It is important when using them to cushion the areas of contact between the patient and the stirrups appropriately.

References

1. Batres F, Barclay DL. Sciatic nerve injury during gynecologic procedures using the lithotomy position. Obstet Gynecol 1983; 62:92s-94s.
2. Capan LM, Bruce DL, Patel KP, Turndorf H. Succinylcholine-induced postoperative sore throat. Anesthesiol 1983; 59:202-206.
3. Loffer FD, Pent D, Goodkin R. Sciatic nerve injury in a patient undergoing laparoscopy. J Reprod Med 1978; 21:371-372.
4. Low LCK, McCruden DC, Ramsay LE. Shoulder-hand syndrome after laparoscopic sterilization. Br J Med 1978; 1:1059-1060.

25

INFORMED CONSENT AND COUNSELING

The importance of informed consent in the patient-practitioner relationship was underscored by its inclusion as a subject of study in the Presidential Commission for the Study of Ethical Problems in Medicine and Biomedical and Behavioral Research. Findings of a 2-year study of informed consent in health care entitled "Making Health Care Decisions" was released in October, 1982. In the letter to the President and Congress that accompanied the report, the Commission stated that "...it did not look to the law as the primary means of bringing about needed changes in attitudes and practices. Rather, it sees informed consent as an ethical obligation that involves a process of shared decision making based upon the mutual respect and participation of patients and health professionals."[6]

A better understanding of the informed consent process, of its origin, of its evolution, and of the controversies that surround it is indispensable for the physician who performs laparoscopies.

IS INFORMED CONSENT A MYTH OR A REALITY?

The principle of providing maximal good to the patient with minimal risk can be found in the Hippocratic Oath: "The regimen I adopt shall be for the benefit of the patients according to my ability and judgment, and not for their hurt or for any wrong." This and other ethical codes in the medical profession are, for the most part, guidelines of intent or purpose. We would like to think that our judgment is always impeccable, and that the limitation of our abilities is always fully known. Such an ideal, if realizable, would make the entire subject of informed consent a superfluous one.

Some physicians believe the whole idea of informed consent to be a "fabricated fictional concept of recent vintage...a term semantically felicitous created by and for the members of the legal system."[3] In support of their contentions they charge that patients do not understand, cannot understand, and do not want to understand. Physicians further point out the ambiguities in the law and claim they reflect expressions of premeditated incompleteness. They see in the law of informed consent an attempt to redefine the doctor-patient relationship in a detrimental way. The demand to transform such a relationship is exemplified by statements such as "...the traditional doctor-patient relationship is seen by lawyers as one in which the doctor and the patient are unequal bargaining partners in a contract for services. It is the doctor's special knowledge that creates the advantage. Informed consent is meant then to force the doctor to give the patient knowledge that will make him or her an equal bargaining partner. Thus, informed consent is meant to transform the essence of the doctor-patient relationship from status to contract."[11]

Immediately we see that the source of such an argument is fallacious. Redefining or transforming is not necessarily detrimental nor is it contrary to medical philosophy. Without change, redefinition, and transformation, we would still be practicing at Hippocrates's level of knowledge.

The essence of the art of medicine still lies in the doctor-patient relationship. Rapport is a basic ingredient in the therapeutic approach of a physician. To imply that a more knowledgeable patient would be a detriment and thereby impair that relation is a contradiction in itself. The law of informed consent as it now stands enshrines two basic principles: (a) every human being of adult years (we will discuss minors separately) and sound mind has a right to determine what shall be done with his body; and (b) an explanation of the procedure, its risks, and alternatives will enable the patient to make an educated choice.

Perhaps room exists for disagreement about how these principles are to be applied. There can be no argument with the concept itself. Free choice of decision is an inalienable right of an individual in a democratic society. Most practicing physicians know that a well informed patient makes a better patient than one who is misinformed or not informed at all. Moreover, there has been a dramatic increase in the number of cases in which lack of information in terms of consent was a primary cause of action against a physician, but in which negligent medical or surgical treatment was not at issue.

CONCEPT OF INFORMED CONSENT

In the medical profession, the concept of informed consent is a recent one. If anything, older traditions such as are laid down in the Corpus Hippocraticum suggest that it is wise for physicians to conceal most things from their patients. It has been alleged that when information is given, many patients have taken a turn for the worse. However, in 1914, Justice Benjamin Cardozo declared that, "Every human being of adult years and sound mind has a right to determine what shall be done with his own body, and a surgeon who performs an operation without his patient's consent commits an assault for which he is liable in damages.''[10] How this simple statement created one of the most troublesome aspects of the doctor-patient relationship is for historians to describe and philosophers to debate. At the present time, it would be unsound for any physician and in particular any surgeon to undertake any procedure without appropriately addressing this statement.

The law of informed consent requires a physician to provide his or her patient with enough information about the condition, the proposed treatment, and the possible risk to allow the patient to make an intelligent decision. Given the ambiguities and uncertainties of the present statutes (Who is to tell what is sufficient information in each particular case?) no specific format of consent would afford physicians fail-safe protection against any liability arising from failure to provide ''complete'' information preoperatively. The quality of information usually prevails over the quantity. Factors to be taken into account are: (a) the measure of duty involved; (b) the scope of disclosure; and (c) the standards of disclosure current at that time and place (state laws). Since one cannot avoid the issue, one should try to minimize the risks inherent in offering incomplete consent. A useful set of guidelines will prove helpful.

The surgeon performing the procedure should discuss the planned treatment with the patient. The scope of the necessary disclosure generally requires the patient to be informed of:

Diagnosis
Contemplated treatment
Risks inherent in such a treatment
Alternative methods of therapy
Prognosis with treatment
Prognosis without treatment

Nevertheless, the session should be more of a dialogue than a monologue intended to provide information. The discussion need only consist of a reasonable explanation of the alternatives and the risks that may ensue. The patient should be given ample time to ask questions and have them thoroughly answered. Not only should she be told, but she must be permitted to understand what is being considered. Whereas one should express the hope that the procedure will most likely be successful, special care should be exercised not to give false assurance that a procedure has no risk or minimal risk.

General consent forms that do not specify the type of treatment consented to and that do not disclose the specific risks are of little value. Phrases such as ''such treatment as deemed necessary'' or ''as advisable in the treatment of this patient'' are so ambiguous in nature as to be considered almost worthless.

In general, the law does not allow a crime to be licensed by a victim's consent. A person may consent to the use of a reasonable degree of force on him or her in circumstances regarded as lawfully justified. Thus, medical and surgical procedures to which a patient consents do not constitute unlawful violence. The ancient legal maxim *volenti non fit injuria* (no injury is done to the man who consents to it) applies only to the intentional injury which is the surgical procedure. Although such a consent includes an assumption of risks present in all medical procedures, it does not offer any defense for an action of negligence.

Two types of tort theories are applicable to the area of lack of informed consent: (a) cause of action in negligence presents itself when a patient has consented to a specific surgical procedure and an undisclosed complication occurs during the operation, providing there is no intentional deviation from the consent; and (b) cause of action for a technical battery exists when a physician obtains consent for one type of medical procedure and then performs a substantially different operation. Since battery is considered an intentional tort, different statutes of limitations and risk for punitive damages apply.

DOCTRINE OF INFORMED CONSENT

The modern informed consent doctrine, based on the case of Nathanson v Kline, reflects the standard professional approach.[5] A physician's duty as it relates to disclosure is determined by the standards of the medical profession. Such an approach would require that any disclosure made to patients conform to the general practice of medicine in a same or a similar community or locality. A variation of this approach was also interpreted as conforming to prevailing medical practice.

Since the early 1970s, a new approach has been gaining acceptance. It defines the physician's duty of disclosure in terms of the information needed by the patient to make an intelligent informed decision about whether or not to undergo the proposed treatment. This requires a physician to disclose any risks that are material to the patient's decision to accept a suggested therapy (Canterbury v Spence).[1] Such an approach is more consistent with the patient's rights of self determination.

The doctrine of informed consent is based on the supposition that a properly informed patient will weigh the risks against the benefits of the proposed treatment and compare them with the risk/benefit ratio of alternative treatments. Such a concept (developed largely by the legal profession) gives more weight to the patient's cognitive understanding of the information disclosed by the physician or nurse. In reality the affective aspects of the physician-patient relationship take precedence over the cognitive aspects of disclosure.

Herbert argues that, "Informed consent has been perverted from an ethical concept to a legalistic one, with the legalisms being used instead of ethics rather than in support of ethics."[2] What was once considered a warm human doctor-patient relationship is now considered by the law to be a contractual relationship in which the physician has the fiduciary duty to make full disclosure. The doctrine of informed consent requires that the physician explain the risks of the procedure and its alternatives and that he or she obtain the competent, voluntary, and understanding consent of the patient before proceeding. This must be done before undertaking any diagnostic or therapeutic procedure that exposes the patient to a reasonable chance of harm. The patient has the right to chart his or her own destiny, and the doctor must supply the patient with the material facts needed to diligently chart that destiny with dignity. A legally competent person has the right to decide what is to be done to his body and thus cannot be compelled to accept a treatment that he does not wish.

The physician is under no obligation to disclose risks when the patient insists or states that she neither wants to be informed nor to discuss the matter. It is, nevertheless, advisable and prudent to document such a situation and to have the patient countersign a waiver. Such a release makes the "prudent person test" inapplicable. Interestingly enough, the rules of disclosure apply only to a procedure that is correctly performed. There is no duty to disclose the untoward results that might occur as a result of an improperly performed procedure. This eventuality is covered by other laws.

Some uncertainty remains in the area of nondisclosure. A physician can invoke "therapeutic privilege" in withholding information when he believes that disclosure of such information would adversely affect the patient's condition. It is clear this privilege would not apply to elective procedures for which full disclosure might affect the patient's decision without incurring adverse consequences.

Lack of disclosure of a risk not known to the physician himself is only acceptable if such ignorance was not by itself a violation of the duty of providing due care. The duty to inform a patient presupposes the duty that the physician should possess the knowledge of a reasonably well-trained colleague practicing under like circumstances. Not to disclose a risk the physician should have known but does not know may make him or her liable for negligent nondisclosure.

DOCUMENTATION

The legal concept of informed consent is considered a contractual relationship in which the physician has the fiduciary duty to make full disclosure. It is immediately obvious that the question of informed consent would only become an issue following a laparoscopy if the outcome of the procedure falls short of the patient's expectations. Complications can encompass many possibilities ranging from a mild degree of dissatisfaction to the most serious of adverse effects. Whereas it would be unwise to standardize the mechanisms by which the patient is informed prior to giving her consent (the doctor-patient relationship is an art), some formalities are important for ensuring that one can fulfill the requirement for documenting the events leading to an informed consent.

The method for providing information to patients can adopt a variety of forms. Recommendations abound in the medical literature. Whichever method is selected, the information one gives to patients not only should be precise and concise, but must be presented in simple terms that are easily understood. The use of medical jargon or acronyms is discouraged as is the use of technical words. Highly scientific information has little place when obtaining informed consent from a lay person. It is as critical to address the patient according to the level of her understanding as it is to utilize a translator when communicating in a foreign language. The ability of a physician to communicate with his or her patient is a primary and intrinsic component of the doctor-patient relationship. It cannot and should not be delegated to auxiliary personnel or to some type of audiovisual aid. This does not preclude using films, tapes, or trained personnel. They can fulfill an important function that supplements recommendations and explanations given by the responsible physician. If used, they should be offered in addition to, and not instead of, the personalized approach by the primary surgeon.

A laparoscopic procedure falls within the aforementioned criteria, thereby universally requiring that an informed consent be obtained. The information provided should include possible hazards related to:

- Anesthesia (usually just mentioned by the gynecologist and left for the anesthesiologist to give a more in-depth discussion)
- Instrumentation for mobilizing the uterus
- Obtaining and maintaining the pneumoperitoneum
- Inserting both primary and secondary trocar
- Nonsurgical intra-abdominal manipulation
- Anticipated surgical procedures (e.g., biopsy, electrocoagulation)
- Instrument failure

The usual hospital or clinic records seldom suffice to document how informed consent was obtained or the content of the information given. However, proper documentation cannot be emphasized too strongly. The physician's own records should contain a summary of recommendations, counseling, and discussion of therapeutic or diagnostic alternatives. The record should state that the patient has opted for a particular therapy of her own volition. If she has taken some time to think it through, that fact should also be documented.

Within the bounds of confidentiality, one should state if a relative was present, was consulted or participated in the decision making process.

The lack of documentation may be interpreted to signify that informed consent was never obtained. Regrettably, I must point out this applies even if it was. Documentation is only a small part of the process of informed consent. Its importance is secondary to the patient's understanding of what is taking place. A signed informed consent form has little value if the patient does not actually have a full understanding of what she is consenting to.

There has been a proliferation of standard formats for informed consent forms (some as extensive as 28 pages) that attempt to fulfill the letter of the law. This raises the question of whether physicians are only modifying the consent form without necessarily modifying how the consent is being obtained. No printed form can ever take the place of the dialogue between the doctor and the patient before she signs that form. At our institution, in addition to the standard *pro forma* operative consent obtained at the time of admission, physicians are required to enter a note in their own handwriting describing the conversation leading to the patient's consent. Although this is surely also subject to legal challenge, it does provide additional evidence that a process of truly informed consent has indeed taken place.

CONSENT IN EMERGENCIES

To perform a surgical procedure in an emergency is perhaps the only situation in which proceeding without manifest written consent is acceptable. This is known an "implied consent." It most commonly involves emergency circumstances in which the patient is a minor (with no responsible adult available) or is an adult who is unconscious or otherwise incapable of consenting. Emergencies are generally understood to include conditions which endanger the life or health of a patient and which require immediate medical or surgical intervention. Before implied consent can be invoked in a purported emergency, efforts should be made to obtain consent from a parent, guardian, or the courts. These efforts should be well documented.

It is strongly recommended that the opinion of another physician be obtained whenever it is not possible to get the patient's consent. When well documented, it helps to show that the decision making, albeit rapid, was both deliberate and carried through without undue haste. It not only offers additional legal protection for the physician and the hospital, but also has an implicit advantage for the patient based on the temperate judgment derived from a team decision.

A clear distinction should be drawn between an emergency procedure and one done for convenience. Although this differentiation is superfluous in clear cut life-and-death situations, it is essential when the physician finds he or she must extend the scope of the planned procedure without first getting informed consent. Measures needed to remedy a complication resulting from an authorized procedure fall within the area of implied consent as it relates to emergency situations. Not as clearly established, yet, generally accepted as a judicious extension of the original procedure, is biopsy for an unexpected finding during a diagnostic laparoscopy, for example. An extension of this type should be recognized as an accepted medical procedure dictated by sound medical practice. However, it must result in a direct benefit to the patient, and it has to be reasonably assumed that if it were feasible the patient would have consented to the procedure of his or her own volition.

To extend the procedure beyond that which was originally consented to by the patient is specifically proscribed. To undertake a sterilization procedure without prior consent at the time of a diagnostic laparoscopy in a patient found to have uterine fibroids or severely diseased fallopian tubes is not an urgent matter, but rather one of convenience, even though a subsequent pregnancy is likely to be hazardous. Such a case could be subject to a cause of action for technical battery.

INFORMED CONSENT IN MINORS AND INCOMPETENT PATIENTS

When laparoscopy has to be performed on a minor, the responsibility for permission is delegated to the patient's closest available relative or legal guardian. In the absence of this individual, the state adopts the right to protect minors under the *parens patriae* doctrine. In emergency cases in which it is impossible or impracticable to contact a responsible adult, the law authorizes the physician to undertake the appropriate treatment or procedure provided it falls within the standard of practice.

In our institution, these cases require administrative concurrence by the hospital administrator on call (usually a lay person). This person acts in the minor's interest, serving as her guardian, until the appropriate legal permits are obtained. Hierarchic departmental authorization by the departmental chairman or chief of service, although not required by law, should be seriously considered. From the viewpoint of the law, an emancipated minor (married minor) is treated as an adult. However, unresolved controversy surrounds some state laws that permit competent minors to consent to medical treatment without the actual consent or even knowledge of their parents or guardian. When a conflict arises between a competent minor and the parent or guardian, the state could invoke the *parens patrie* doctrine to assert the rights of the minors. Once the court has assumed jurisdiction, a parent or guardian cannot subsequently grant permission. When no conflict exists, the consent provided by the parent or guardian is binding.

Most of the statutes protecting minors also apply to incompetent adults. Some exceptions are worth nothing. A mentally retarded adult, who has sufficient basic skills to be considered a functional adult, should be considered competent. The constitutional right of privacy for an incompetent patient should always be respected. The right to consent or withhold consent to medical treatment is included in that right of privacy. Some procedures, such as sterilization, require consent even by the incompetent patient; the guardian has only limited authority to give consent in such a case.

INFORMED CONSENT IN RESEARCH

Contributions to knowledge in medicine often take the form of experiments (research) on patients. As a consequence of the atrocities performed by the Nazis on their prisoners during World War II, the Nuremberg Convention established a code of practice that should always be followed by those performing experiments on patients.[13]

In June, 1964, the World Medical Association adopted the final draft of the code of ethics on human experimentation; this became known as the Declaration of Helsinki. It recognizes the distinction between clinical research, in which the aim is essentially therapeutic, and purely scientific clinical research, in which the aim is not therapeutic.

By virtue of its recent widespread acceptance, laparoscopy is a procedure involving active research. New instrumentation is constantly being developed to satisfy actual and anticipated needs. In order to prove that these are effective and safe, each of them has to be evaluated in real-life situations involving patients. Substitution of laparoscopy for more extensive surgical procedures requires confirmation of benefit over risk in every instance.

The guidelines laid down by the Declaration of Helsinki prevent patients from being subjected to deplorable abuse under the excuse of research. However, there is some degree of conflict between the guidelines and the requirements of informed consent as understood at the present time. An experiment on humans is performed to answer unresolved questions. We should remember, however, that the law does not allow a crime (harm) to be licensed by the victim's consent. Moreover, in the case of research, not even the physician knows all the risks (side effects and complications) that might occur. Thus, we see why consent to research is an important aspect of informed consent.

To address this particular issue, most institutions in the United States have created some type of committee which bears the responsibility to protect patient's rights by assuming the role of advocate. It brings together lay people and physicians who possess the medical knowledge that the patient presumably lacks. It attempts to fulfill a dual role: (a) to adhere to the recommendations of the Declaration of Helsinki, and (b) to minimize the potential risks a patient is exposed to if she participates in a research protocol. It would be fair to question the wisdom of carrying out a laparoscopic procedure that is not yet established and accepted without prior consultation with and approval by such a committee.

At our institution, the informed consent form for a research protocol includes information as to the purpose of the study, an explanation of the procedure and the risks and discomforts which can be anticipated. In addition, we include explanations concerning what is the current accepted standard of treatment for that condition. Protection of confidentiality and any cost or payment available for participating in the study is also stated. A copy of the consent is given to the patient. The original signed form becomes part of her hospital medical record.

An amendment to the definition of informed consent for injured research subjects was issued by the United States Department of Health, Education and Welfare in November, 1978.[8] This regulation, which is currently in effect, states that research subjects must be told whether compensation and medical treatment would be available to them in case of physical injury resulting from their participation in a research protocol. Although the regulation was intended to be applied to protocols in federally supported research projects, experience has shown that the extension of this policy to nonfederally funded protocols is advisable.

ETHICAL DIMENSIONS OF INFORMED CONSENT

As previously discussed, an informed consent should include factors such as proposed treatment, possible risks, alternative modalities of treatment, and their inherent risks and prognosis. Regardless of the prevailing standard of disclosure in a given area, informed consent requires frank, open, and careful communication between the doctor and the patient. Disclosure implies that information and knowledge are shared by the parties involved. In the case of informed consent, the flow is usually unidirectional from the doctor to the patient. This educational process is undoubtedly influenced by the physician's opinions and prior experience and can often lead consciously or subconsciously to the introduction of some bias with respect to the information offered. Some of the physician's recommendations are based more on personal experience and habit of practice than on hard factual data.

The situation is complex and as medicine advances presents an ethical dilemma of increasingly greater proportions. Developments in medical technology require that physicians receive constant training to update their skills. New developments cause some techniques to become outdated or obsolete. This poses a moral dilemma that raises the following questions: should the physician propose an older plan of management because he or she is experienced with it and excels at it? or alternatively should the outcome be potentially compromised by undertaking a more desirable procedure that he or she has not yet completely mastered? The issue can be resolved by referring the patient to a colleague who has already mastered the newer technique. This idealistic resolution may not be realistic but it does address the ethics of the matter.

To illustrate an instance applicable to laparoscopy, let us analyze a case involving consideration of abdominal exploration to rule out the presence of an ectopic pregnancy. Physician A is an experienced, skilled, and dextrous surgeon who can perform an exploratory laparotomy expeditiously with a low incidence of complications. His experience with diagnostic laparoscopy is limited, and he is not enthusiastic about undertaking the procedure. By contrast, physician B is an experienced laparoscopist who could visually explore the abdomen by means of diagnostic laparoscopy in less time and with lower morbidity than could physician A perform a laparotomy. If the patient did not have an ectopic gestation, can physician A justify the prolonged hospitalization, increased discomfort and morbidity, future surgical hazards, and cosmetic impact of the exploratory laparotomy he recommends? This example depicts a typical case of potential manipulation of the consent process based on a physician's bias favoring one procedure over another even though apparently contrary to the patient's interests.

COUNSELING

Counseling is an integral part of the informed consent process. It assumes greater importance when it applies to an elective surgical procedure. In regard to laparoscopy, particularly as it relates to sterilization, counseling is an essential component of the evaluation of a patient as to her suitability for the procedure (see Chapter 5).

The surgeon must ensure that the patient understands not only the technical aspects of the procedure and its possible risks and complications, but also the need for the operation. In emergency situations, one should encourage the participation of relatives or close friends. For elective procedures, the patient must be offered as much time as she requires to give her consent for surgery.

Timing of the informed consent is also important. In elective laparoscopic procedures, a consent signed several days prior to the procedure implies, at the very least, that the patient had sufficient time to ask additional questions or to change her mind. Any addendum to a previously signed consent form should be initialled and witnessed anew. It is improper to obtain consent or to make additions after the patient has been premedicated by the anesthesiologist or is under the influence of a psychodynamic drug.

The law of informed consent is an example of case law (which is law developed by and based upon precedent). Although precedents will most likely be considered in each particular case, there is always a possibility that an innovative judgement will be made which deviates from the preexisting law, and thus becomes a precedent itself. Therefore, just as in other matters with medicolegal implications, nothing replaces a well established, warm and trusting relationship between the doctor and the patient. The physician's integrity and strict adherence to the ethical codes continues to represent the most effective guarantee of patient rights.

FAILED CONTRACEPTION

Pregnancy following sterilization may give rise to a variety of legal actions. For the most part, wrongful gestation is the parent's cause of action against a physician for the negligent performance of a sterilization that results in the birth of a healthy child. Wrongful life is the cause of action in which a child alleges the injury of being born despite having been born healthy. Finally, wrongful birth is a parental cause of action based on the economic loss and expense incurred by the birth and upbringing of an unplanned and unwanted child.

Of particular concern to the laparoscopist are the first and the last of these. Indisputably, a wrongful gestation in which negligence on the part of the operator can be proved is generally considered to constitute malpractice. The courts have no reluctance to grant damages for cases associated with misidentification of pelvic structures or incompletely performed operations. However, assessing awards for damages is often a dilemma. Courts across the country have been inconsistent in regard to weighing the extent of injury inflicted upon parents by the birth of a normal child.

When disallowing recovery for damages based on the costs of raising the purportedly unwanted child, courts have resorted to a variety of arguments. One court stated "The satisfaction, joy and companionship which normal parents have in rearing a child make such economic loss worthwhile...Who can place a price tag on a child's smile, or the parental pride in a child's achievement?...Public sentiment recognizes that these benefits to the parents outweigh their economic loss in rearing and educating a healthy, normal child."[12] Another said "...to permit the parents to keep their child and shift the entire cost of its upbringing to the physician would be to create a new category of surrogate parent...We hold that such result would be wholly out of proportion to the culpability involved, and that allowance of recovery would place too unreasonable a burden upon physicians, under the facts and circumstances alleged."[7]

Still others have applied the so called "Benefits Rule." This rule (expressed by the American Law Institute in their Restatement of the Law of Torts 920 states "Where defendant's wrongful conduct has had a two-sided effect insofar as the consequences have been harmful and beneficial to the plaintiff's interest, the value of the benefit conferred sometimes is considered in mitigation of damages. When the Benefits Rule is used, damages are limited and usually less extreme.'' In Mason v Western Pennsylvania Hospital, action was brought against a physician and a hospital following the birth of a normal child after an unsuccessful tubal ligation.[4] The judge rejected the notion that damages assessing the value of human life against its costs was at best speculative and conjectural. The jury was allowed to make such a determination.

Some courts have rejected the aforementioned Benefits Rule as being too speculative and difficult to apply. In turn, they sustained the rights of parents to recover damages for the cost of raising a child born following a failed sterilization. In Raja v Tulsky and Michael Reese Hospital and Medical Center, a patient delivered a healthy child 5 years after a tubal cauterization was performed.[9] Parents were seeking to recover expenses of raising and educating the child. The court stated that a couple has a legally protectable right to determine whether they will have a child. It further reasoned that emotional rewards of parenthood cannot be used to offset its financial costs.

References

1. Canterbury v Spence. 464 F 2d 772 (DC Circ 1972).
2. Herbert V. Informed consent: A legal evaluation. Cancer 1980; 46:1042-1044.
3. Laforet EG. The fiction of informed consent. JAMA 1976; 235:1579-1585.
4. Mason v Western Pennsylvania Hospital. 286 PaS 354, 428 A. 2d 1366 (1981).
5. Nathanson v Kline. 186 Kan 393,350 P. 2d 1093 (1960).
6. President's commission for the study of ethical problems in medicine and biomedical and behavioral research: Making health care decision. A report on the ethical and legal implications of informed consent in the patient-practitioner relationship. Washington DC, US Government Printing Office 1982:147.
7. P v Portandin. 179 NJ Super 465,432 A. 2d 556 (1981).
8. Protection of human subject: Informed consent: Definition amended to include advice on compensation. Fed Regist November 3, 1978; 43(214):51559.
9. Raja v Tulsky and Michael Reese Hospital and Medical Center. 99 Ill. App 3d 271,425 N.E. 2d 968 (1981).
10. Schloendorff v Society of New York Hospital. 211 N.Y. 125,105 N.E. 92 (1914).
11. Stone AA. Informed consent: Special problems for psychiatry. Hosp Commun Psych 1979; 30:321-327.
12. Terrell v Garcia. 94 S. Ct. 1434,496 S.W. 2d 124 (1973).
13. The Nuremberg code. In: Trials of war criminals before the Nuremberg military tribunals under control council law No 10 Vol 2. Washington DC US Government Printing Office 1949; 181-182.

26 TRANSLAPAROSCOPIC PHOTOGRAPHY

Many surgeons seem reluctant to prolong the surgical procedure for a few additional minutes to obtain endoscopic pictures. They consider this to be a superfluous exercise that adds little if anything to what they have already seen with their own eyes. Nothing can be further from the truth. Without pictorial documentation, the surgeon must rely on the operative report for recall. Dictated operative notes are usually done in a hurry and are subjective at best. At a later time, inadequate description of the findings leads to limited interpretation, even by the surgeon who did the procedure.

ADVANTAGES

Advantages of endoscopic photography are not limited to the teaching aspects of the technique or to the creation of a photographic collection. Direct patient care can also be affected beneficially by proper documentation. Photographic records permit (a) better explanation of the findings to the patient; (b) more precise and detailed description of the findings for use when referring the patient to another physician; and often, (c) avoidance of a repeat laparoscopy to establish a correct plan of management.

Explanation to Patient

Experience has shown repeatedly that an informed patient is a better patient. Aside from the medicolegal implications of adequate informed consent, proper understanding of the nature of any disorder found at laparoscopy permits the patient to make an educated decision concerning the care she is to receive. As physicians, we cannot assume that patients are familiar with, or clearly understand, anatomical landmarks and pathologic processes. A detailed explanation is facilitated by photographs that depict the conditions affecting a particular patient.

Referral to Another Physician

Frequently, a patient who has undergone a diagnostic laparoscopy by her primary physician is referred for treatment to another specialist. Personally, on more than one occasion, I have found myself faced with a discrepancy between the findings I encountered at the surgical exploration and the description of abnormalities reportedly found at an earlier laparoscopy by the referring physician. Lack of precise documentation, such as afforded by endoscopic photography, places both the treating physician and the patient at a disadvantage.

Avoidance of a Repeat Laparoscopy

Recent advances in the fields of gynecologic surgery (particularly as regards the introduction of microsurgical techniques) and infertility care (especially with in vitro fertilization) have already had an impact on the choice of management plans for an infertile patient. Similarly, they have influenced the decisions that patients make after appropriate counseling. Adequate information is essential to make such a determination. Because of poor prior documentation, before major surgery is undertaken an inordinate number of repeat laparoscopies need to be performed to clarify whether newer techniques are applicable. The opportunity to evaluate photographs of the findings would certainly avoid most, if not all, of them.

EQUIPMENT

In the past, good quality endoscopic photographic pictures depended heavily on the experience of the photographer (i.e., the endoscopist). The advent of modern photographic technology provides the laparoscopist with new, highly automated equipment that permits excellent pictures to be obtained even by the average photographically unsophisticated surgeon. Nevertheless, knowledge about some basic photographic principles and an understanding of the capabilities of some of the new equipment proves extremely helpful and allows for consistently good endoscopic photographs.

The equipment used to obtain the photographs presented in this book consisted of a light source with flash capabilities, a single-lens reflex camera, an automatic exposure endoscopic adapter, and a laparoscope of either 5 mm or 10 mm diameter.

Light Source

The Olympus CLE-F or CLE-F10 (Figures 26.1 and 26.2) cold light supply with flash provides in a single unit the necessary light source to carry out laparoscopy, a flash unit for high speed flash photography, and through-the-lens (TTL) automatic exposure. Appropriate illumination to perform the investigative portion of the endoscopic procedure is provided by a 150-watt tungsten halogen mirrored lamp. The degree of brightness can be regulated according to the different laparoscopic requirements.

Photographic flash capabilities originate from a xenon flash tube with a short recycling time (2 to 3 sec) that allows it to be fired at short intervals. The high intensity xenon light permits accurate exposures at fast speeds of between 1/100 and 1/3,000 sec, thus preventing blurred pictures due to movement of the surgeon or the patient.

The solid-state TTL automatic exposure relies on a series of signals which are measured by a photoelectric cell within the laparoscopic adapter. The signal is processed to provide the correct amount of light for proper exposure. The surgeon can override this automatic TTL light measuring circuit, if he or she desires to operate the system manually, using expertise based on personal photographic experience.

Automatic Exposure Endoscope Adapter

The SM-EFR 2 is the adapter instrument that couples the laparoscope with the photographic camera (Olympus OM2) (Figure 26.3). It fulfills the dual function of synchronizing the flash illumination with the time of film exposure and serves as an automatic exposure meter index. Once attached, the surgeon needs only adjust the focus to clearly delineate the area to be photographed.

Technically, the SM-EFR 2 adapter is a 110 mm macro lens with an approximate 1:1 ratio. It does not have an effective F stop (diaphragm). Its focal distance extends from 5 mm to infinity, with the upper range limited only by the focal length of the laparoscope used. A photoelectric cell measures the reflected light and relays the signal to the illumination source which emits the correct amount of light for adequate exposure.

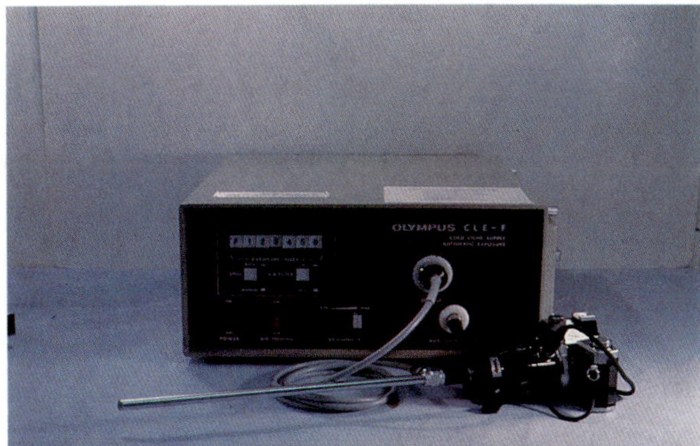

Figure 26.1 Olympus CLE-F light source. Camera, adapter and laparoscope are assembled and connected.

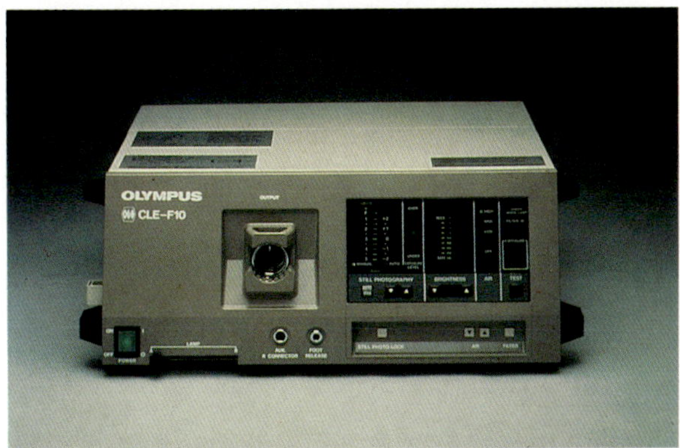

Figure 26.2 Olympus CLE-F10 light source. Settings can be locked after adjustment to avoid accidental changes. Shutter speed can be increased to 2/100,000 to 5/1,000 sec.

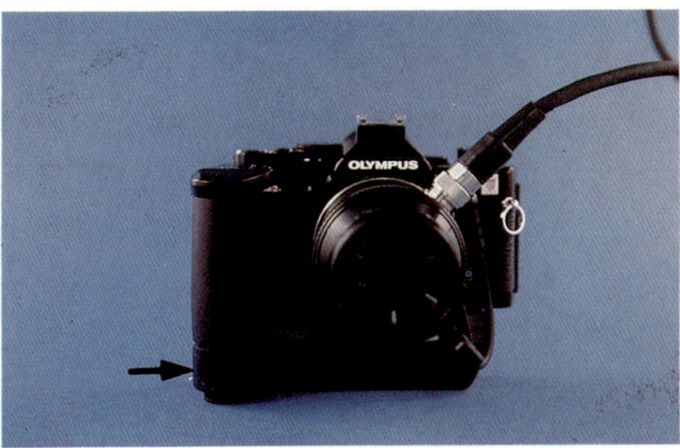

Figure 26.3 Olympus OM2 camera. Motor drive (arrow) advances the film automatically. This facilitates one-handed operation.

Single-Lens Reflex Camera

The 35 mm single-lens reflex camera used to obtain the photographs for this book was an Olympus OM2. When using the light source with flash capabilities as previously described, one should switch the camera to its manual mode. This enables the flash generator to automatically adjust the amount of light required. The shutter speed is set on 4 (¼ sec).

To facilitate accurate focusing of the object to be photographed, a clear double cross hair screen (Olympus 1-12) is used. Each line of the double cross should be seen clearly and separately from each other. Additionally, the fully clear screen permits the endoscopist to see the entire visual field that will be reproduced on the film.

Care should be exercised when handling the film and camera. The film should never be loaded or unloaded while wearing surgical gloves or immediately after ungloving. The starch powder that covers both sides of the gloves is detrimental to the proper functioning of the camera and film emulsions.

Laparoscope

Best photographic results are obtained when using a 10 mm 0° to 5° angle of view laparoscope. Good quality pictures can also be obtained with a 5 mm laparoscope with similar angles of view. The main differences are the smaller image size and the lower light intensity that reach the photographic film in the latter.

The size of the endoscopic image can be calculated by multiplying the diameter of the field stop by the magnification of the ocular lens. Taylor reported the apparent images of 5 mm and 10 mm laparoscopes to be 32 mm and 64 mm in diameter, respectively.[1] Although a smaller image provides sufficient resolution for diagnostic purposes, the smaller number of fiberoptic fibers transmitting light requires a higher flash intensity to properly expose the film used. This is discussed later.

DEFOGGING THE LENS

Usually, the initial view seen through the laparoscope upon entering the peritoneal cavity is blurred. This is a direct result of the fogging of the laparoscope's front lens. Under normal circumstances, when a piece of glass is exposed to a large temperature difference, water condensation accumulates on its warmer side. Routinely, the laparoscope is prepared for use on the operating room instrument table. It thus adapts to the operating room temperature which varies between 71° and 76° (22° to 24° C). The body temperature in afebrile individuals fluctuates in the range of 96° to 99° F (35° to 37° C). Such a differential temperature is sufficient to fog the front lens of the laparoscope, which obliterates the clear view of intraperitoneal structures.

Various means have been devised to achieve defogging of the laparoscopic lens. They are divided into physical and chemical methods. Physical methods are based on the principle of temperature equalization; chemical methods seek to cover the lens with anticondensation solutions.

Physical Methods

The easiest and most economical mode of defogging the forward lens of the laparoscope is to appose it to any intra-abdominal structure. Contact between the organ (usually the uterus or bowel) and the front lens warms the lens and thus prevents condensation. This maneuver if done blindly does carry a risk of damage to the organ being contacted.

For purposes of taking translaparoscopic pictures, however, such contact between an intraperitoneal organ and the front lens is not recommended. While the contact accomplishes the desired defogging, it also leaves a thin layer of peritoneal fluid on the lens. The human eye is capable of self correcting the resulting image distortion. However, the photographic camera lacks this capability and, therefore, it registers the image as blurred and out of focus.

A simpler method to prevent fogging of the lens is to warm the instrument prior to inserting it into the peritoneal cavity. This can be accomplished by means of electrical warmers which are highly efficient but rather expensive. Similar results can also be obtained by immersing the laparoscope or just its forward end in warm saline solution. When using this method prior to translaparoscopic photography, one should carefully dry the laparoscope before placing it into the abdominal cavity to avoid leaving any residual solution on the lens because this might blur the pictures.

The warmed front lens retains its elevated temperature for several minutes within the peritoneal cavity. Immersion in warm saline may have to be repeated several times over the course of the procedure according to its duration. Cooling of the instrument is the result of continued contact with the cold distending gas that invests it within the trocar sleeve. It is advisable, therefore, to discontinue insufflation of gas when introducing the laparoscope through its sleeve and especially while taking photographs. Ideally, if the initial pneumoperitoneum is being maintained, insufflation of gas can be completely discontinued.

Chemical Methods

Anticondensation solutions have been used successfully to prevent the fogging of photographic lenses. These solutions have detergent capabilities that, by coating the external surface of the lens, prevent accumulation of condensed water droplets. Utilization for laparoscopy has been facilitated by the commercial production of sterile, multidose vials. Unfortunately, repeated applications create a thick coating on the laparoscope's front lens. This has the disadvantage of requiring periodic cleansing.

VISUAL FIELD

The extent of the area that can be visualized laparoscopically varies according to the size of the laparoscope, its angle of view, and the distance from the desired region to be explored. A small diameter laparoscope provides a more constricted visual field than a larger size instrument. This proves to be important when translaparoscopic photography is to be undertaken. The amount of light reaching the film is the result of the amount of light reflected from the area to be photographed. The intensity of the light falling on an object is inversely proportional to the square of the distance between the source of the light and the object illuminated. The reflected light is a function of the light intensity of the flash and the distance between the laparoscope and the area to be recorded. Small size laparoscopes have proportionally fewer fiberoptic bundles than have larger size instruments. Therefore, because they can transmit less light the instrument has to be moved closer to the structures being studied in order to obtain adequate illumination. Thus, the size of the visual field is correspondingly reduced.

The distance from the object to be photographed also varies according to its color. As previously mentioned, the illumination reaching the film plane depends on the light reflecting off the area to be photographed. Ovaries have a white, shiny capsule that reflects most of the light it receives. It is, therefore, necessary to maintain a distance of no less than 5 cm between the laparoscope and the ovary in order to avoid overexposure. By way of contrast, photography of the right upper quadrant requires a short distance from the liver, gallbladder or spleen since the dark backround does not reflect light adequately.

The automatic exposure control establishes the amount of light required for proper film exposure by means of internal measurement (photoelectric cell). The Olympus system comes equipped with an alarm that emits an audible sound during flash recharge. The duration of the sound emitted gives the laparoscopist a measure of the adequacy of illumination. A sound lasting less than 2 sec is appropriate for good quality pictures. Those of longer duration require the laparoscope to be moved closer to the object to be photographed. Alernatively, one can use more sensitive film. Types of film are discussed later.

IMAGE SHARPNESS

The most common difficulties encountered during translaparoscopic photography are the lack of sufficient light and poor picture definition. Introduction of suitable light sources and film, as described previously, has solved most of the problems relating to adequacy of illumination. With respect to the clarity and sharpness of the photographs, however, certain recommendations will prove valuable.

Clarity and sharpness of a laparoscopic photograph depend upon a variety of factors: focal length of the lens, depth of field, and accuracy of focusing. The focal length and depth of field are fixed by the type of laparoscope and adapter lens used and are not under the operator's control. This leaves focusing as the only variable that affects the quality of picture obtained.

Focusing means accommodating the lens-to-film distance to adjust for the lens-to-subject distance so as to produce the sharpest image. This is done by rotating the focusing ring of the adapter lens. The laparoscopist must be the best judge as to when an image is in focus.

Because the adapter lens can serve as a corrective lens for the operator's myopia or hyperopia, it is important that the operator's vision be corrected before focus adjustment is attempted. If the surgeon ordinarily wears corrective glasses, he or she must wear them while taking pictures through the laparoscope. Failure to do so will focus the image in the operator's retina, but the film will register a blurred picture.

The adapter lens acts as a single focus zoom lens. Therefore, best focusing is achieved by first adjusting the focal plane at the shortest distance to the object being photographed. Minimal adjustments are required following slight withdrawal of the laparoscope for a more panoramic view.

Wearing glasses during laparoscopy may, at times, be cumbersome. Spectacles tend to fog and collide with the laparoscopic eyepiece. The use of contact lenses or a dioptric corrective lens applied to the camera's viewfinder overcomes this difficulty. To avoid fogging the viewfinder lens by the operator's expired warm air, the upper border of the surgical mask should be taped to the bridge of the nose and the suborbital area (Figure 26.4).

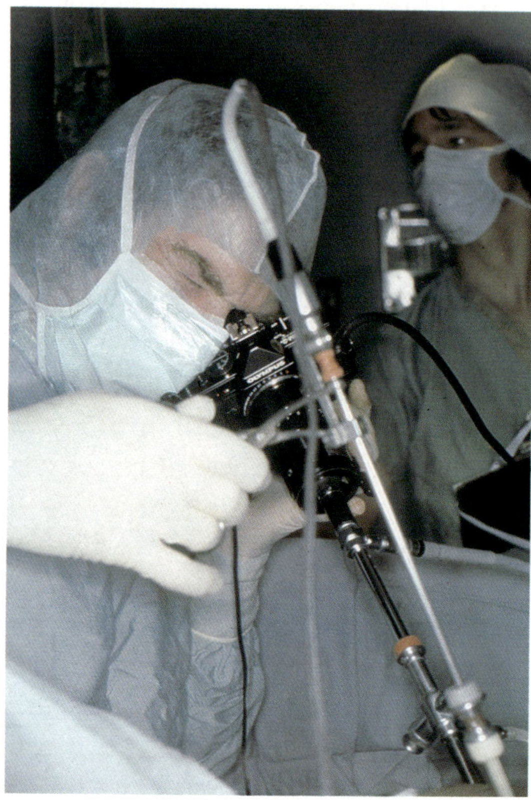

Figure 26.4 Camera attached to laparoscope in operation. Holding the camera and focusing can be accomplished by means of one hand. The surgical mask is taped to the bridge of the operator's nose to prevent fogging the viewfinder lens.

TYPE OF FILM

Standard 35 mm film has become the most acceptable medium for biomedical photography. Color print or slide film can be used according to the operator's preference. It has been my experience that color slide film is easier to manipulate, develop, catalogue, and file. Therefore, it is the only one I use and recommend.

The ideal film for translaparoscopic photography must possess good definition, high contrast, and accurate color balance. The better the definition of a film, the more detail can be distinguished in the final picture. The contrast or sharpness is influenced by the thickness of the film emulsion; thinner emulsions produce sharper photographs. Satisfactory color balance is obtained with panchromatic film. Because it is sensitive to all colors and ultraviolet light, this type of film proves especially suitable for biomedical photography.

Photographic film is broadly categorized according to its sensitivity to light (light speed). High sensitivity films are known as high speed or fast. Faster films allow one to obtain sharply defined photographs with less exposure to light. Film sensitivity is determined by the manufacturer according to standards established by the American Standards Association (ASA). Film sensitivity is expressed in terms of ASA speed numbers. Films rated ASA 250 to 640 are considered high speed; those rated ASA 800 to 1600 are designated as very high speed. In continental Europe, the Deutsche Industrie Norm (DIN) sensitivity figures are still preferred. Recently, the International Standards Organization (ISO) combined ASA and DIN ratings and issued ISO figures (e.g., ISO 400/27°).

Sharpness of the photograph is inversely proportional to the density of the film emulsion grain. The finer the grain, the greater the detail capable of being distinguished on the final picture. A counterbalancing principle is the direct correlation that exists between the grain of the emulsion and the film speed. The higher the film speed, the grainier the photograph will be, resulting in decreased sharpness.

All the color photographs shown in this book were obtained using Ektachrome 400 ASA daylight film routinely developed by Kodak processing (Eastman-Kodak Co, Rochester, NY). Although the sensitivity of the film can be boosted by presetting the camera to a lower ASA position or altering the developing process, best results have been obtained by adhering to standard exposure and developing processes.

A recently introduced film (Ektachrome P800/1600) has proved capable of producing good quality pictures with much less available light. Special processing permits this 400 ASA film to be developed as if it had 800 or 1600 ASA characteristics (by process E-6P/push). Even though it has a slightly grainier appearance, the resolution is excellent for documentation purposes. This film is particularly suitable for use with smaller size (5 mm) endoscopes.

NUMBER OF EXPOSURES

The number of pictures to be taken in any given case varies according to the particular findings. Adequate documentation may be obtained with as few as three photographs. Based on my personal experience, however, it is preferable to get no less than 10 to 12 exposures per case to ensure all details are properly recorded.

For a process strictly confined to one adnexal region or to the center of the pelvis (such as the uterus or posterior cul-de-sac), a set of three exposures is usually sufficient. For documentation of more extensive abdominopelvic abnormalities, three pictures per area are recommended. The short recharging time of the xenon flash lamps (2 to 3 sec) enables the laparoscopist to obtain a full series of pictures in a relatively short time (2 to 3 min).

It is advisable to use short rolls of film unless several laparoscopies are being performed seriatim. This avoids prolonged delays between the time the film is exposed and the time it is developed. Furthermore, it facilitates correct cataloguing of the pictures while the operative findings are still fresh in the surgeon's mind.

STERILE FIELD

Sterility of the operating field is paramount to all surgical procedures. Nevertheless, breaks in sterile technique are essentially unavoidable during laparoscopy. Contact beween the operator's periorbital area and the laparoscopic eyepiece contaminates that section of the instrument. Care to avoid contamination of any portion of the instrument likely to enter the peritoneal cavity, in conjunction with the natural defenses of the peritoneum, helps keep infectious morbidity associated with laparoscopy at a low rate.

Decontamination of the equipment for translaparoscopic photography is not easily accomplished. The camera can be gas sterilized between procedures, but the process is expensive and cumbersome. Loading the film into the camera would contaminate it anyway. No experience is available concerning the effects of gas sterilization on the emulsion of photographic film.

A simpler method for maintaining sterility of the photographic equipment required on the surgical field is the use of sterile plastic camera covers. Some commercially available covers have been designed to fit a particular camera with diverse lense openings, but these prove to be expensive since they cannot be resterilized. A product readily at hand in most operating suites can fulfill the purpose. This is the intestinal bag used by general surgeons to encompass the small bowel during major abdominal procedures. After the camera is dropped into the bag, sterile scissors are used to cut out an appropriate sized opening to accommodate the laparoscope's eyepiece. A similar opening is made for the camera's visor.

Experience has shown that when translaparoscopic photography is to be done after the diagnostic and/or operative aspects of the procedure have been completed, complicated aseptic maneuvers are generally unnecessary. It is acceptable to don a second pair of sterile gloves over the contaminated ones or to change gloves if any further manipulations are required.

Alternatively, the use of a foot shutter release restricts contamination to the hand holding the camera. The other hand can remain sterile and serve to manipulate the accessory probe or instruments, as needed. An automatic film advance mechanism is provided by a motor drive attached to the base of the camera (see Figure 26.3).

OPERATIVE REPORT

Documentation of findings at laparoscopy ought not to be limited to photographs alone. Verbal description in the form of a detailed dictated operative report is required for a number of compelling reasons. They include communication of findings, dynamic impression, and medicolegal aspects.

Communication of Findings. The importance of a fully descriptive narrative report cannot be overestimated. A report offers information during the immediate postoperative period before any photographs are available. Furthermore, it becomes the only record available in the event of a photographic failure. Although infrequent, equipment may not function properly, the film may be defective, the developing process may malfunction, or film may be lost in transit.

The narrative report is best prepared immediately following the procedure. This ensures that all pertinent details are described while they are still fresh in one's mind. Future usefulness of the report is directly related to how complete and thorough it is. The descriptive report of the laparoscopic findings should be written or dictated by the surgeon and not delegated to a junior member of the team. This recommendation is based on the need for the report to reflect not only the findings encountered but also a prognostic and therapeutic assessment as to future management.

Dynamic Impression. Notwithstanding the importance of translaparoscopic photographs, they can never fully replace the narrative report of the procedure. Difficulties encountered during the procedure can only be described verbally. Similarly, maneuvers performed to facilitate visualization or operative procedures, such as lysis of adhesions, require a thorough description. Any untoward intraoperative events or complications have to be described, as well.

Medicolegal Reasons. The main function of the medical record is to communicate to others (physicians, nurses, and nonmedical persons) specific findings related to a particular patient. No less important is its function for purposes of verifying the need for the procedure, for detailing any unexpected difficulties encountered, and for documenting one's thought process as can only be thoroughly expressed in words.

Reference

1. Taylor HW. A comparative evaluation of the 5 mm laparoscope in gynecological endoscopy. J Reprod Med 1975; 15:65-68.

INDEX

Note: Page numbers followed by *f* indicate figures.